Methods in Molecular Biology

Series Editor
John M. Walker
School of Life and Medical Sciences
University of Hertfordshire
Hatfield, Hertfordshire, UK

For further volumes:
http://www.springer.com/series/7651

For over 35 years, biological scientists have come to rely on the research protocols and methodologies in the critically acclaimed Methods in Molecular Biology series. The series was the first to introduce the step-by-step protocols approach that has become the standard in all biomedical protocol publishing. Each protocol is provided in readily-reproducible step-by step fashion, opening with an introductory overview, a list of the materials and reagents needed to complete the experiment, and followed by a detailed procedure that is supported with a helpful notes section offering tips and tricks of the trade as well as troubleshooting advice. These hallmark features were introduced by series editor Dr. John Walker and constitute the key ingredient in each and every volume of the Methods in Molecular Biology series. Tested and trusted, comprehensive and reliable, all protocols from the series are indexed in PubMed.

Manuscript Instructions https://drive.google.com/file/d/1K4Az5vpAFVzYadJ3jKx2-QSo7Dqa_SNA/view?usp=sharing

Biomolecular Display Technologies

Edited by

Huan Peng

College of Life Science and Technology, Huazhong University of Science and Technology, Wuhan, Hubei, China

Theam Soon Lim

Institute for Research in Molecular Medicine, Universiti Sains Malaysia, Pulau Pinang, Malaysia

Humana Press

Editors
Huan Peng
College of Life Science and Technology
Huazhong University of Science and Technology
Wuhan, Hubei, China

Theam Soon Lim
Institute for Research in Molecular Medicine
Universiti Sains Malaysia
Pulau Pinang, Malaysia

ISSN 1064-3745 ISSN 1940-6029 (electronic)
Methods in Molecular Biology
ISBN 978-1-0716-5248-0 ISBN 978-1-0716-5249-7 (eBook)
https://doi.org/10.1007/978-1-0716-5249-7

This work was supported by National Natural Science Foundation of China (Grant No. 32201100). Dr. Lim is grateful for the support from the Ministry of Higher Education of Malaysia (Grant No. FRGS/1/2024/STG01/USM/02/10).

This Humana imprint is published by the registered company Springer Science+Business Media, LLC, part of Springer Nature.
The registered company address is: 1 New York Plaza, New York, NY 10004, U.S.A.

Preface

Biomolecular display technologies are foundational to modern molecular biology, synthetic biology, and translational research, linking genetic information (genotype) to molecular function (phenotype) seamlessly. Spanning phage, yeast, mRNA, and cDNA platforms, these tools revolutionize biomolecule generation, screening, and engineering, driving breakthroughs in drug discovery, antibody development, and peptide/protein engineering. Unlike traditional methods limited by throughput or specificity, display technologies allow researchers to mine vast, diverse libraries for functional variants, bridging molecular design and real-world application.

Over decades, cross-disciplinary innovations have advanced display technologies, from optimized library construction to tailored display systems, enabling answers to complex biological questions. Today, auxiliary tools (AI for protein function prediction and hit optimization, high-performance computing for mass spectrometry analysis, and protein engineering for intracellular functionality) amplify these advances, transforming display technologies from niche techniques into essential assets for researchers across disciplines.

This book, *Biomolecular Display Technologies*, captures this dynamic field's breadth, encompassing all major display platforms and their applications. Organized into four thematic parts, it brings together practical protocols, cutting-edge methods, and translational insights from experts, supporting researchers at all career stages. Part 1 (Library Construction and Modification) covers foundational techniques for diverse, functional libraries (phage antibody, cyclic peptide, and chemically modified), key to successful screening. Part 2 (Display System Optimization) explores tailored yeast, phage, and cDNA display strategies to boost efficiency, modulate binding, and engineer scaffolds for specialized needs. Part 3 (Ligand Discovery and Application) showcases display-driven identification of macrocyclic ligands, nanoparticle-binding peptides, epitopes, and functional proteins, focusing on in vitro selection and real-world use cases. Part 4 (Auxiliary Tools and Post-Selection Optimization) integrates computational advances, protein engineering, and post-selection analysis to refine hits and accelerate translation.

We thank the contributing authors, whose hard-won expertise and dedication to knowledge-sharing made this volume possible. Their work reflects the field's collaborative spirit, where diverse researchers unite to push boundaries. Fueled by synthetic biology, computational science, and molecular engineering innovations, future advances will include more efficient libraries, high-throughput screening, and novel display-based therapeutics.

This book targets students, early-career scientists, and seasoned investigators looking to expand their technical toolkit. Whether constructing your first library, optimizing yeast display, leveraging AI for analysis, or engineering proteins, these chapters offer practical guidance and insight into display technologies' transformative potential.

The coming years will be dynamic for biomolecular display as we refine methods and explore new frontiers. It is our privilege to share this journey, and we hope this book fuels your research and the next generation of breakthroughs.

Wuhan, China *Huan Peng*
Penang, Malaysia *Theam Soon Lim*

Contents

Contributors

AZIMAH AHMAD • *Institute for Research in Molecular Medicine, Universiti Sains Malaysia, Penang, Malaysia*
WATARU AOKI • *Department of Biotechnology, Graduate School of Engineering, Osaka University, Osaka, Japan*
ANGELA CHIEW WEN CH'NG • *Institute for Research in Molecular Medicine, Universiti Sains Malaysia, Penang, Malaysia*
FA-JIE CHEN • *College of Chemistry, Fuzhou University, Fuzhou, Fujian, P. R. China*
TAO CHEN • *State Key Laboratory of Medical Proteomics, National Center for Protein Sciences(Beijing), Beijing, China*
YEE SIEW CHOONG • *Institute for Research in Molecular Medicine, Universiti Sains Malaysia, Penang, Malaysia*
JAIME FERNÁNDEZ DE CÓRDOBA • *Advanced Optical Microscopy Facility, Centro Nacional de Biotecnología-CSIC, Madrid, Spain*
GOPAL DUBEY • *Texas A&M Drug Discovery Center and Department of Chemistry, Texas A&M University, College Station, TX, USA*
ZONGYUAN FAN • *College of Life Science and Technology, Huazhong University of Science and Technology, Wuhan, Hubei, China*
SOFÍA FRAILE • *Department of Systems Biology, Centro Nacional de Biotecnología-CSIC, Madrid, Spain*
JULIA GOBL • *LoopLab Bio GmbH, Vienna, Austria*
PIOTR GOLEC • *Department of Molecular Virology, Institute of Microbiology, Faculty of Biology, University of Warsaw, Warsaw, Poland*
YUKI GOTO • *Department of Chemistry, Graduate School of Science, Kyoto University, Sakyo, Kyoto, Japan; Department of Chemistry, Graduate School of Science, The University of Tokyo, Bunkyo, Tokyo, Japan; Toyota Riken Rising Fellow, Toyota Physical and Chemical Research Institute, Sakyo, Kyoto, Japan*
J. TRAE HAMPTON • *Texas A&M Drug Discovery Center and Department of Chemistry, Texas A&M University, College Station, TX, USA*
QIANG HE • *School of Computer Science and Technology, Huazhong University of Science and Technology, Wuhan, China*
ZHIJIE HU • *College of Life Science and Technology, Huazhong University of Science and Technology, Wuhan, Hubei, China*
ZIYUE HUANG • *College of Life Science and Technology, Huazhong University of Science and Technology, Wuhan, Hubei, China*
COLIN M. LEAF • *Department of Chemistry, University of Southern California, Los Angeles, CA, USA*
CHUANG LI • *School of Computer Science, Hunan University of Technology and Business, Changsha, China*
DAIRONG LI • *College of Life Science and Technology, Huazhong University of Science and Technology, Wuhan, Hubei, China*

THEAM SOON LIM • *Institute for Research in Molecular Medicine, Universiti Sains Malaysia, Penang, Malaysia; Analytical Biochemistry Research Centre, Universiti Sains Malaysia, Penang, Malaysia*

BELLE LI LING • *Institute for Research in Molecular Medicine, Universiti Sains Malaysia, Penang, Malaysia*

ANNIKA DE SOUSA LINHARES • *LoopLab Bio GmbH, Vienna, Austria*

WENSHE R. LIU • *Texas A&M Drug Discovery Center and Department of Chemistry, Texas A&M University, College Station, TX, USA; Institute of Biosciences and Technology and Department of Translational Medical Sciences, College of Medicine, Texas A&M University, Houston, TX, USA; Department of Biochemistry and Biophysics, Texas A&M University, College Station, TX, USA; Department of Cell Biology and Genetics, College of Medicine, Texas A&M University, College Station, TX, USA; Department of Pharmaceutical Sciences, Texas A&M University, College Station, TX, USA*

VÍCTOR DE LORENZO • *Department of Systems Biology, Centro Nacional de Biotecnología-CSIC, Madrid, Spain*

ESTEBAN MARTÍNEZ-GARCÍA • *Department of Systems Biology, Centro Nacional de Biotecnología-CSIC, Madrid, Spain*

GUODONG MIN • *School of Computer Science and Technology, Huazhong University of Science and Technology, Wuhan, China*

NAOTO NEMOTO • *Graduate School of Science and Engineering, Saitama University, Sakura-ku, Saitama, Japan*

RUTENDO NYAMADZAWO • *Texas A&M Drug Discovery Center and Department of Chemistry, Texas A&M University, College Station, TX, USA*

SOPHEA PA • *Texas A&M Drug Discovery Center and Department of Chemistry, Texas A&M University, College Station, TX, USA*

HUAN PENG • *College of Life Science and Technology, Huazhong University of Science and Technology, Wuhan, China*

NICOLE PINNETTE • *Department of Chemistry, Merkert Chemistry Center, Boston College, Chestnut Hill, MA, USA*

PEARL QI • *Mork Family Department of Chemical Engineering and Materials Science, University of Southern California, Los Angeles, CA, USA*

RICHARD W. ROBERTS • *Department of Chemistry, University of Southern California, Los Angeles, CA, USA; Mork Family Department of Chemical Engineering and Materials Science, University of Southern California, Los Angeles, CA, USA; USC Norris Comprehensive Cancer Center, University of Southern California, Los Angeles, CA, USA*

SEIJI SHIBASAKI • *Laboratory of Natural Science, Faculty of Economics, Toyo University, Hakusan, Bunkyoku, Tokyo, Japan*

KATHARINA STADLBAUER • *Institute for Molecular Biotechnology, Department of Biotechnology and Food Sciences, BOKU University, Vienna, Austria*

JOCHEN STRITZKER • *LoopLab Bio GmbH, Vienna, Austria*

HIROAKI SUGA • *Department of Chemistry, Graduate School of Science, The University of Tokyo, Bunkyo, Tokyo, Japan*

ELISE SYLVANDER • *Institute of Biochemistry, BOKU University, Vienna, Austria*

TERRY T. TAKAHASHI • *Department of Chemistry, University of Southern California, Los Angeles, CA, USA*

MICHAEL W. TRAXLMAYR • *Institute of Biochemistry, BOKU University, Vienna, Austria; CD Laboratory for Next Generation CAR T Cells, Vienna, Austria*
SOTA UCHIDA • *Department of Chemistry, Graduate School of Science, Kyoto University, Sakyo, Kyoto, Japan; Department of Chemistry, Graduate School of Science, The University of Tokyo, Bunkyo, Tokyo, Japan*
MITSUYOSHI UEDA • *Office of Institutional Advancement and Communications (IAC), Kyoto University, Yoshidahonmachi, Sakyoku, Kyoto, Japan*
WOLFGANG WALLNER • *LoopLab Bio GmbH, Vienna, Austria*
XUANLIANG WANG • *College of Life Science and Technology, Huazhong University of Science and Technology, Wuhan, Hubei, China*
ZISHAN WANG • *College of Life Science and Technology, Huazhong University of Science and Technology, Wuhan, Hubei, China*
GRZEGORZ WĘGRZYN • *Department of Molecular Biology, Faculty of Biology, University of Gdansk, Gdansk, Poland*
YANHUA WEN • *School of Computer Science, Hunan University of Technology and Business, Changsha, China*
CECILIA WICK • *Institute for Molecular Biotechnology, Department of Biotechnology and Food Sciences, BOKU University, Vienna, Austria*
GORDANA WOZNIAK-KNOPP • *Institute for Molecular Biotechnology, Department of Biotechnology and Food Sciences, BOKU University, Vienna, Austria*
JUNPEI YAMASHITA • *Graduate School of Science and Engineering, Saitama University, Sakura-ku, Saitama, Japan*
JIA XUAN YEOH • *Institute for Research in Molecular Medicine, Universiti Sains Malaysia, Penang, Malaysia*

Part I

Library Construction and Modification

Chapter 1

Incorporation of Butyryl-Lysine into Phage-Displayed Peptide Libraries

Sophea Pa, Rutendo Nyamadzawo, Gopal Dubey, J. Trae Hampton and Wenshe R. Liu

Abstract

There are several epigenetic reader proteins that recognize butyrylated lysine residues, yet the majority peptide probes have been limited to histone-based substrates. Development of selective peptide substrates will play a key role in studying these proteins and in developing inhibitors of therapeutic potential. We have previously reported a strategy to incorporate N^{ε}-butyryl-L-lysine into phage-displayed peptide libraries that was used to identify inhibitors for the ENL YEATS domain. Here, we describe the production of phage-displayed peptide libraries that contain butyrylated lysine residues and their subsequent use to direct phage selections toward the active sites of epigenetic proteins. We envision the technique can be applicable to performing phage selections toward many different epigenetic readers, writers, and erasers implicated in a variety of cellular processes and diseases.

Keywords Phage display, Epigenetic proteins, N^{ε}-butyryl-L-lysine, Phage biopanning, YEATS domain

1 Introduction

Phage display is a powerful tool for producing large peptide libraries (>10^9 sequences) that can be used to identify high-affinity peptide ligands for relevant biological targets [1]. However, these libraries are typically only composed of the 20 canonical amino acids, thus hindering selections by limiting the ability to explore new chemical spaces for certain targets. Nearly simultaneous to the development of phage display libraries in the 1990s, genetic code expansion also emerged as a tool to efficiently introduce noncanonical amino acids (ncAAs) into ribosomally-encoded peptides [2]. In the past 20 years, the technique has been optimized to incorporate over 200 different ncAAs using mutant pyrrolysyl tRNA/tRNA^{CUA} pairs that incorporate amino acids at amber (UAG) stop codons [3, 4]. Recently, we have combined genetic code expansion with phage display to

Huan Peng and Theam Soon Lim (eds.), *Biomolecular Display Technologies*, Methods in Molecular Biology, vol. 3030,
https://doi.org/10.1007/978-1-0716-5249-7_1,

efficiently incorporate lysine post-translational modifications into peptide libraries [5–8]. This has proven useful to target epigenetic reader proteins that recognize or modify lysine residues by directing phage selections toward active sites of proteins. Through incorporation of N^{ε}-butyryl-L-lysine (BuK) into phage-displayed peptide libraries, we have recently identified peptide inhibitors of a histone deacetylase (SIRT2) and epigenetic reader protein (ENL) [5, 6]. As lysine butyrylation continues to be an emerging landscape in disease development and cellular processes, the development of selective peptide probes will prove to be crucial in better understanding epigenetic readers that interact with BuK residues [9]. This chapter provides detailed instructions for preparing phage-displayed peptide libraries that contain butyrylated lysine residues and their subsequent use in selections toward epigenetic proteins.

2 Materials

All solutions are prepared using high-purity water (MilliQ Water with a resistance of 18.2 MΩ-cm at 25°C) and stored at room temperature unless otherwise noted. Solutions should be handled with sterile techniques during phage expressions and selections. To prevent phage contaminations, all flasks and containers should be thoroughly sterilized with 10% bleach prior to use and autoclaved. Waste should be properly sterilized and disposed of in accordance with local regulations.

2.1 Buffers, Reagents, and Supplies

1. 5× Phage Precipitation Buffer: 2.50 M NaCl, 20% PEG8000. Dissolve 200 g PEG8000 and 146 g NaCl in 1 L MilliQ water and autoclave prior to use (*see* **Note 1**).
2. Phage Binding Buffer: 10 mM HEPES, 150 mM NaCl, 10 mM $MgCl_2$, 1 mM KCl, pH 7.4. Autoclave prior to use.
3. 5× Blocking Buffer: Phage Binding Buffer with 5% BSA and 0.5% Tween-20. Filter using a 0.2 μm filter prior to use.
4. Neutralization Buffer: 1 M Tris, pH 8.0. Autoclave prior to use.
5. Phage Elution Buffer: 50 mM glycine, pH 2.2. Autoclave to sterilize prior to use.
6. 2×YT Medium: Weigh out 16 g of tryptone, 10 g of yeast extract, and 5 g of NaCl. Dissolve solids in 1 L of water, then autoclave to sterilize prior to use.
7. Kanamycin stock solution: 25 mg/mL kanamycin sulfate in MilliQ water. Sterilize via filtration prior to use.
8. Tetracycline stock solution: 10 mg/mL tetracycline in 70% ethanol.
9. Ampicillin stock solution: 100 mg/mL ampicillin sodium salt in MilliQ water. Sterilize via filtration prior to use.

10. Chloramphenicol stock solution: 34 mg/mL chloramphenicol in ethanol.
11. Plasmid and Gel Extraction Kit (Epoch Life Sciences Gencatch miniprep kit).
12. N^{ε}-butyryl-L-lysine hydrochloride (BuK-HCl): Prepare a 100 mM stock solution in water and sterilize by filtration with a 0.2 μm filter. Large amounts (gram-scale quantities) can be readily synthesized following published protocols [5] (*see* **Note 2**).
13. Lysis Buffer: 50 mM Tris, 300 mM NaCl, 10 mM imidazole, pH 7.8.
14. Wash Buffer 1: 50 mM Tris, 300 mM NaCl, 30 mM imidazole, pH 7.8.
15. Wash Buffer 2: 50 mM Tris, 300 mM NaCl, 60 mM imidazole, pH 7.8.
16. Ni-NTA Elution Buffer: 50 mM Tris, 300 mM NaCl, 250 mM imidazole, pH 7.8.
17. Storage Buffer: 50 mM Tris, 300 mM NaCl, 5 mM DTT, pH 7.8.

2.2 Helper Phages, Cell Lines, and Plasmids

1. CM13 Helper Phage (Antibody Design Labs)
2. CM13d3 Helper Phage (Antibody Design Labs)
3. M13KO7 Helper Phage (Antibody Design Labs)
4. Top10 (ThermoFisher Scientific)
5. ER2738 (New England Biolabs)
6. Top10F' (ThermoFisher Scientific)
7. pBirAcm (Avidity LLC)
8. BL21 (DE3) (ThermoFisher Scientific)

2.3 Primers

1. M13KO7-g3TAA-F: 5′-gttgaaagtt gtttagcaTa accccataca gaaaattc-3′
2. M13KO7TAA-R: 5′-gaattttctg tatggggttA tgctaaacaa ctttcaac-3′
3. pADL-AAKAA-NGS-F: 5′TCGTCGGCAGCGTCAGATGTGTATAAGAGACAGGCCCAGCCGGCCATG3′
4. pADL-AAKAA-NGS-R: 5′GTCTCGTGGGCTCGGAGATGTGTATAAGAGACAGCGGCCGCTTTCGCCGC3′
5. NGS-i7: 5′CAAGCAGAAGACGGCATACGAGAT[i7]GTCTCGTGGGCTCGG3′
    a. [i7] corresponds to any unique index of ten base pairs. We recommend ordering four different i7 indices, but this can be increased or decreased depending on total samples.

6. NGS-i5: 5′AATGATACGGCGACCACCGAGATCTACAC[i5] TCGTCGGCAGCGTC3′
   a. [i5] corresponds to any unique index of ten base pairs. We recommend ordering four different i5 indices, but this can be increased or decreased depending on total samples.

3 Methods

Carry out all procedures at room temperature and in a sterile environment unless otherwise specified. Verify all plasmids and libraries for high quality through sequencing prior to beginning any experiments.

3.1 Preparation of M13KO7TAA (pIII Deficient Helper Plasmid)

1. Introduce a TAA nonsense mutation at position K10 of gene III in the M13KO7 helper phage through a polymerase chain reaction on the phage DNA using primers **M13KO7-g3TAA-F** and **M13KO7TAA-R**.
2. Following PCR amplification, transform the purified PCR product into *E. coli* Top10 F′ and confirm proper mutagenesis through whole plasmid sequencing of a single clone.
3. To validate pIII deficiency, express the helper phage overnight from the confirmed stock by incubation at 37°C in 2× YT supplemented with 25 μg/mL kanamycin.
4. Pellet cells by centrifugation at 5251×*g*, 20 min for 15 min and incubate the supernatant at 65°C for 15 min to kill residual bacteria.
5. Spot 10 μL of heat-killed supernatant onto an overlay of *E. coli* Top10 F′ in top agar on agar supplemented with 10 μg/mL tetracycline.
6. Incubate plates at 37°C overnight and observe zones of delayed growth.
7. As a positive control, express wild-type M13KO7 and observe zones of delayed growth.
8. Interpret Results:
   a. No plaque formation with M13K07TAA indicates that the absence of pIII prevents phage expression.
   b. Plaques with the wild-type M13KO7 demonstrate the pIII requirement in phage expression.
9. To confirm that M13K07TAA does not produce any phages without amber suppression; cotransform *E. coli* Top10F′ with M13KO7(pIII^{-}) and pADLg3-amber which encodes pIII with an in-frame amber mutation.
10. Grow transformed cultures in 2×YT supplemented with 100 μ g/mL ampicillin and 25 μg/mL kanamycin to log-phase.

11. Add 20% arabinose to induce pIII expression and incubate cultures overnight at 37°C.
12. Pellet cells by centrifugation at 5251×*g* for 20 min and incubate the supernatant at 65°C for 15 min to kill residual bacteria.
13. Infect 90 µL of log-phase *E. coli* Top10F′ with 10 µL of heat-killed supernatant for 45 min.
14. Plate infected cultures onto agar supplemented with 100 µg/mL ampicillin and incubate overnight at 37°C.
15. Interpret results:

    a. No growth from pADLg3-amber supernatant indicates that both phagemid and helper phage carry nonsense mutations in pIII.

3.2 Sequencing and Analysis to Verify Amber Content of Library

1. Isolate plasmid DNA encoding a randomized peptide library that contains amber codons within the library region. Methods to develop such libraries are readily available [6, 7].
2. Amplify the library region from the phagemid DNA using primers **pADL-AAKAA-NGS-F** and **pADL-AAKAA-NGS-R** (*see* **Note 3**).
3. Separate PCR amplicons on a 3% agarose gel and gel-extract the desired band.
4. Perform a second PCR using primers **NGS-i7** and **NGS-i5** to attach unique index sequences for sample identification.
    a. Assign a unique i7/i5 index combination to each unique sample library to allow for demultiplexing during NGS sequencing. The indices are any unique ten base pair sequences.
5. Gel-extract the indexed PCR products from a 3% agarose gel.
6. Submit purified, indexed libraries for paired-end sequencing on an Illumina MiSeq platform (2 × 150 bp, 1 million reads per sample).
7. Analyze sequencing data for amber content using custom R scripts designed for the specific library region [6]. At least 95% of sequences should contain at least one amber codon for a successful expression.

3.3 Cloning of M13k07(pIII⁻) and BuKRS into Top10

1. To verify incorporation of BuK, transform the library into Top10 cells containing M13KO7(pIII⁻) helper phage and pEVOL-CloDF-BuKRS (pEVOL-PylT-BuKRS with a CloDF origin of replication). See reference for construction of the BuKRS plasmid [6, 10]. Refer to Fig. 1 for the expression system necessary for production of phage libraries containing BuK residues.

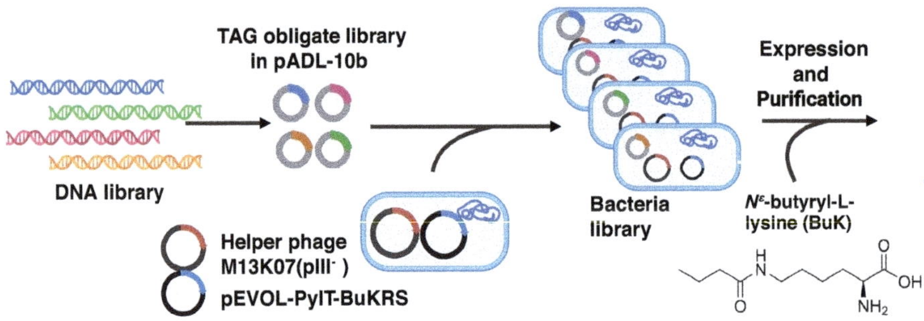

Fig. 1 Expression system for producing phage-displayed peptide libraries that contain butyryl-lysine residues

2. Incubate at 37°C, 250 rpm for 1 h and perform a titer with some of the transformed cells to ensure library coverage.
3. Pellet down the remaining transformed cells at 3750×*g* for 15 min.
4. Resuspend the pellet in 2×YT medium supplemented with 100 μg/mL ampicillin, 34 μg/mL chloramphenicol, and 25 μg/mL kanamycin and grow to OD_{600} = 0.4–0.6.
5. Add 1 mM IPTG and 0.2% arabinose, then divide culture into two flasks, one with a volume 10× than the other.
6. To the flask with 10× volume, add BuK (100 mM in H_2O) to a final concentration of 4 mM (+BuK).
7. Leave the second flask without BuK as a control (−BuK) expression.
8. Express phages at 30°C with shaking for 18–24 h.
9. Distribute the cells into 36 mL portions in 50 mL falcon tubes and pellet cells by centrifugation at 5251×*g*, 20 min for 15 min.
10. Transfer each supernatant to prechilled 9 mL of 5× phage precipitation solution in 50 mL falcon tubes.
11. Mix tubes by inversion and precipitate the phages overnight in 4°C (*see* **Note 4**).
12. Pellet down phages at 11,000×*g* for 25 min and discard the supernatant.
13. Resuspend pellets in 2 mL phage binding buffer per 50 mL falcon tube and combine them to one tube.
14. Add phages to the phage precipitation buffer accordingly based on volume and precipitate overnight at 4°C.
15. Pellet down phages at 11,000×*g* for 25 min and discard the supernatant.
16. Resuspend pellets in 1 mL of phage binding buffer per 50 mL falcon tube.

17. Remove residual cells by pelleting down at 16,873×*g* for 10 min and kill any remaining cells by incubating the phage supernatant at 65°C for 15 min.
18. Titer both −BuK and +BuK phages (protocol described in Step 3.4).
19. Interpret Results:
    a. No difference between the titers means a significant number of nonamber clones were expressed or improper functioning of the amber suppression machinery.
    b. ≥Ten-fold difference between the titers means successful BuK incorporation and higher proportion of amber clones.

3.4 Phage Titer

1. Prepare an overnight culture of ER2738 stock in 2×YT with tetracycline (10 μg/mL) along with the negative control culture containing 2×YT with ampicillin (100 μg/mL) and tetracycline (10 μg/mL), and a 2×YT culture with kanamycin (25 μg/mL) with tetracycline (10 μg/mL).
2. Dilute the overnight culture 100-fold in 2×YT + tetracycline, 2×YT + tetracycline + ampicillin, and 2xYT + tetracycline + kanamycin and grow at 37°C. The culture containing ampicillin and kanamycin should not grow.
3. Prepare ten-fold serial dilutions of purified phage in phage binding buffer medium or 2×YT (90 μL of buffer, 10 μL of phage for each dilution). Use filtered tips when handling the phage solutions.
4. When the ER2738 culture reaches the mid-log-phase (OD_{600} ≈ 0.5), transfer 90 μL of the culture into 0.6 Eppendorf tubes labeled for each of the phage dilutions. Add 10 μL of each of the phage dilutions to the corresponding tube. Vortex and incubate at 37°C for 45 min.
5. While the phages infect the ER2738, make and dry the LB agar plates containing the appropriate antibiotics (tetracycline and ampicillin for pADL).
6. After incubation, spot 10 μL in triplicate onto the plate, noting the dilution factor. Use filtered tips when plating to avoid contamination of phages into the pipet.
7. Place the plate in the 37°C incubator overnight once all the spots are dry.
8. Count the number of colonies at a single dilution and calculate the phage concentration (pfu/mL). The phage concentration (pfu/mL) = average number of colonies at the single dilution * $10^{(x+3)}$, where x is the phage dilution factor.

9. Compare titers from BuK-supplemented cultures with the negative control to verify amber suppression and ncAA-dependent display efficiency. Phage yields from the BuK-supplemented cultures should be at least 20× higher than the negative control.

3.5 Preparation of Cells for Large-Scale Phage Expression

1. Thaw aliquots of electrocompetent TOP10 *E. coli* cells containing:
   a. pEVOL-CloDF-PylT-BuKRS encoding the orthogonal aminoacyl-tRNA synthetase/tRNA pair for BuK incorporation.
   b. M13K07(pIII⁻) helper phage carrying a nonsense TAA mutation in gIII to prevent functional pIII expression in the absence of amber suppression.
2. Prechill the electroporation cuvettes on ice and preincubate 50 mL of 2×YT at 37°C.
3. Transfer 200 μL of Top10 electrocompetent cells into each cuvette and add the amber-containing pADL library into the cuvette. Gently mix and incubate on ice for 15–20 min. The amount of DNA added should be around 150–300 ng for each transformation.
4. Remove the cuvette from the ice and wipe off with a Kimwipe for any of the remaining ice and condensation around the cuvette. Make sure that the solution is between the electrodes.
5. Put the cuvette in the electroporator and shock the cells using the 2 mm *E. coli* method, which has the following conditions:
   a. Voltage: 2500 V
   b. Resistance: 200 Ω
   c. Capacitance: 25 μF
   d. Number of Pulses: 1
   e. Pulse Interval: 0.0 s
   f. Electrode Gap: 2.0 mm
6. Immediately after electroporation, add 1 mL of 37°C 2×YT to the cuvette and mix gently. Transfer the solution to another flask with 50 mL of 2×YT media.
7. Recover the cell solutions by placing the flask in the 37°C shaker, shaking at 250 rpm for 45 min.
8. Take out 1 mL of the recovered cells to perform serial dilutions. Transfer the rest of the culture to a fresh new 1 L 2×YT containing the appropriate antibiotics and let it grow overnight at 37°C, shaking at 250 rpm.
9. For the serial dilutions, prepare a series of sterile microcentrifuge tubes labeled with the dilution factors (at least eight tubes). For each of the tubes, add 90 μL of 2×YT. For the first

dilution factor, add 10 μL of the recovered cell. Continue the dilution series by pipetting 10 μL from the first dilution to the second and from the second to the third, till all the dilution factors are covered.

10. Plate serial dilutions of the transformants on LB agar containing the appropriate antibiotics (ampicillin 100 μg/mL, chloramphenicol 34 μg/mL, kanamycin 25 μg/mL) and incubate overnight at 37°C to maintain all three genetic elements. Calculate the titer and make sure the library size is covered (*see* **Note 5**).
11. Inoculate a single colony into 10 mL 2×YT medium with antibiotics and grow overnight at 37°C, 250 rpm.

3.6 Expression of BuK-Containing Phage Libraries

1. Dilute the overnight culture 200-fold into 1.1 L of 2×YT medium containing antibiotics. Grow at 37°C and shake at 250 rpm.
2. Once the OD_{600} reaches 0.5–0.8, induce the expression through the addition of 1 mM IPTG, 5 mM nicotinamide, and 0.2% arabinose.
3. Take out 100 mL of cells and add to a sterile flask to express the negative control.
4. Add 5 mM of BuK-HCL to the remaining 1 L of cells.
5. Resume shaking at 250 rpm and incubate the culture at 30°C for 16–20 h.
6. Transfer cells into 50 mL Falcon tubes (36 mL aliquots). Separate and label 50 mL centrifuge tubes for the BuK expression and the negative control.
7. Harvest the culture by centrifugation at 5251×*g* for 20 min at 4°C.
8. Transfer 36 mL of the supernatant into fresh 50 mL Falcon tubes and add 9 mL of 5× precipitation buffer.
9. Mix thoroughly and precipitate at 4°C for at least 2 h.
10. Centrifuge at 11,000×*g* for 25 min at 4°C to pellet the phage. Discard the supernatant and for the best recoveries, do a quick spin at 5251×*g* for 1 min to bring the phage pellet to the bottom.
11. Resuspend the pellet in 2 mL sterile phage binding buffer for each tube. Vortex vigorously to ensure that most of the phages are not sticking to the wall of the tube. Let the phage resuspend in the buffer for 15–20 min before continuing.
12. Perform a quick spin at 5251×*g* for 1 min to bring the phage solution to the bottom and use the serological pipette to combine the phage solution to one tube of the same expression. For this expression, there should be two tubes, one for the BuK expression and one for the negative control.

13. Add appropriate amounts of 5× phage precipitation buffer to each of the tubes (final concentration of the buffer to the volume of the phage solution should be 1×) for the second round of precipitation and incubate at 4°C for at least 1 h to remove residual contaminants.
14. Harvest the phage by centrifugation at 11,000×*g* for 25 min at 4°C.
15. Decant the supernatant and dissolve the phage pellet with 1 mL phage binding buffer.
16. Centrifuge the phages at 16,873×*g* for 10 min at room temperature to clarify.
17. Transfer the phage solution into a new Eppendorf and heat-shock the phages at 65°C for 15 min to kill any remaining bacteria. Store the phages at 4°C.
18. Titer the phage solutions as in Sect. 3.4. Successful expressions at 1 L scale typically yield more than 10^{10} total phages and 20-fold increases in titers dependent on BuK supplementation.

Following the generation of a phage library encoding butyrylysine residues, the next crucial step is the selection of target specific binders using phage-assisted, active site-directed ligand evolution (PADLE). Figure 2 gives a brief overview of PADLE and the selection process. PADLE is particularly suited for libraries incorporating chemically reactive or structurally unique unnatural amino acids, enabling the identification of covalent or high-affinity noncovalent binders that engage defined surface pockets or functional sites on the target protein.

To demonstrate this method, the ENL protein (eleven-nineteen leukemia protein), a chromatin reader domain implicated in leukemogenesis, was used as a representative target [11]. The following protocols describe this PADLE-based selection process in detail and can be applied for other proteins that recognize or interact with butyrylated lysine residues. For selections using phage display, the target protein must be immobilized to allow for enriching specific interactions with the peptide library. As such, the target protein is recombinantly expressed with affinity tags such as His_6, GST, or biotin to facilitate immobilization on magnetic beads. This protocol provides details for producing and performing a selection against biotinylated ENL YEATS domain, but the concepts discussed may be applied generally using other proteins with complementary tags.

3.7 Production of Biotinylated ENL YEATS Domain

1. For biotinylation of an Avi-tagged protein, clone the target protein fused with an N- or C-terminal AviTag (GLNDIFEAQKIEWHE). We used pET28a-AviSUMO-ENL for the ENL YEATS domain (residues 1–148) fused with an Avi-SUMO tag for in vivo biotinylation [5].

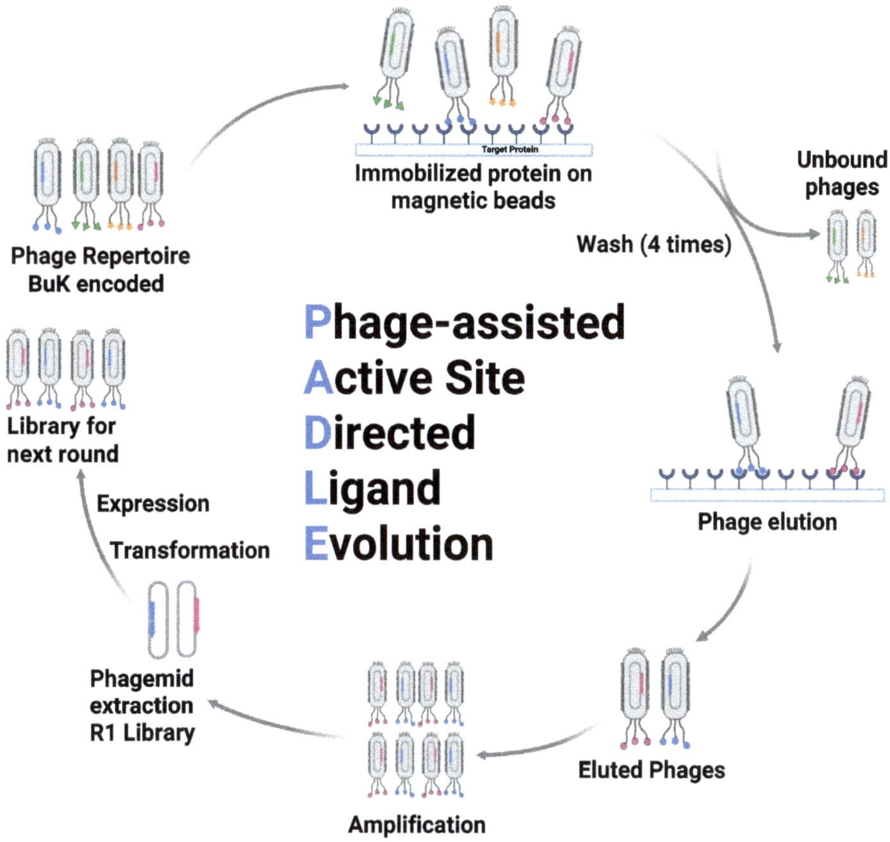

Fig. 2 Through iterative biopanning of phage displayed peptide libraries, sequences that bind to the desired protein target are enriched. Incorporation of BuK into phage libraries allows for phage-assisted active site-directed ligand evolution (PADLE) toward proteins that recognize BuK

2. Cotransform pET28a-AviSUMO-ENL and pBirAcm into BL21(DE3) competent cells.
3. Plate transformants on LB agar containing kanamycin (50 μg/mL) and chloramphenicol (34 μg/mL), then incubate overnight at 37°C.
4. Inoculate a single colony into 1 L of 2×YT broth with the same antibiotics and grow at 37°C with shaking until OD_{600} reaches 0.5–0.8.
5. Induce protein expression through addition of 0.4 mM IPTG and 50 μM Biotin.
6. Grow the cells at 16°C for 18 h with shaking.
7. Harvest cells by centrifugation at 4000×*g* for 10 min at 4°C.
8. Resuspend the pellet in 50 mL of cold lysis buffer supplemented with 0.1 mM PMSF.
9. Lyse cells by sonication on ice and centrifuge at 16,000×g for 30 min at 4°C.

10. Collect the supernatant and transfer it to a tube containing pre-equilibrated Ni-NTA resin.
11. Incubate at 4°C for 45 min with gentle rotation.
12. Transfer the Ni-NTA resin onto a column and wash the resin with gravity flow as follows:
    a. 3× with Wash Buffer 1
    b. 3× with Wash Buffer 2
13. Elute bound protein with 10 mL of Ni-NTA Elution Buffer.
14. Dialyze the eluted protein overnight at 4°C into storage buffer.
15. Concentrate the protein solution at 4000×*g* using a 10 kDa Amicon ultracentrifugal filter as needed and aliquot.
16. Store at −80°C. Avoid repeated freeze-thaw cycles.

3.8 Immobilization of Target Protein and Selections

1. For 10 μg of target protein, use 50 μL of appropriate magnetic beads that correspond to the protein tags. For biotinylated proteins, streptavidin magnetic beads can be used for the selection (*see* **Note 6**).
2. Wash magnetic beads three times with 1 mL of phage binding buffer using a magnetic stand.
3. Resuspend beads in 500 μL of binding buffer and incubate with the purified tagged target protein for 30–60 min at RT or 4°C with gentle rotation.
4. Wash beads 3× with 1 mL of binding buffer to remove unbound protein.
5. Block nonspecific sites by incubating beads with 1× blocking buffer for 30–60 min at RT or 4°C with gentle rotation.
6. Dilute appropriate amounts of phage library with 5× blocking buffer to achieve a 1× blocking buffer solution and incubate for 30 min at RT. Typical input: 10^{11}–10^{12} phage particles.
7. Incubate the blocked, protein-coated beads with phage solution for 1 h at RT or 4°C with gentle rotation.
    a. For a negative selection (optional) against the resin, preincubate phage with control beads (without target immobilized) for 30 min to remove nonspecific binders (*see* **Note 7**).
8. Wash the phage-bound beads 3–5× with wash buffer (PBS + 0.1% Tween-20).
    a. Increase stringency by adding more washes, higher detergent concentration or lower pH of wash buffer in later rounds (*see* **Note 8**).

9. Elute bound phage by adding 100 μL of phage elution buffer and incubate with beads for 10–15 min at RT
   a. Alternatively, a competitive ligand can be used to selectively elute phages from proteins if available. This should be done at a high concentration (>10× the K_D) to avoid enrichment of low-affinity clones.
10. Separate the beads magnetically and collect the supernatant, then neutralize the elution through addition of 50 μL of neutralization buffer.

3.9 Amplification of Eluted Phages

1. Calculate the selection output by performing a phage titer of the neutralized eluted phages (see Sect. 3.4).
2. Inoculate 10 mL of ER2738 with tetracycline (10 μg/mL) to mid log phase to OD ~ 0.5 and infect eluted phages.
3. Incubate at 37°C for 45 min for infection with shaking.
4. Centrifuge the cells after 45 min (4000×*g*, 15 min) and resuspend the pellet in 50 mL fresh 2YT media with antibiotics ampicillin (100 μg/mL) and tetracycline (10 μg/mL).
5. Grow the cells overnight at 37°C and shake at 250 rpm.
6. Extract phagemid DNA from overnight culture using a miniprep kit according to manufacturer's instructions and transform into cells containing pEVOL-CDF-BuKRS and M13k07(pIII$^-$) as described in Sects. 3.5–3.6.
7. Express and purify phages for the next round of panning (see Sect. 3.6).
8. Perform three to five rounds of biopanning with increasing stringency in each round (e.g., negative selections, more washes, less target protein, or use of competitive elution).
9. Calculate percentage enrichment from each round. If the enrichment profile is satisfactory, proceed for identification of sequences using next-generation sequencing (NGS) (*see* **Note 9**).

3.10 Sequencing and Analysis

1. Amplify the library region of phagemid DNA from different rounds of selections by performing a four-step PCR cycle using primers pADL-AAKAA-NGS-F and pADL-AAKAA-NGS-R, as described in Sect. 3.2.
2. Separate the PCR products on a 3% agarose gel and purify the desired amplicons using a GenCatch Gel Extraction Kit.
3. Attach index sequences to the amplicons by performing an additional PCR using NGS-i7 and NGS-i5 primers. Assign a unique combination of i7 and i5 indices to each selection round for identification.
4. Purify the indexed PCR products using a GenCatch Gel Extraction Kit.

5. Submit purified, indexed libraries for sequencing on an Illumina MiSeq platform (1 M reads, paired-end 2 × 150 bp).
6. Analyze sequencing data for enrichment of peptide sequences throughout the rounds of selection. See [5, 7] for the R scripts that can be used for analysis.

4 Notes

1. After autoclaving, the precipitation buffer separates into two phases. This should be thoroughly mixed immediately after autoclaving. If it is not mixed and solidifies, the PEG8000 can be redissolved through sonication, but insoluble fragments may still be observed in the solution.
2. While we typically use BuK-HCl for experiments, there is a commercially available BuK derivative that does not include the hydrochloride salt (MedChemExpress Cat. No. HY-W048217) that will likely function well for these experiments.
3. These primers are designed for a library encoded within a pADL-10b plasmid and can be customized to produce library amplicons through standard PCR techniques.
4. Typically, phages will sufficiently precipitate after 1.5 h at 4°C. However, yields can increase ~2–5-fold when extending precipitation times beyond 10 h.
5. We recommend covering the library size at least ten-fold to ensure phage diversity. It is useful to perform several test conditions for electroporating the plasmid into cells prior to replicating transformations to cover the library size. Typically, for libraries composed of 10^9 peptides, 20 transformations are sufficient to produce enough transformants for proper coverage.
6. Integrity of the protein is essential to phage selections. This may require testing different tags to make sure the protein retains desirable activity when immobilized to the resin. We also recommend using alternative resins during the selection to prevent enrichment of parasitic phage clones that interact with the backbone support (Streptavidin, Ni-NTA, glutathione, etc.). Consider the loading capacity of the resin and desirable stringency of selection to determine the amount of protein to load.
7. Always include a negative selection step if the target is expressed with common affinity tags to reduce tag-specific binders. It also may help to sequence the peptides that bind and elute from the resin scaffold using next-generation sequencing.
8. To prevent undesired enrichment of peptides that bind to the plastic, it is useful to switch microcentrifuge tubes during the

wash steps. Typically, we switch tubes at least three times during a selection.

9. Monitor enrichment by phage titration (percent of phages bound to resin) or phage ELISA after each round.

Acknowledgments

Research in the Liu Lab was supported in part by the Welch Foundation (grant A-1715 to W.R.L.), National Institutes of Health (grants R35 GM145351 and R01 CA291968 to W.R.L.), Cancer Prevention and Research Institute of Texas (Grant RP230345), and the Harry E. Bovay, Jr. Foundation.

References

1. Smith GP, Petrenko VA (1997) Phage display. Chem Rev 97:391–410. https://doi.org/10.1021/cr960065d
2. Wang L, Brock A, Herberich B, Schultz PG (2001) Expanding the genetic code of Escherichia coli. Science 292:498–500. https://doi.org/10.1126/science.1060077
3. Wan W, Tharp JM, Liu WR (2014) Pyrrolysyl-tRNA synthetase: an ordinary enzyme but an outstanding genetic code expansion tool. Biochim Biophys Acta (BBA)–Proteins Proteom 1844:1059–1070. https://doi.org/10.1016/j.bbapap.2014.03.002
4. Koch NG, Budisa N (2024) Evolution of pyrrolysyl-tRNA synthetase: from methanogenesis to genetic code expansion. Chem Rev 124:9580–9608. https://doi.org/10.1021/acs.chemrev.4c00031
5. Chen P-HC, Guo XS, Zhang HE, Dubey GK, Geng ZZ, Fierke CA, Xu S, Hampton JT, Liu WR (2024) Leveraging a phage-encoded noncanonical amino acid: a novel pathway to potent and selective epigenetic reader protein inhibitors. ACS Cent Sci 10:782–792. https://doi.org/10.1021/acscentsci.3c01419
6. Tharp JM, Hampton JT, Reed CA, Ehnbom A, Chen P-HC, Morse JS, Kurra Y, Pérez LM, Xu S, Liu WR (2020) An amber obligate active site-directed ligand evolution technique for phage display. Nat Commun 11: 1392. https://doi.org/10.1038/s41467-020-15057-7
7. Hampton JT, Cho C-CD, Coleman DD, Geng ZZ, Chen P-HC, Dubey GK, Sylvain LD, Xu S, Liu WR (2023) An amber-encoding helper phage for more efficient phage display of noncanonical amino acids. Nucleic Acids Res 51:6566–6577. https://doi.org/10.1093/nar/gkad488
8. Morse JS, Sheng YJ, Hampton JT, Sylvain LD, Das S, Alugubelli YR, Chen P-HC, Yang KS, Xu S, Fierke CA, Liu WR (2022) Phage-assisted, active site-directed ligand evolution of a potent and selective histone deacetylase 8 inhibitor. Protein Sci 31:e4512. https://doi.org/10.1002/pro.4512
9. Xue Q, Yang Y, Li H, Li X, Zou L, Li T, Ma H, Qi H, Wang J, Yu T (2023) Functions and mechanisms of protein lysine butyrylation (Kbu): therapeutic implications in human diseases. Genes Dis 10:2479–2490. https://doi.org/10.1016/j.gendis.2022.10.025
10. Wang Y-S, Fang X, Wallace AL, Wu B, Liu WR (2012) A rationally designed pyrrolysyl-tRNA synthetase mutant with a broad substrate spectrum. J Am Chem Soc 134:2950–2953. https://doi.org/10.1021/ja211972x
11. Wan L, Wen H, Li Y, Lyu J, Xi Y, Hoshii T, Joseph JK, Wang X, Loh Y-HE, Erb MA, Souza AL, Bradner JE, Shen L, Li W, Li H, Allis CD, Armstrong SA, Shi X (2017) ENL links histone acetylation to oncogenic gene expression in acute myeloid leukaemia. Nature 543:265–269. https://doi.org/10.1038/nature21687

Chapter 2

Construction and Functional Validation of a High-Diversity Naive Phage Antibody Library

Angela Chiew Wen Ch'ng, Azimah Ahmad, Yee Siew Choong and Theam Soon Lim

Abstract

Phage display technology has emerged as an indispensable and highly successful platform for the in vitro generation of monoclonal antibodies (mAbs) against a vast spectrum of targets, ranging from disease biomarkers and native biologically important proteins to small molecules. The critical determinant for constructing a high-quality library capable of yielding high-affinity antibodies is the diversity of the source antibody genes. Naïve antibody libraries, the most common type, are typically derived from the IgM repertoire of healthy human donors, using B-cells isolated from peripheral blood mononuclear cells (PBMCs). The preferred format for these displayed antibodies is the single-chain fragment variable (scFv) due to its smaller size and functional suitability for the phage display system. This chapter details the technical workflow for harnessing this power, which involves a robust two-step cloning method for constructing the high-diversity library, followed by the iterative process of biopanning for the efficient selection and isolation of target-specific, high-affinity clones.

Keywords Naïve antibody, scFv, Phage display, Phagemid, Monoclonal antibodies

1 Introduction

Monoclonal antibodies (mAbs) stand as one of the most significant classes of therapeutic and diagnostic agents developed in modern biotechnology, forming the bedrock of precision medicine. For decades, the gold standard for mAb production relied on the hybridoma technique, a groundbreaking yet often laborious and time-consuming approach that yields murine antibodies [1]. These mouse-derived antibodies are xenogeneic and frequently require subsequent expensive and complex humanization engineering steps to mitigate their immunogenicity (the tendency to provoke an adverse immune response) when administered to patients [2].

The advent of antibody phage display technology has fundamentally revolutionized the landscape of therapeutic antibody discovery

Huan Peng and Theam Soon Lim (eds.), *Biomolecular Display Technologies*, Methods in Molecular Biology, vol. 3030,
https://doi.org/10.1007/978-1-0716-5249-7_2,

by offering a powerful, entirely in vitro alternative for selecting high-affinity human antibodies. This revolutionary system functions by creating a physical link between an antibody gene (genotype) and its corresponding antibody protein (phenotype) on the surface of a harmless filamentous bacteriophage (a virus that infects bacteria). This process transforms a genetic library into a massive screening tool [3].

At the core of this technology are different types of antibody libraries, but the most versatile is the naïve library. A naïve antibody library is constructed using immunoglobulin (Ig) genes isolated from the B-cells of healthy, nonimmunized human donors. By sourcing the genetic material from peripheral blood mononuclear cells (PBMCs), this library captures the complete, unprimed repertoire of the human immune system, representing the full, uneducated genetic potential of the immune system before it has encountered any specific antigens [4].

The critical measure of success for any phage display effort is maximizing the library's diversity. This requires constructing a library of colossal size, often encompassing 10^9–10^{11} unique antibody clones, which is necessary to ensure that a binder exists for virtually any conceivable antigen. This extreme diversity is the sine qua non of a high-quality naïve library; it ensures functional breadth and serves as a universal starting point for antibody discovery against novel or recalcitrant targets without the need for prior animal immunization [5].

Achieving this staggering level of diversity relies heavily on the cloning strategy used to assemble the antibody genes. Antibody fragments are typically expressed in the preferred single-chain fragment variable (scFv) format, which links the variable regions of the heavy (VH) and light (VL) chains using a flexible peptide linker. For creating high-diversity antibody phage libraries, several cloning strategies are employed, each with distinct advantages for assembling the variable heavy (VH) and variable light (VL) chain genes into the single-chain fragment variable (scFv) format. The classical approach is Restriction Enzyme-Based Cloning [6], which uses specific restriction sites engineered into the gene fragments to sequentially insert them into the phage display vector; while reliable, it demands meticulous selection of enzymes to prevent unintended cleavage within the natural, diverse immunoglobulin (Ig) sequences. This is a robust and widely favored technique for naïve libraries is the Two-Step Cloning Strategy, which maximizes scFv pairing and functional display by sequentially inserting the VL genes first, followed by a second, high-efficiency ligation step to introduce the VH genes [6].

This chapter provides a detailed, practical guide to the creation of these essential genetic resources. We will systematically walk through the critical steps involved in naïve library generation, starting with the crucial isolation and preparation of the genetic source material. This is followed by the design and molecular cloning of the diverse Ig heavy and light chain genes into the preferred scFv format, specifically detailing the robust two-step cloning strategy often favored for its efficiency in generating vast combinatorial diversity. Finally, we will cover the creation of the phage display library itself, culminating in the foundational genetic resource necessary for the subsequent selection of high-affinity binders via the iterative process of biopanning. The content of this chapter is derived from a protocol that appeared earlier in this series with slight modifications.

2 Materials

2.1 Isolation of B-Cells

1. Ficoll-Paque™ PLUS (Cytiva, USA).
2. QIAamp® RNA Blood Mini Kit (QIAGEN, Germany).
3. Phosphate buffered saline (PBS), pH 7.4: 8 g NaCl, 0.2 g KCl, 1.44 g $Na_2HPO_4 \cdot 2H_2O$, 0.24 g KH_2PO_4 in 1 L dH_2O, autoclave and store at room temperature.

2.2 First Strand cDNA Synthesis

1. Approximately 500 ng RNA from each donor.
2. SuperScript First-Strand Synthesis System for RT-PCR (Invitrogen, USA).

2.3 Amplification of Heavy Chain (HC) and Light Chain (LC) Gene Repertoire

1. Vent® DNA Polymerase (NEB, USA) (*see* **Note 1**).
2. *Pfu* DNA Polymerase (Thermo Scientific, USA) (*see* **Note 1**).
3. 10 mM dNTP mixture.
4. Forward and reverse primers for first amplification of VH and VL (*see* Table 1).
5. Forward and reverse primers for second amplification of VH and VL with restriction endonuclease sites (*see* Table 2).
6. QIAquick® Gel Extraction Kit (QIAGEN, Germany).
7. Agarose.
8. 10× TBE buffer, pH 8.0: 108 g Tris, 55 g boric acid, and 7.4 g EDTA in 1 L dH_2O, autoclave and store at room temperature.

2.4 Two-Step Cloning

1. Antarctic Phosphatase.
2. T4 DNA Ligase.
3. QIAGEN Plasmid Maxi Kit (QIAGEN, Germany).
4. QIAquick® PCR Purification Kit (QIAGEN, Germany).
5. pLABEL phagemid vector.
6. Ampicillin stock solution (50 mg/mL): 2.5 g ampicillin sodium salt in 50 mL of 50% (v/v) ethanol, filter sterilize and store at −20°C.

Table 1
Primers for first amplification of VH and VL gene repertoire

Primer name	Primer sequence
VH amplification	
VH1 Fw	5′- CAGGTCCAGCTKGTRCAGTCTGG -3′
VH157 Fw	5′- CAGGTGCAGCTGGTGSARTCTGG -3′
VH2 Fw	5′- CAGRTCACCTTGAAGGAGTCTG -3′
VH3 Fw	5′- GAGGTGCAGCTGKTGGAGWCY -3′
VH4 Fw	5′- CAGGTGCAGCTGCAGGAGTCSG -3′
VH4 DP63 Fw	5′- CAGGTGCAGCTACAGCAGTGGG -3′
VH6 Fw	5′- CAGGTACAGCTGCAGCAGTCA -3′
Human scFv IgM CH1 Rv	5′- AAGGGTTGGGGCGGATGCACT -3′
VL amplification	
Vλ1 Fw	5′- CAGTCTGTSBTGACGCAGCCGCC -3′
Vλ1459 Fw	5′- CAGCCTGTGCTGACTCARYC -3′
Vλ15910 Fw	5′- CAGCCWGKGCTGACTCAGCCMCC -3′
Vλ2 Fw	5′- CAGTCTGYYCTGAYTCAGCCT -3′
Vλ3 Fw	5′- TCCTATGWGCTGACWCAGCCAA -3′
Vλ3 DPL16 Fw	5′- TCCTCTGAGCTGASTCAGGASCC -3′
Vλ338 Fw	5′- TCCTATGAGCTGAYRCAGCYACC -3′
Vλ6 Fw	5′- AATTTTATGCTGACTCAGCCCC -3′
Vλ78 Fw	5′- CAGDCTGTGGTGACYCAGGAGCC -3′
Vκ1 Fw	5′- GACATCCRGDTGACCCAGTCTCC -3′
Vκ246 Fw	5′- GATATTGTGMTGACBCAGWCTCC -3′
Vκ3 Fw	5′- GAAATTGTRWTGACRCAGTCTCC -3′
Vκ5 Fw	5′- GAAACGACACTCACGCAGTCTC -3′
scFv Fab Lambda CL1 Rv	5′- TGAACATTCTGTAGGGGCCACTG -3′
scFv Fab Lambda CL2 Rv	5′- TGAACATTCCGTAGGGGCAACTG -3′
scFv Fab Kappa CL Rv	5′- ACACTCTCCCCTGTTGAAGCTCTT -3′

7. 3 M sodium acetate, pH 5.2: sodium acetate in 800 mL dH_2O, adjust pH to 5.2 with glacial acetic acid, top up to 1 L with dH_2O and store at room temperature.
8. 40% (w/v) glucose: 40 g D-(+)-glucose in 100 mL of dH_2O, autoclave and store at 4°C.

Table 2
Primers with restriction endonucleases site for second amplification

Primer name	Primer sequence
VH amplification	
VH1 NcoI Fw	5′- CCC AGC CGG CCA TGG CC CAG GTC CAG CTK GTR CAG TCT GG -3′
VH157 NcoI Fw	5′- CCC AGC CGG CCA TGG CC CAG GTG CAG CTG GTG SAR TCT GG -3′
VH2 NcoI Fw	5′- CCC AGC CGG CCA TGG CC CAG RTC ACC TTG AAG GAG TCT G -3′
VH3 NcoI Fw	5′- CCC AGC CGG CCA TGG CC GAG GTG CAG CTG KTG GAG WCY -3′
VH4 NcoI Fw	5′- CCC AGC CGG CCA TGG CC CAG GTG CAG CTG CAG GAG TCS G -3′
VH4 DP63 NcoI Fw	5′- CCC AGC CGG CCA TGG CC CAG GTG CAG CTA CAG CAG TGG G -3′
VH6 NcoI Fw	5′- CCC AGC CGG CCA TGG CC CAG GTA CAG CTG CAG CAG TCA -3′
Human scFv IgM CH1 XhoI Rv	5′- ACCG CTC GAG AC AAG GGT TGG GGC GGA TGC ACT -3′
VL amplification	
Vλ1 SalI Fw	5′- TGT GAC AAA GTC GAC G CAG TCT GTS BTG ACG CAG CCG CC -3′
Vλ1459 SalI Fw	5′- TGT GAC AAA GTC GAC G CAG CCT GTG CTG ACT CAR YC-3′
Vλ15910 SalI Fw	5′- TGT GAC AAA GTC GAC G CAG CCW GKG CTG ACT CAG CCM CC -3′
Vλ2 SalI Fw	5′- TGT GAC AAA GTC GAC G CAG TCT GYY CTG AYT CAG CCT -3′
Vλ3 SalI Fw	5′- TGT GAC AAA GTC GAC G TCC TAT GWG CTG ACW CAG CCA A -3′
Vλ3 DPL16 SalI Fw	5′- TGT GAC AAA GTC GAC G TCC TCT GAG CTG AST CAG GAS CC -3′
Vλ338 SalI Fw	5′- TGT GAC AAA GTC GAC G TCC TAT GAG CTG AYR CAG CYA CC -3′
Vλ6 SalI Fw	5′- TGT GAC AAA GTC GAC G AAT TTT ATG CTG ACT CAG CCC C -3′
Vλ78 SalI Fw	5′ - TGT GAC AAA GTC GAC G CAG DCT GTG GTG ACY CAG GAG CC -3′

(continued)

Table 2
(Continued)

Primer name	Primer sequence
Vκ1 SalI Fw	5′- TGT GAC AAA GTC GAC G GAC ATC CRG DTG ACC CAG TCT CC -3′
Vκ246 SalI Fw	5′- TGT GAC AAA GTC GAC G GAT ATT GTG MTG ACB CAG WCT CC -3′
Vκ3 SalI Fw	5′- TGT GAC AAA GTC GAC G GAA ATT GTR WTG ACR CAG TCT CC -3′
Vκ5 SalI Fw	5′- TGT GAC AAA GTC GAC G GAA ACG ACA CTC ACG CAG TCT C -3′
scFv Lambda NotI Rv	5′- ATG ATG ATG TGC GGC CGC AGA GGA SGG YGG GAA CAG AGT GAC -3′
scFv Kappa NotI Rv	5′- ATG ATG ATG TGC GGC CGC GAA GAC AGA TGG TGC AGC CAC AGT -3′

9. 2× YT medium: 16 g tryptone, 10 g yeast extract, and 5 g NaCl in 1 L dH_2O, autoclave and store at room temperature.
10. 2× YT agar: 16 g tryptone, 10 g yeast extract, 5 g NaCl, and 15.5 g agar in 1 L dH_2O, autoclave.
11. 2× YT-amp medium: 2× YT medium, 0.1 mg/mL ampicillin, and 2% (v/v) glucose.
12. 2× YT-amp agar plate: 2× YT agar, 0.1 mg/mL ampicillin, and 2% (v/v) glucose.
13. 80% (v/v) glycerol: 40 mL glycerol in 10 mL dH_2O, autoclave and store at room temperature.
14. Sterile Petri Dish, 90 mm.
15. Nunc™ Square BioAssay Dish, 25 mm (Thermo Scientific, USA).
16. MicroPulser™ Electroporator (Bio-Rad, USA).

2.4.1 First Step Cloning (VL)

1. SalI.
2. NotI.
3. ElectroMAX™ DH10β Cells (Invitrogen, USA), genotype: F^- *mcrA* Δ(*mrr-hsdRMS-mcrBC*) Φ80*lacZ*Δ*M15* Δ*lacX74 recA1 endA1 araD139*Δ(*ara, leu*)*7697 galU galK* λ^- *rpsL nupG*.

2.4.2 Second Step Cloning (VH)

1. NcoI.
2. XhoI.
3. XL1-Blue MRF' Competent Cells (Agilent Technologies, USA), genotype: *recA1 endA1 gyrA96 thi-1 hsdR17 supE44 relA1 lac* [F′ *proAB lacI*^{q} *Z*Δ*M15* Tn*10* (Tet^r)].

2.5 Colony PCR

1. DreamTaq DNA Polymerase (Thermo Scientific, USA).
2. Forward primer, LMB3: 5′ - CAG GAA ACA GCT ATG AC - 3′
3. Reverse primer, pIII: 5′ - TTA GAT CGT TAC GCT AAC - 3′

2.6 scFv Phage Library Packaging

1. M13K07 helper phage (Invitrogen, USA).
2. Hyperphage (Progen)
3. 2× YT medium: 16 g tryptone, 10 g yeast extract, and 5 g NaCl in 1 L dH_2O, autoclave and store at room temperature.
4. 2× YT agar: 16 g tryptone, 10 g yeast extract, 5 g NaCl, and 15.5 g agar in 1 L dH_2O, autoclave.
5. Ampicillin stock solution (50 mg/mL): 2.5 g ampicillin sodium salt in 50 mL of 50% (v/v) ethanol, filter sterilize and store at −20°C.
6. Kanamycin stock solution (30 mg/mL): 1.5 g kanamycin sulfate in 50 mL of dH_2O, filter sterilize and store at −20°C.
7. 40% (w/v) glucose: 40 g D-(+)-glucose in 100 mL of dH_2O, autoclave and store at 4°C.
8. 2× YT-amp medium: 2× YT medium, 0.1 mg/ mL ampicillin, and 2% (v/v) glucose.
9. 2× YT-amp/kan medium: 2× YT medium, 0.1 mg/mL ampicillin, and 0.06 mg/mL kanamycin.
10. 2× YT-amp agar: 2× YT agar, 0.1 mg/mL ampicillin, and 2% (v/v) glucose.
11. 2× YT-kan agar: 2× YT agar and 0.06 mg/mL kanamycin.
12. PEG/NaCl solution: 200 g polyethylene glycol 6000 (PEG 6000) and 146 g NaCl in 1 L dH_2O, autoclave and store at room temperature.
13. Phosphate buffered saline (PBS), pH 7.4: 8 g NaCl, 0.2 g KCl, 1.44 g $Na_2HPO_4{\cdot}2H_2O$, 0.24 g KH_2PO_4 in 1 L dH_2O, autoclave and store at room temperature.

2.7 Phage Titration

1. TG1 Electrocompetent Cells (Lucigen, USA), genotype: *supE thi-1 Δ(lac-proAB) Δ(mcrB-hsdSM)5(rK - mK -)* [F' *traD36 proAB lacI^{q}Z ΔM15]*.
2. 2× YT medium: 16 g tryptone, 10 g yeast extract, and 5 g NaCl in 1 L dH_2O, autoclave and store at room temperature.
3. 2× YT agar: 16 g tryptone, 10 g yeast extract, 5 g NaCl, and 15.5 g agar in 1 L dH_2O, autoclave.
4. 2× YT-amp agar: 2× YT agar, 0.1 mg/mL ampicillin, and 2% (v/v) glucose.
5. 2× YT-kan agar: 2× YT agar and 0.06 mg/mL kanamycin.

6. Phosphate buffered saline (PBS), pH 7.4: 8 g NaCl, 0.2 g KCl, 1.44 g $Na_2HPO_4 \cdot 2H_2O$, 0.24 g KH_2PO_4 in 1 L dH_2O, autoclave and store at room temperature.

2.8 scFv Library Biopanning

2.8.1 scFv Selection

1. Coating buffer, pH 9.6: 1.59 g Na_2CO_3 and 2.93 g $NaHCO_3$ in 1 L dH_2O, store at 4°C.
2. Phosphate-buffered saline (PBS), pH 7.4: 8 g NaCl, 0.2 g KCl, 1.44 g $Na_2HPO_4 \cdot 2H_2O$, 0.24 g KH_2PO_4 in 1 L dH_2O, autoclave and store at room temperature.
3. PBST: 1 mL Tween 20 in 1 L PBS.
4. PTM blocking buffer: 2 g skim milk in 100 mL PBST (*see* **Note 2**).
5. Trypsin (10 μg/mL): 10 μg trypsin in 1 mL dH_2O, store at −20°C.
6. Ampicillin stock solution (50 mg/mL): 2.5 g ampicillin sodium salt in 50 mL of 50% (v/v) ethanol, filter sterilize and store at −20°C.
7. Kanamycin stock solution (30 mg/mL): 1.5 g kanamycin sulfate in 50 mL of dH_2O, filter sterilize and store at −20°C.
8. 40% (w/v) glucose: 40 g D-(+)-glucose in 100 mL of dH_2O, autoclave and store at 4°C.
9. 2× YT medium, pH 7.2: 16 g tryptone, 10 g yeast extract and 5 g NaCl in 1 L dH_2O, autoclave and store at room temperature.
10. 10× amp: 1 mg/mL ampicillin and 20% (v/v) glucose in PBS.
11. 2× YT-amp: 2× YT medium with 0.1 mg/mL ampicillin and 2% (v/v) glucose.
12. 2× YT-amp/kan: 2× YT medium with 0.1 mg/mL ampicillin and 0.06 mg/mL kanamycin.
13. XL1-Blue Competent Cells (Agilent Technologies, USA), genotype: *recA1 endA1 gyrA96 thi-1 hsdR17 supE44 relA1 lac* [F′ *proAB lacI^q ZΔM15* Tn*10* (Tet^r)].
14. Corning® 96-well clear polystyrene high bind Stripwell™ microplate (Corning, USA).

2.8.2 Polyclonal and Monoclonal Phage ELISA

1. PBST: 1 mL Tween-20 in 1 L PBS.
2. PTM blocking buffer: 2 g skim milk in 100 mL PBST (*see* **Note 2**).
3. Anti-M13 horseradish peroxidase (HRP): Prepare at 1:5000 dilution in PTM blocking buffer.

4. Bovine serum albumin (BSA) Fraction V (Sigma-Aldrich, USA).
5. 2,2'-azino-bis(3-ethylbenzothiazoline-6-sulphonicacid)(ABTS) Tablets (Roche, USA).
6. ABTS buffer (Roche, USA).

3 Methods

3.1 Total Lymphocyte Isolation

The antibody repertoire used to build the human naïve library comes from blood samples collected from healthy donors. Specific donor inclusion and exclusion criteria are detailed in the notes (*see* **Note 3**).

1. Dilute the EDTA-treated fresh blood and PBS in equal volumes (1:1 dilution).
2. Carefully layer 10 mL of whole blood onto 7.5 mL of Ficoll-Paque™ PLUS (*see* **Note 4**). Centrifuge the layered solution at 1200×*g* for 15 min (min) at 18°C.
3. Gently remove the lymphocytes from the interface separating the Ficoll-Paque™ PLUS and the plasma. Place the aspirated layer into a sterile 50 mL polypropylene tube.
4. Dilute the isolated lymphocytes are with PBS to a final volume of 50 mL. Centrifuge the lymphocytes at 250×*g* for 10 min at 18°C.
5. The supernatant is removed using a clean filter-tip.
6. Perform one additional wash using PBS.
7. Using a total RNA extraction kit, the isolated lymphocytes are subjected to RNA extraction as specified by the kit manufacturer (*see* **Note 5**).
8. Store the extracted total RNA at −80°C until use.

3.2 First Strand cDNA Synthesis

1. First-strand cDNA synthesis is performed with SuperScript™ II Reverse Transcriptase, as per the manufacturer's protocol.
2. The cDNA is stored at −20°C until use.

3.3 Amplification of Heavy Chain and Light Chain Gene Repertoire

The scFv fragment is composed of the heavy chain variable region (VH) and the light chain variable region (VL), joined by a flexible peptide linker. The cDNA serves as the template to amplify these VH and VL genes for subsequent library cloning. Duet to the diversity in the V gene repertoires for both VH and VL, a variety of primers are required for this amplification. A set of primers consisting of 7 VH primers, 9 Vλ primers, and 4 Vκ primers are used for this purpose (*see* Table 1).

1. Each 20 μL PCR reaction is prepared by mixing 200 ng of cDNA, 200 μM dNTPs, 0.2 μM Fw and Rv primers (Table 1),

2 µL of *Pfu* buffer with $MgSO_4$, and 0.5 U *Pfu* DNA Polymerase. The remaining volume is filled with dH_2O.

2. The PCR cycling begins with an initial denaturation step at 95°C for 2 min. This is followed by 30 amplification cycles, each consisting of denaturation at 95°C (30 s/cycle), annealing at 55°C or 62°C (30 s), elongation at 72°C (45 s). The program concludes with a final elongation at 72°C (5 min) (*see* **Note 6**).
3. The PCR products are first separated by gel electrophoresis (1% TBE agarose, 110 V for 50 min). The bands of interest (~400 bp for VH and ~650 bp for LC) are then excised and the DNA purified using the QIAquick® Gel Extraction Kit per the provided instructions (*see* **Note 7**).
4. After purifying the first PCR product, quantify its concentration. Use this purified product in the second amplification step, which is designed to add the necessary restriction sites. If you do not proceed immediately, store the DNA at −20°C.
5. For the second amplification, each PCR reaction is prepared with 20 µg of the purified VH or LC, 200 µM dNTPs, 0.2 µM Fw and Rv primers (Table 2), 2 µL of ThermoPol® buffer and 0.4 U Vent® DNA Polymerase. Top up the reaction to 20 µL using dH_2O. At this stage, the LC will be amplified with the Rv primers to shorten the fragment to yield only the VL domain.
6. The PCR program is as follows: initial denaturation at 95°C (2 min), 30 cycles of amplification with denaturation at 95°C (30 s/cycle), annealing at 55°C or 62°C (30 s), elongation at 72°C (45 s), and a final elongation at 72°C (5 min) (*see* **Note 6**).
7. Separate the amplified PCR product using gel electrophoresis on a 1% TBE agarose gel at 110 V for 50 min. Excise the band corresponding to the desired size (~400 bp for both VH and VL) and extract the DNA from the gel slice using the QIAquick® Gel Extraction Kit following the manufacturer's protocol.
8. The purified DNA products are then pooled according to the subfamilies in a set of five donors each. Determine the concentration and store the DNA at −20°C until use.

3.4 Two-Step Cloning

The library is constructed using a two-step cloning strategy. The first step creates a mini library (containing both and repertoires) by cloning into cells. The second step then introduces the repertoire into this mini library, resulting in the final library, which is hosted in cells.

3.4.1 First Step Cloning (VL)

1. Double digest the pLABEL vector and pooled Vλ or Vκ with SalI and NotI overnight at 37°C. Heat-inactivate the reaction at 65°C for 20 min (*see* **Note 8**).

2. Add 5 U of alkaline phosphatase only to the double digested pLABEL vector and incubate at 37°C for 1 hour (h). Incubate the reaction at 80°C for 2 min for heat inactivation.
3. The digested vector is first resolved on a 1% TBE agarose gel via electrophoresis (110 V, 50 min). The target band is then excised, and the DNA purified using the QIAquick® Gel Extraction Kit as instructed by the manufacturer.
4. The digested Vλ and Vκ fragments are purified using QIAquick® PCR Purification Kit according to the manufacturer's protocol.
5. Ligate digested pLABEL and digested Vλ or Vκ pools at 1:2 ratio using T4 DNA Ligase (*see* **Note 9**). Incubate the ligation reaction overnight at 16°C. Heat-inactivate the reaction at 65°C for 10 min.
6. Precipitate the ligated DNA by adding 2.5 volumes of ethanol and 0.1 volume of 3 M sodium acetate. Incubate the mixture at −80°C for 1 h (or, alternatively, flash-freeze it in liquid nitrogen). Finally, pellet the DNA by centrifuging for 20 min at 14,000×*g*.
7. Wash the DNA pellet with 500 μL of 70% (v/v) ethanol and centrifuge again at 14,000×*g* for 20 min.
8. Dissolve the DNA pellet with 4 μL dH_2O per ligation reaction.
9. Thaw DH10β cells on ice for 2 min and mix with 2 μL DNA.
10. Transfer the mixture to a prechilled 0.1 cm electroporation cuvette. Transform the mixture at 1.7 kV using an electroporator.
11. Add 1 mL of prewarmed 2× YT medium to the electroporated sample to resuspend it. Immediately move the resulting suspension into a 1.5 mL microcentrifuge tube. Incubate the cell suspension for 1 h at 37°C and 700 rpm.
12. Pool the cell suspension according to subfamilies and take 10 μL of cells to determine the cloning efficiency. Dilute the 10 μL cells in 90 μL 2× YT-amp and plate out on 2× YT-amp agar plates in 90 mm petri dish.
13. Plate out the remaining pooled cell suspension on 30 BioAssay Dish with 2× YT-amp agar. Incubate the agar plates overnight at 37°C.
14. Scrape the colonies on the BioAssay Dish with 2× YT-amp.
15. Estimate the library diversity by titrating the scraped library stock (see Sect. 3.4.3).
16. Prepare glycerol stocks of the VL-mini library (see Sect. 3.4.4).

17. Perform a colony PCR using colonies on the 90 mm petri dish to confirm successful cloning of the VL repertoire (see Sect. 3.5) (*see* **Note 10**).

3.4.2 Second Step Cloning (VH)

1. Culture a tube of VL-mini library glycerol stock overnight in 500 mL of 2× YT-amp at 37°C with shaking at 200 rpm.
2. Perform plasmid extraction using the QIAGEN Plasmid Maxi Kit per the manufacturer's protocol.
3. Perform an overnight double digestion of the VL mini library and VH repertoire at 37°C with the enzymes NcoI and XhoI. The reaction is then stopped by heat-inactivating the enzymes at 65°C for 20 min (*see* **Note 8**).
4. Perform the digestion and ligation as in the first step cloning procedure (see Sect. 3.4.1).
5. Transform the scFv library into XL1-Blue MRF' cells.
6. Pool the cell suspension according to its subfamilies. Take a 10 µL aliquot from the pool to determine the cloning efficiency. Dilute this 10 µL aliquot in 90 µL of 2× YT-amp and plate the mixture onto a 90 mm petri dish containing 2× YT-amp agar.
7. Plate out the remaining pooled cell suspension on 40 BioAssay Dish with 2× YT-amp agar. Incubate the agar plates overnight at 37°C.
8. Scrape the colonies on BioAssay Dish with 2× YT-amp.
9. Titrate the scraped library stock to estimate the library diversity (see Sect. 3.4.3) (*see* **Note 11**).
10. Prepare glycerol stock of the scFv library (see Sect. 3.4.4).
11. Perform a colony PCR using colonies on the 90 mm petri dish to confirm successful cloning of the VH repertoire (see Sect. 3.5) (*see* **Note 10**).

3.4.3 Library Size Estimation

1. Take 10 µL of cells from the scraped library suspension to perform a ten-fold serial dilution to 10^{-13}.
2. Spot 10 µL of the dilution on the 2× YT-amp agar plate and incubate overnight at 37°C.
3. Count the library size based on the formula:

$$\text{Library size} = \frac{\text{number of colonies} \times \text{dilution factor}}{\text{total volume}}$$

3.4.4 Preparation of Bacteria Library Stock

1. Pellet down the colonies scraped from the BioAssay Dish at 4500×*g*, 10 min.

2. Resuspend the pellet with adequate amount of 2× YT-amp and add 80% (v/v) glycerol to the cells suspension to make a 20% glycerol library stock (*see* **Note 12**).
3. Aliquot the final library suspension into 2 mL cryogenic vial and keep in −80°C until use.

3.5 Colony PCR

1. Pick single colonies randomly and resuspend in 10 μL dH_2O.
2. Set up the PCR reaction using 2 μL of colony supernatant, 200 μM dNTPs, 0.5 μM LMB3 Fw and pIII Rv primers, 1× DreamTaq buffer and 0.5 U DreamTaq DNA Polymerase. Top up the reaction to 20 μL with dH_2O.
3. Set the PCR program as follows: initial denaturation at 95°C (5 min), 20 cycles of amplification with denaturation at 95°C (30 s/cycle), annealing at 55°C (30 s), elongation at 72°C (2 min), and a final elongation at 72°C (5 min).
4. Separate the amplified PCR product on 1% TBE agarose gel using gel electrophoresis run at 110 V for 50 min (*see* **Notes 10 and 13**).
5. Send the colonies with the correct band size for sequencing.
6. Analyze the DNA sequences for V,D,J gene usage and mutations using IMGT/V-quest (www.imgt.org/IMGT_vquest/vquest) (*see* **Note 14**).

3.6 scFv Phage Library Packaging

1. Thaw a tube of the library glycerol stock and inoculate into 500 mL of 2× YT-amp. Culture at 37°C with shaking at 200 rpm until OD_{600} ~0.5.
2. Infect 250 mL of the culture with 10^{12} M13KO7 helper phage, following the multiplicity of infection (MOI) of 1:20. Incubate the culture static at 37°C for 30 min.
3. Pellet down the culture at 3500×*g* for 10 min. Remove the supernatant (*see* **Note 15**).
4. Resuspend the pellet with 300 mL 2× YT-amp/kan. Culture overnight at 30°C, 200 rpm.
5. Pellet down the cells at 10,000×*g* for 10 min. Transfer the phage-containing supernatant to a new 50 mL polypropylene tube.
6. Add 1/5 volume of PEG/NaCl solution to 4/5 volume of supernatant. Mix well and incubate on ice for 1 h (*see* **Note 16**).
7. Centrifuge the mixture at 10,000×*g* for 30 min at 12°C, remove the supernatant and resuspend the phage pellet in 8 mL PBS.
8. Add 2 mL PEG/NaCl solution, mix well and incubate on ice for 20 min.

9. Centrifuge the mixture at 10,000×*g* for 30 min at 12°C. Remove the supernatant, short spin briefly and pipette out remaining PEG/NaCl solution.
10. Resuspend the phage pellet in 2 mL PBS.
11. Centrifuge at 10,000×*g* for 10 min to remove remaining bacterial cells from the phage precipitation. Repeat centrifugation until no bacteria pellet is observed.
12. Take 10 μL of the phage to check the titer of the packaged scFv library (see Sect. 3.7).
13. Store the scFv antibody library at 4°C until use (*see* **Note 17**).

3.7 Phage Titration

1. Dilute 10 μL of scFv phage library in 90 μL of PBS and perform a ten-fold serial dilution.
2. Add 100 μL of TG1 or XL1-Blue MRF' cells at OD_{600} ~0.5 to the diluted phage.
3. Spot 10 μL of the infected cells on 2× YT-amp agar plate and 2× YT-kan agar plate. Incubate overnight at 37°C (*see* **Note 18**).
4. Calculate the phage titer using the formula:

$$\text{Phage titer (cfu/mL)} = \frac{\text{number of colonies} \times \text{dilution factor}}{\text{total volume spotted}}$$

3.8 scFv Library Biopanning

The displayed protein fragments are screened through biopanning. The number of biopanning rounds required is determined by the rate of phage discovery, which typically increases with each subsequent round. Usually, three to four rounds are enough to produce a suitably enriched subpopulation of display phages [6].

3.8.1 scFv Selection

1. Coat a microtiter well with 100 μL of coating buffer containing 1–10 μg of antigen. For subsequent biopanning rounds, reduce the amount of antigen to increase the selection stringency. Incubate the well overnight at 4°C (*see* **Note 19**).
2. Wash the antigen-coated well three times with 300 μL of PBST per wash, using an ELISA plate washer (*see* **Note 20**).
3. The antigen-coated well is blocked using 300 μL of PTM blocking buffer and breathable tape. Incubate for 1 h at room temperature with constant shaking. Afterwards, wash the wells three times with 300 μL of PBST each time.
4. Concurrently, dilute 10^{11} phage particles in 200 μL of PTM blocking buffer. Incubate the mixture on a blocked microtiter well for 1 h to allow for pre-absorption (*see* **Note 21**).
5. Add 100 μL of the preabsorbed phage to the antigen-coated well for binding. Perform the incubation for 2 h at room temperature with constant shaking at 700 rpm.

6. Remove unbound and unspecific phages by performing ten washes with PBST. Increase the washing stringency in subsequent biopanning rounds by adding an extra ten washes (e.g., 20×, 30×, etc.).
7. Elute the bound phages with 100 μL of 10 μg/mL trypsin and incubate static at 37°C for 30 min (*see* **Note 22**).
8. Transfer the eluted phages to a new 2 mL microcentrifuge tube and add 100 μL of XL1-Blue MRF' cells at OD_{600} ~0.5. Incubate the cells static at 37°C for 30 min followed by 30 min of incubation with shaking at 700 rpm.
9. Take 10 μL of infected culture to determine the rescued phage titer (see Sect. 3.7).
10. Add 20 μL of 10× amp to the remaining culture and culture overnight at 37°C, 700 rpm.
11. Inoculate 190 μL of 2× YT-amp with 10 μL of the overnight culture. Culture at 37°C with shaking at 700 rpm for 2.5 h.
12. Mix the remaining overnight culture with 65 μL of 80% (v/v) glycerol and store the glycerol stock in −80°C.
13. Infect the culture with 10^{11} M13KO7 helper phage and incubate static at 37°C for 30 min.
14. Pellet down the culture at 3500×*g* for 10 min. Resuspend the cell pellet with 230 μL of 2× YT-amp/kan. Culture overnight at 30°C with shaking at 700 rpm.
15. Pellet down the overnight culture at 3500×*g* for 10 min.
16. Move the supernatant into a fresh tube. The resulting phage preparation is divided: 100 μL is used for the subsequent biopanning round, and the remainder is stored at 4°C for polyclonal ELISA. The amplified phage titer must be determined for each round of biopanning (see Sect. 3.7) (*see* **Note 23**).

3.8.2 Polyclonal and Monoclonal Phage ELISA

A key indicator of successful biopanning is a distinct and increasing enrichment signal that is readily observable in the polyclonal ELISA results with each successive screening round. This progressive increase confirms that the library is successfully concentrating phage particles that specifically bind to the target antigen, effectively separating them from nonbinders.

However, the process is not simply about achieving the highest possible enrichment. It is critical to select the optimal biopanning round—not necessarily the last one—before proceeding to monoclonal screening. This strategic selection is vital for two reasons: to ensure the eventual isolation of monoclonal antibodies with high specificity, and to maximize the recovery of a diverse panel of unique binding clones. Choosing a round that is too late may lead to the selection of only the fastest-growing or highest-affinity clones, potentially sacrificing the overall diversity of the final antibody repertoire.

1. Coat the required number of microtiter wells with 1–10 µg of antigen in 100 µL of coating buffer. Incubate these wells overnight at 4°C. Simultaneously, prepare an equal number of negative control wells by coating them with the same amount of BSA to monitor for nonspecific binding.
2. Wash the coated wells 3× with PBST using ELISA plate washer (*see* **Note 20**).
3. Block the coated wells with 300 µL of PTM blocking buffer for 1 h at room temperature shaking at 700 rpm and then wash 3× with PBST.
4. Dilute 50 µL phage with 50 µL PTM blocking buffer, add the 100 µL mixture to corresponding antigen coated wells and the control wells. Incubate for 2 h at room temperature with shaking at 700 rpm.
5. Wash the wells 3× with PBST.
6. Add 100 µL of anti-M13-HRP to each antigen coated wells and control wells. Incubate for 1 h at room temperature with shaking at 700 rpm.
7. Wash the wells 3× with PBST.
8. Develop the wells with 100 µL ABTS solution for 30 min in the dark. Measure the readings at 405 nm using a microtiter plate spectrophotometer.
9. After determining the biopanning round for monoclonal selection, take 10 µL of the remaining phage to perform a ten-fold serial dilution and infect 100 µL of XL1-Blue MRF' cells of OD_{600} ~ 0.5 at 37°C, static. Plate out the infected cell on 2× YT-amp agar plate.
10. Pick 92 monoclonal antibody clones randomly to inoculate 200 µL of 2× YT-amp. Culture overnight at 37°C, 1250 rpm.
11. Package the monoclonal scFv antibody as described in Steps 11–15 in Sect. 3.8.1.
12. Perform monoclonal phage ELISA using the procedures as described in Steps 1–8 in this section.
13. Identify positive clones with good signal/noise ratio for colony PCR (see Sect. 3.5) and send for DNA sequencing analysis.

4 Notes

1. An alternative high-fidelity proofreading polymerase may also be utilized.
2. Alternative blocking agents such as bovine serum albumin (BSA), casein, ovalbumin, or gelatin can be used. It is

required that the blocking agent be freshly prepared for each use to effectively prevent microbial contamination.

3. Sampling requirement:

   a. Inclusion criteria: Donors with healthy backgrounds, received standard common vaccination, no infection in the past 6 months prior to collection date, not on immunosuppressors or other medications.

   b. Exclusion criteria: Donors with family backgrounds of severe illnesses, suffering from autoimmune disorder, having on-going infection, experiencing symptoms of infection or on medication including antibiotics and immunosuppressors within a month from date of blood collection.

   The requirements may vary depending on the disease or library being generated.

4. Exercise care to prevent the blood layer from mixing with the Ficoll-Paque™ PLUS solution. Mixing can cause erythrocyte aggregation, which traps lymphocytes and leads to their sedimentation, thereby reducing the final lymphocyte yield.

5. The integrity and concentration of the total RNA extracted from lymphocytes should be analyzed using a Bioanalyzer Instrument (Agilent, USA) or any other comparable instrumentation.

6. To prevent bias and loss of repertoire that might be caused by sample pooling, the VH and VL repertoire is amplified independently from each donor. This process is crucial for ensuring better repertoire diversity.

7. The VH fragment is expected to be approximately 400 base pair (bp), though V-gene rearrangement may produce bands of slightly varying sizes around this 400 bp mark. Care must be taken to accurately excise the targeted band.

8. To ensure enough DNA for cloning, the number of digestion reactions can be scaled up. When using restriction enzymes with differing buffer requirements, sequential digestion is necessary because the salt concentration of the buffer can significantly impact digestion efficiency.

9. Since the variable heavy chain (VH) is the primary region for antigen binding, a naïve library must contain at least 10^7–10^9 unique clones or more. To ensure such a highly diverse library size, you may need to perform multiple ligation reactions.

10. The expected band size of colony PCR is approximately 750 bp for the first step cloning and 1200 bp for the second step cloning.

11. The final naïve library size should be between 10^9 and 10^{12} or higher.

12. The library stocks with starting OD_{600} ~ 0.1 are prepared when the tube of stock is thawed into 500 mL of 2× YT-amp during library packaging.
13. The goal is to achieve a cloning efficiency exceeding 80% for the inserts used in both the VL mini library and the full scFv library construction.
14. Alternatively, deep sequencing can be utilized as a method for analyzing the diversity within the library repertoire.
15. To prevent the suppression of scFv::pIII fusion protein expression, the cells must be pelleted and the glucose-containing medium removed to discard the excess glucose.
16. The enhancement of the number of phage particles precipitated by the PEG/NaCl solution can be done by extending the ice-cold incubation period to 2 h.
17. Limit phage storage to a maximum of four weeks at 4°C. It is crucial to use freshly packaged phage to avoid the loss of antibody binding activity caused by proteolysis of the displayed proteins.
18. The colony count on the ampicillin agar plate should be at least twice the count on the kanamycin plate. This ratio indicates that fewer helper phages are being produced alongside the main phage library. Additionally, these colonies can be used to estimate the size of the final phage library before starting biopanning.
19. SDS-PAGE and Western-blot are used to determine the purity of the antigens before proceeding to biopanning to ensure total isolation of specific scFv antibody binders.
20. As an alternative washing method, fill the wells with PBST using a squirt bottle. After shaking to discard the wash buffer, remove any residual liquid by tapping the plate on a dry paper towel. Take special care to prevent bubbles from contaminating the next step.
21. The first biopanning round should employ 100 times as much phage as the total library size. For a library size of 10^9, a total of 10^{11} phage particles should be used.
22. Other suitable elution buffers or methods can be substituted here. Examples include competitive elution (with free antigens) or acid elution (glycine-HCl, pH 2.2). The ideal method will be determined by user requirements.
23. The phage recovery value (rescued titer/input titer) serves as the metric for success. A successful biopanning process, indicating the enrichment of binding clones, is confirmed by a gradually increasing phage recovery across each cycle.

Acknowledgments

The authors would like to acknowledge the support of Malaysian Ministry for Higher Education through the Fundamental Research Grant Scheme (FRGS/1/2024/STG01/USM/02/10).

References

1. Madej B, Tomaszewski F, Szmajda-Krygier D, Świechowski R, Jeleń A, Mirowski M (2025) Monoclonal antibodies: historical perspective and current trends in biological drug development. Int J Mol Sci 26(18):8794
2. Foltz IN, Gunasekaran K, King CT (2016) Discovery and bio-optimization of human antibody therapeutics using the XenoMouse® transgenic mouse platform. Immunol Rev 270(1):51–64
3. Zhang Y (2023) Evolution of phage display libraries for therapeutic antibody discovery. Mabs 15(1):2213793
4. Lai JY, Corona A, Ng CL, Tramontano E, Choong YS, Lim TS (2023) Naïve antibody library derived monoclonal antibody against VP35 of Ebola virus. Int J Biol Macromol 245:125571
5. Bashir S, Paeshuyse J (2020) Construction of antibody phage libraries and their application in veterinary immunovirology. Antibodies 9(2):1–13.
6. Ruschig M, Heine PA, Führer V, Zilkens KJK, Steinke S, Schubert M, Bertoglio F, Hust M (2023) Construction of human immune and naive scFv phage display libraries. Methods Mol Biol 2702:15–37

Check for updates

Chapter 3

Construction of a Cyclic Peptide Library for Phage Display

Nicole Pinnette and Fa-Jie Chen

Abstract

Phage display is a powerful high-throughput screening technique used to screen diverse peptide libraries against therapeutically relevant protein targets. Compared to linear peptides, cyclic peptides have improved stability and binding characteristics. There are various methods to construct cyclic peptide phage display libraries, which can be screened against targets to identify cyclic peptide candidates. These peptides can then be optimized to enhance potency and specificity. In this chapter, we outline a strategy to generate cyclic peptide phage display libraries using a bischlooroxime crosslinker.

Keywords Phage display, Cyclic peptides, Cysteine crosslinking, Peptide screening, Peptide therapeutics

1 Introduction

Phage display is a widely used screening technique for discovering peptide ligands with high affinity and specificity for protein targets [1–3]. In addition to linear genetically encoded libraries (GELs), traditional phage display techniques use disulfide-bridged libraries for screening cyclic peptides [4]. However, disulfide bonds are unstable under reducing conditions, which can limit their structural integrity and practical use in biological applications [5]. To overcome these limitations, covalent crosslinking cyclization strategies have been developed to create monocyclic and multicyclic peptides [6, 7]. These approaches introduce a stable and permanent covalent linkage that enhances the peptide's rigidity and improves the thermodynamic properties, which are critical for high-affinity binding and can lead to improved binding affinity and specificity.

In our laboratory, we have developed a range of chemical crosslinkers, such as chlorooximes, that can generate monocyclic and bicyclic phage display libraries. The general workflow of the construction of a phage library precursor for cyclization is the same as that of the conventional linear or disulfide-bridged library.

Huan Peng and Theam Soon Lim (eds.), *Biomolecular Display Technologies*, Methods in Molecular Biology, vol. 3030,
https://doi.org/10.1007/978-1-0716-5249-7_3,

However, optimizations of the reaction conditions, including the crosslinker concentration, reaction time, and incubation temperature, are required for the cyclization of peptide libraries on phage with a specific crosslinker. This chapter focuses on the construction and validation of a bischlorooxime (BC)-cyclized peptide library for phage display [8].

Generally speaking, constructing a chemically modified cyclic phage library involves two main steps: (i) genetically encoding of the peptide library into the phage and (ii) chemical modification of the displayed peptide library (Fig. 1). In this chapter, the phage library was designed to incorporate a randomized ACX$_n$C sequence at the N-terminal of the M13 phage minor coat (pIII) protein (Fig. 2). This sequence carries an N-terminal alanine (A) and incorporates two cysteine residues (C) flanking a region of randomized amino acids (X$_n$). The cysteines act as the reactive sites for the covalent attachment of the BC-crosslinker to form the cyclic peptides displayed on the phage surface. The phage library was also designed to include a tobacco etch virus (TEV) protease recognition site, which can be used to cleave the peptide from the phage for LC–MS analysis and in covalent phage display screenings.

The library construction begins with the digestion of a commercially synthesized DNA library and the engineered M13KE phage vector, followed by ligation and transformation into Top10 *E. coli* cells (Fig. 3) [9]. The phage library was then amplified in ER2738 *E. coli* cells, which allow for phage infection and propagation. Once the library is constructed, the phages were precipitated and pelleted to remove the library storage buffer. During the library construction, the two cysteine bonds will naturally form a disulfide-cyclized peptide. To construct the BC-cyclized phage library, the disulfide bond was chemically reduced, and the excess reducing reagent was removed by precipitating and pelleting the phage. Then, the BC-crosslinker was used to react with the thiol groups to form a cyclic peptide on the phage surface (Fig. 4). A final precipitation and pelleting step were performed to remove excess reagents, and then the phages were ready to be used in a screening against the target.

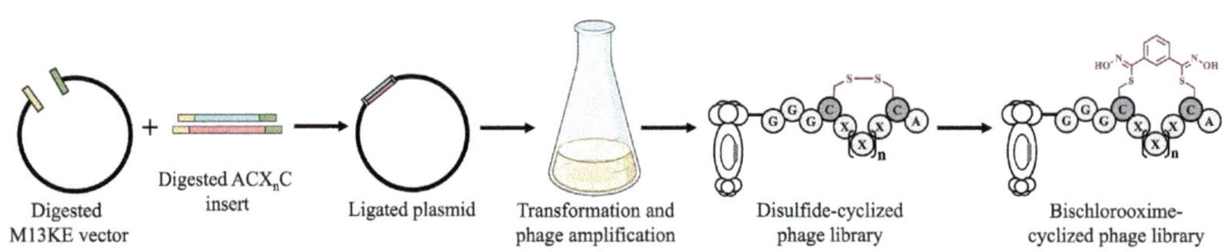

Fig. 1 Overview of the construction of a bischlorooxime-cyclized phage library. The digested library insert and vector are ligated and transformed, followed by phage amplification. The phage library is precipitated, and the disulfide bond is reduced using TCEP and modified with the bischlorooxime crosslinker

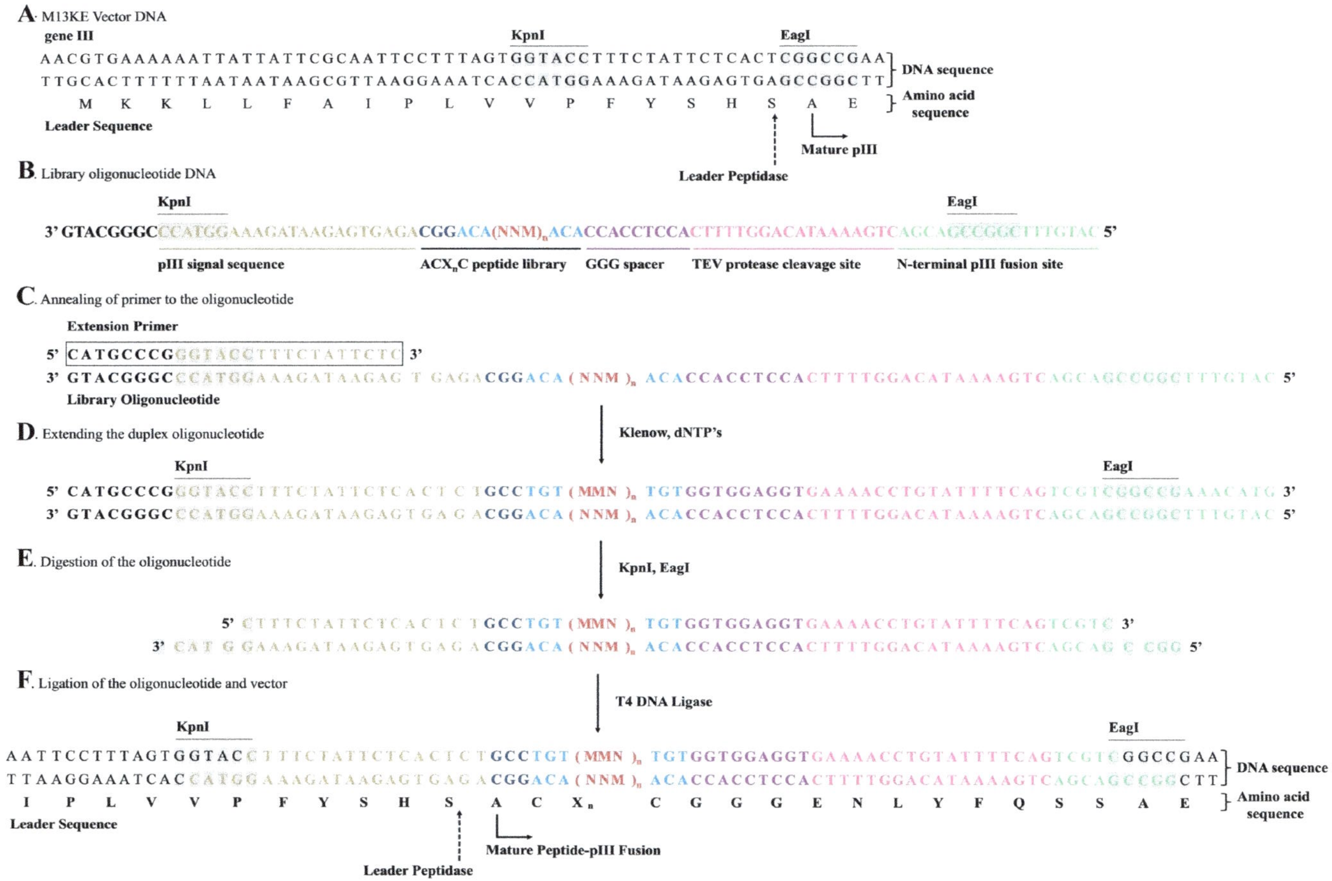

Fig. 2 Design of the library oligonucleotide. (**A**) DNA and amino acid sequence of the engineered M13KE vector. (**B**) DNA sequence of the library oligonucleotide, where the red NMM portion can be adjusted to the desired number of randomized amino acids. (**C**) Annealing of the extension primer to the oligonucleotide. (**D**) Extension of the oligonucleotide duplex. (**E**) DNA sequence that results from the digestion of the oligonucleotide duplex with KpnI and EagI. (**F**) Final DNA sequence of the oligonucleotide ligated with the M13KE vector

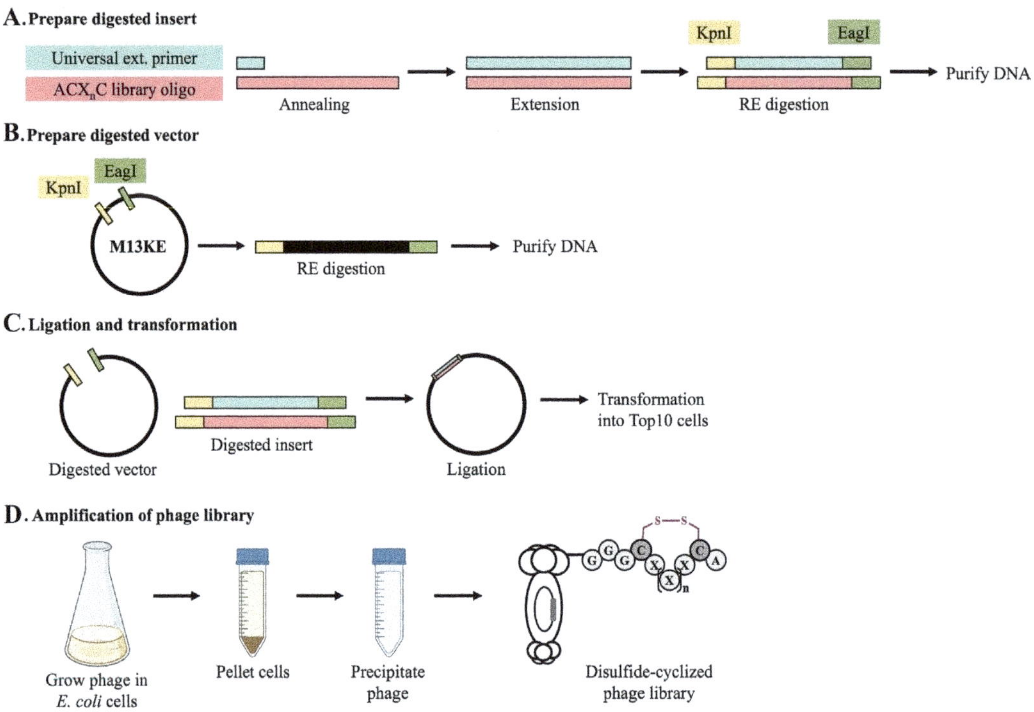

Fig. 3 Schematic of phage display library construction. (**A**) The library oligonucleotide is prepared by annealing the universal extension (ext.) primer, extending the duplex, digesting with restriction enzymes (RE), and purifying the DNA. (**B**) The vector is prepared by RE digestion followed by DNA purification. (**C**) The digested insert and vector are ligated and transformed into *E. coli* Top10 cells. (**D**) The transformed phage is amplified in *E. coli* ER2738 cells to generate the final phage library

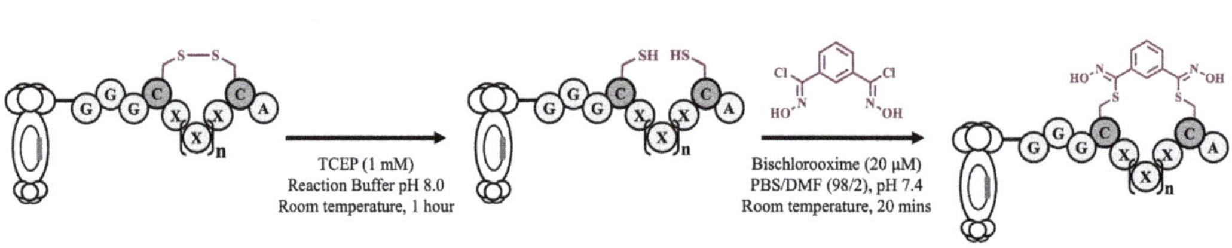

Fig. 4 Construction of an oxime-bridged cyclic peptide library for phage display. The disulfide bond is reduced by TCEP, and the free thiols are reacted with the bischlorooxime crosslinker to form the cyclic peptide

To validate the efficiency of peptide cyclization on phage, a liquid chromatography-mass spectrometry (LC–MS) based analytical method was developed [10]. Once the phages were modified with the BC-crosslinker, the TEV protease was used to cleave the peptide from the phage. The cleaved peptide was separated from the phage and then analyzed by LC–MS (Fig. 5). The percentage of cyclic peptide was determined by comparing the mass of the peptide before and after modification.

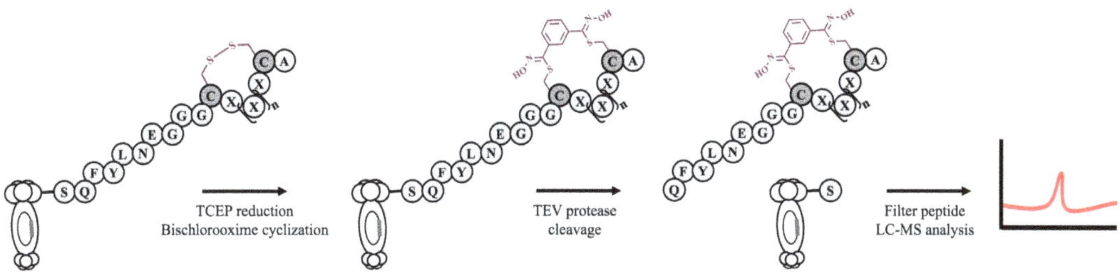

Fig. 5 Schematic for validating the efficiency of bischlorooxime cyclization on phage using an LC–MS based approach. The phage is modified with the bischlorooxime crosslinker, and the peptide is cleaved from the phage using the TEV protease. The cleaved peptide is filtered and analyzed by LC–MS

2 Materials

The solutions were prepared using Nanopure Ultrapure water and sterilized using an autoclave (exhaust 20 min at 121°C) and stored at room temperature unless otherwise stated. The chemicals used in the experiments were commercially purchased and used without further processing.

2.1 Media and Solutions

1. TE buffer:
   - 10 mM Tris-HCl, 1 mM ethylenediaminetetraacetic acid (EDTA), pH. 8.0.
2. 5× Tris-borate-EDTA (TBE) buffer:
   - Measure 800 mL of water and weigh 54 g Tris base, 27.5 g boric acid, and 20 mL 0.5 M EDTA (pH 8.0), adjust water to 1 L.
3. 10× Tris-acetate-EDTA (TAE) buffer:
   - Measure 800 mL of water and weigh 48.5 g Tris base, 11.4 mL glacial acetic acid, and 20 mL of 0.5 M EDTA (pH 8.0), adjust water to 1 L.
4. DNA elution buffer:
   - 100 mM sodium acetate, pH 4.5, 1 mM EDTA, 0.1% sodium dodecyl sulfate (SDS). Sterile filter.
5. Lysogeny broth (LB) medium:
   - Measure 1 L of water and weigh 10 g of tryptone, 5 g of yeast extract, and 5 g of NaCl.
6. IPTG/Xgal Stock and LB plates:
   - Dissolve 0.25 g of isopropyl-β-D-thiogalactoside (IPTG) and 0.20 g of 5-bromo-4-chloro-3-indolyl-β-D-galactoside (Xgal) in 5 mL of dimethylformamide (DMF). Do not autoclave this solution. Store the solution at −20°C protected from light.

- To prepare plates, make 1 L of LB medium with 15 g of agar, and sterilize by autoclaving. Allow the solution to cool to below 70°C, then add 1 mL of the IPTG/Xgal stock solution. Pour the plates with around 20 mL per plate and store them at 4°C in the dark.

7. Tetracycline stock and LB plates:
   - Measure 20 mg of tetracycline and dissolve in 0.5 mL ethanol and 0.5 mL water (*see* **Note 1**). Do not autoclave this solution. Store the stock at −20°C.
   - To prepare plates, make 1 L of LB medium with 15 g of agar, and sterilize by autoclaving. Allow the solution to cool to below 70°C, then add 1 mL of the tetracycline stock solution and store the plates at 4°C in the dark.
8. Top agar:
   - Measure 50 mL of water and weigh 0.5 g tryptone, 0.25 g yeast extract, 0.25 g NaCl, and 0.35 g agar. Autoclave and store solid at room temperature.
   - When ready to use, microwave to melt the agar.
9. Super optimal broth (SOC) medium:
   - Measure 1 L of water and add 20 g of tryptone, 5 g of yeast extract, and 0.5 g of NaCl. Mix thoroughly, then divide into 100 mL portions and sterilize by autoclaving.
   - Once the medium has cooled to room temperature, add 0.5 mL 2 M $MgCl_2$ and 2 mL 1 M glucose (filter sterilized separately) per 100 mL of solution. Store the prepared medium at 4°C.
10. Tris-buffered saline (TBS):
    - 50 mM Tris-HCl and 150 mM NaCl adjusted to pH 7.5.
11. Phosphate-buffered saline (PBS):
    - 137 mM NaCl, 2.7 mM KCl, 10 mM Na_2HPO_4, and 1.8 mM KH_2PO_4 adjusted to a pH of 7.4.
12. Polyethylene glycol (PEG)/NaCl solution:
    - Prepare a solution containing 20% (w/v) PEG-8000 and 2.5 M NaCl. After autoclaving, mix thoroughly while the solution is still warm to ensure combination of the separated phases.
13. Reaction buffer:
    - 20 mM ammonium bicarbonate pH 8.0 and 5 mM EDTA.
14. TEV cleavage buffer:
    - 50 mM Tris and 0.5 mM EDTA adjusted to pH 8.0.

2.2 ER2738 Plate

- *E. coli* K12 ER2738 were purchased from New England Biolabs (NEB), Catalog # E4101.
- Streak the *E. coli* K12 ER2738 cells onto the tetracycline LB agar plates.
- Incubate at 37°C for 12–16 h.

2.3 Oligonucleotide

1. Library insert (Fig. 1):
   - Purchased commercially on a minimum of 0.2 μM scale and purified by PAGE.
   - Ordered as the reverse complement strand (Fig. 2B).
   - Contains the VPFYSHS sequence of the pIII signaling/leader peptidase sequence (Fig. 2A).
   - Designed with the same restriction sites (KpnI and EagI) as the vector to allow for later ligation (Fig. 2A, B).
   - Includes a GGG spacer to separate the displayed peptide from the pIII protein, as well as an ENLYFQS sequence that corresponds to a TEV protease cleavage site (Fig. 1B).
   - Additionally, contains 21 complementary bases to anneal with the universal extension primer (Fig. 2B, C).
2. Universal extension primer:
   - Purchased through the New England Biolabs (NEB) Ph.D.™ Peptide Display Cloning System Catalog #E8101S.
   - The extension primer can also be purchased through commercial sources with the sequence being 5′-d(CATGCCCGGGTACCTTTCTATTCTC)-3′.
3. Preparation of double stranded insert:
   - dNTPs purchased from NEB, Catalog #N0447.
   - Klenow fragment purchased from NEB, Catalog #M0210.

2.4 M13KE Vector

- Purchased through the NEB Ph.D.™ Peptide Display Cloning System, Catalog #E8101S.

2.5 Cells and Enzymes

1. ER2738:
   - *E. coli* K12 ER2738 was purchased from NEB, Catalog #E4101.
   - To prepare the ER2738 plate, streak the *E. coli* K12 ER2738 cells onto the tetracycline LB agar plates and incubate at 37°C for 12–16 h. Make a new ER2738 plate every 3–4 weeks.
   - To prepare an overnight ER2738 sample, inoculate 1 ER2738 colony in 5 mL LB medium with 5 μL of tetracycline stock. Incubate overnight at 37°C with shaking at 250 rpm.

2. Top10:
   - Can be commercially purchased from ThermoFisher Scientific, Catalog #C404050, or be prepared in the lab.
3. Restriction enzymes:
   - EagI-HF purchased from NEB, Catalog #R3505.
   - KpnI-HF purchased from NEB, Catalog #R3142.
4. Ligation enzyme:
   - T4 DNA ligase purchased from NEB, Catalog #M0202.

2.6 8% Nondenaturing Polyacrylamide Gel

1. Assemble a 1.5 mm thick gel cast.
2. In a 15-mL Falcon tube, mix reagents in this order: 3.2 mL of 30% acrylamide, 6.4 mL of water, 2.4 mL of 5× TBE, 200 μL of 10% ammonium persulfate (APS), and 10 μL of *N,N,N',N'*-tetramethylethylenediamine (TEMED).
3. The APS and TEMED will initiate the polymerization of the gel, and therefore, transfer the liquid quickly to the gel cast.
4. Place the comb into the gel and let solidify at room temperature for at least 30 min.
5. After solidified, place the gel into a vertical gel electrophoresis chamber and fill the chamber with 1× TBE.
6. Add the samples and ladder and run the gel at 90 V for at least 90 min.
7. Remove the gel from the chamber and glass plates. Stain the gel with 0.5 μg/mL of ethidium bromide (EtBr) in 1× TBE with gentle mixing for 15 min. Image the gel and excise the DNA if required.

2.7 1% Agarose Gel

1. Assemble the gel cast.
2. Prepare the gel in an Erlenmeyer flask with 500 mg of agarose in 50 mL of 1× TAE buffer.
3. Microwave the solution to fully dissolve the agarose.
4. Add 25 μg of EtBr and swirl slowly to mix. Pour the solution into the gel cast, add the comb, and let it solidify at room temperature.
5. After solidifying, place the gel into a horizontal gel electrophoresis chamber and fill with 1× TAE.
6. Load the samples and ladder and run the gel at 90 V for 40–60 min.
7. Remove the gel from the chamber and image the gel. Excise the DNA if required.

3 Methods

The phage library is constructed through a modified procedure adapted from the NEB Ph.D.™ Phage Display Libraries Instruction Manual [9]. All procedures must be performed using autoclaved pipette tips and sterile Eppendorf tubes. When working with *E. coli*, it is important to maintain sterile conditions by working near a flame or in a biosafety cabinet.

3.1 Preparing the Oligonucleotide Duplex

1. Make a 100 μM stock of the insert in sterile water (*see* **Note 2**).
2. Mix 5 μg of the insert with 3 molar equivalents of the universal extension primer in a total volume of 50 μL TE buffer containing 100 mM NaCl (Fig. 2C).
3. Heat the reaction to 95°C in a thermocycler, then slowly cool to 4°C over 30 min to allow annealing.
4. Extend the duplex by adding the reagents in this order: 119 μL of sterile water, 20 μL of NEBuffer 2 (10×), 50 μL of duplex, 8 μL of dNTPs (10 mM), and 3 μL of DNA Polymerase I (Klenow) Fragment (5 units/μL) (Fig. 2D).
5. Incubate at 37°C for 10 min in a heat block or water bath, then inactivate the enzyme at 65°C for 15 min. Save 4 μL of the sample for later gel analysis.
6. Digest the insert by combining 196 μL of the duplex with 154 μL of H_2O, 40 μL of rCutSmart Buffer (10×), 5 μL of KpnI-HF (20 units/μL), and 5 μL of EagI-HF (20 units/μL) (*see* **Note 3**) (Fig. 2E).
7. Mix the sample by gently flicking the tube multiple times and incubate at 37°C for approximately 3.5 h.
8. Purify the digested DNA using phenol/chloroform extraction followed by ethanol precipitation, as described by ThermoFisher Scientific [11].
9. Resuspend the digested insert in 20–50 μL of TE buffer (*see* **Note 4**).
10. Purify the digested insert by running an 8% polyacrylamide gel using no SDS gel loading dye. Add a low molecular weight ladder to the first lane, the undigested insert to the second lane, and the digested insert in an additional four to eight lanes.
11. Excise the doubly digested insert bands and mince the gel using a pipette tip.

12. Add 500 µL of DNA elution buffer and incubate overnight at 37°C, mixing at 250 rpm.
13. Centrifuge the sample for 2 min at maximum speed and carefully remove as much of the supernatant as possible into a new Eppendorf tube.
14. Repeat the phenol/chloroform extraction and ethanol precipitation as described by ThermoFisher Scientific [11].
15. Resuspend the purified digested insert in approximately 20 µ L of TE buffer. Measure the DNA concentration using a Nanodrop spectrophotometer.

3.2 Preparing the M13KE Vector

1. Transform the M13KE vector by electroporating 1 µL of the vector into Top10 electrocompetent cells.
2. Outgrow the cells by adding 250 µL of SOC medium and incubating for 40 min at 37°C, 250 rpm.
3. Plate the transformed cells on IPTG/Xgal agar plates. For plating, use dilutions of 10^6, 10^7, and 10^8 with 200 µL of ER2738 cells (OD_{600} ~0.5), and 790 µL of top agar. Incubate the plates overnight at 37°C.
4. Amplify the phage by growing one plaque in 5 mL of LB medium with 50 µL of overnight grown ER2738 cells for around 8–16 h (*see* **Note 5**).
5. Extract the DNA using a plasmid miniprep kit. Combine the extracted M13KE DNA samples and determine the DNA concentration using a Nanodrop spectrophotometer.
6. Digest the vector by combining 10 µg of vector with 40 µL of rCutSmart Buffer (10×), 10 µL of KpnI-HF (20 units/µL), 10 µL of EagI-HF (20 units/µL), and up to 400 µL of water (Fig. 3B).
7. Gently mix the sample by flicking the tube multiple times and incubate at 37°C for 3–5 h.
8. Add 80 µL of 6× purple loading dye (NEB, Catalog #B7024) to stop the reaction and store at −20°C until purification.
9. Purify the digested vector by loading 40–50 µL of the sample onto a 1% agarose gel with 5 µL of 1 kb Plus DNA Ladder (NEB, Catalog #N3200).
10. Using a UV transilluminator and a razor blade, excise the band corresponding to the doubly digested vector and transfer the gel slice into a new Eppendorf tube.
11. Extract the DNA using the Monarch Spin DNA Gel Extraction Kit (NEB, Catalog #T1120). Measure the DNA concentration using a Nanodrop spectrophotometer.
12. Dephosphorylate the 5' and 3' ends of the digested vector using 1 µL of Quick CIP (NEB, Catalog #M0525), with 2 µg

digested M13KE vector, 2 μL rCutSmart Buffer, and sterile water to a final volume of 20 μL.

13. Incubate the sample for 10 min at 37°C and then inactivate the enzyme at 80°C for 2 min.
14. The digested vector can be used directly or buffer-exchanged into TE buffer using a Bio-Spin P-6 Gel Column (Bio Rad, Catalog #7326227), according to the manufacturer's protocol [12]. Determine the DNA concentration with a Nanodrop spectrophotometer.

3.3 Optimizing the Ligation and Transformation Conditions

1. Test a range of insert-to-vector ratios (5:1, 10:1, 20:1, and 30:1) to determine the best conditions.
2. Combine 50 ng of digested vector, the corresponding amount of digested insert, 2 μL T4 DNA ligase buffer (10×), 1 μL of T4 DNA ligase (400,000 μ/mL), and sterile water to a final volume of 20 μL (Fig. 2F).
3. Incubate the sample for 2 h at room temperature, and then inactivate the ligase for 15 min at 65°C.
4. Electroporate 1 μL of ligated sample into Top10 cells.
5. Outgrow in 250 μL of SOC medium for 40 min at 37°C.
6. Titer the transformed cells and plate 10 μL of the diluted sample with 200 μL of overnight ER2738 and 790 μL of top agar onto IPTG/Xgal plates. Incubate the plates overnight at 37°C.
7. Determine the transformation efficiency by using this equation: (Transformation Efficiency = (PFU × dilution factor × total resuspended volume)/electroporated DNA (μg)).
8. Sequence approximately ten plaques to evaluate the diversity of the library.

3.4 Large-Scale Library Construction

1. Use the optimized ligation conditions to scale up the reaction to generate the phage library.
2. Add 1 μg of vector, the corresponding amount of insert, 10 μL of T4 DNA ligase, and 20 μL of T4 DNA ligase buffer (10×), with water in a total volume of 200 μL.
3. Incubate the ligation at room temperature for 2 h, flicking the tube every 30 min, and heat inactivate at 65°C for 15 min.
4. Purify the ligated sample by phenol/chloroform extraction and precipitation using the ThermoFisher Scientific procedure [11].
5. Resuspend the DNA in 10–20 μL of TE buffer and measure the DNA concentration using a Nanodrop spectrophotometer.
6. Perform a final test electroporation by electroporating 50 ng of the ligated sample into Top10 cells.

7. Perform additional large-scale ligations if more DNA is required to reach the target diversity.
8. Electroporate ~1 μL of ligated sample per aliquot of Top10 cells. Depending on the diversity needed, it may be necessary to perform between 50 and 100 electroporation's (Fig. 3C).
9. Group the electroporation's into pools of five to ten transformations each.
10. Outgrow each electroporated sample by adding 250 μL of SOC medium and incubate for 40 min at 37°C, 250 rpm.
11. Save 5 μL from each pool to titer later to determine the final library diversity.
12. Combine the remaining transformed cells from each pool and transfer them into 1 L of LB medium with 10 mL of an overnight culture of ER2738 cells (Fig. 3D).
13. Incubate the culture for 4 h at 37°C, shaking at 250 rpm to amplify the phage (*see* **Note 6**).
14. Centrifuge the sample for 20 min at 4°C, 5000 g to pellet the cells.
15. Carefully transfer the supernatant into new tubes and add 1/6 of the total volume of the PEG/NaCl solution. Invert the tubes several times to mix thoroughly and then store the samples at 4°C overnight to precipitate the phage.
16. Centrifuge the samples for 45 min at 4°C, 5000 g to pellet the phage particles.
17. Discard the supernatant and resuspend the phage pellet in 100 mL of TBS buffer. Rock the sample at 4°C overnight to allow the phage to go fully into solution.
18. Centrifuge the resuspended phage sample for 10 min at 4°C, 5000 g to pellet any remaining cell debris.
19. Transfer the supernatant to new tubes, add 1/6 total volume of PEG/NaCl solution, and precipitate the phage on ice for 1–2 h or overnight at 4°C.
20. Centrifuge the samples for 20 min at 4°C, maximum speed to pellet the phage.
21. Carefully discard the supernatant and resuspend the final phage pellet in 20 mL of TBS buffer. Allow the phage suspension to rock at 4°C for 24–48 h to ensure complete solubilization.
22. Store the phage library with an equal volume of 100% glycerol in the phage suspension (*see* **Note 7**). Ensure thorough resuspension, aliquot the library into appropriate storage tubes and store at −20°C.

3.5 Bischlorooxime-Mediated Cyclization on Phage

1. Add 20 μL of the prepared phage library (10^{12} pfu/mL), 80 μL of PBS, and 20 μL of PEG/NaCl solution to a 1.5-mL Eppendorf tube and either place on ice for 1 h or place at 4°C overnight. Pellet the phage by centrifugation at 4°C, 14,000 rpm for 20 min (*see* **Note 8**).
2. Precipitate the phage library by taking 20 μL of the library (~10^{12} pfu/mL), 80 μL of PBS, and 20 μL of PEG/NaCl solution to a 1.5-mL Eppendorf tube. Incubate on ice for 1 h or at 4°C overnight.
3. Pellet the phage by centrifugation at 4°C, 14,000 rpm for 20 min. Remove the supernatant.
4. Resuspend the phage pellet in 99 μL of reaction buffer with 1 μL of 100 mM tris(2-carboxyethyl)phosphine (TCEP) in reaction buffer (*see* **Note 9**) (Fig. 4). Incubate at room temperature for 1 h, shaking at ~200 rpm.
5. Precipitate the reduced phage particles using 20 μL of the PEG/NaCl solution and place on ice for 1 h. Pellet the phage by centrifugation at 4°C, 14,000 rpm for 20 min.
6. Remove the supernatant and resuspend the phage pellet in 98 μL of PBS and add 2 μL of the BC-crosslinker (1 mM in DMF) (Fig. 4). Incubate the reaction at room temperature for 20 min, shaking at ~200 rpm.
7. Quench the reaction by adding 1 μL of free cysteine (100 mM in PBS pH 7.4) and incubating at room temperature for 20 min, shaking at ~200 rpm.
8. Precipitate the cyclic phage particles by adding 20 μL of the PEG/NaCl solution to the sample and incubating on ice for 1 h. Pellet the phage by centrifugation at 4°C, 14,000 rpm for 20 min.
9. Remove the supernatant and resuspend the phage pellet in buffer used for screening. The cyclic phage can then be used for selection against the target protein.

3.6 Validation of the Bischlorooxime-Mediated Cyclization on Phage

1. Titer the phage library by diluting 10 μL of the phage (~10^{12}pfu/mL) into 990 μL of LB medium. Perform serial dilutions in LB to get the final dilutions of 10^8 and 10^9pfu/mL (*see* **Note 10**).
2. Add 10 μL of the diluted sample into 200 μL of ER2738 cells (OD_{600} ~0.5), and then 790 μL of microwaved top agar. Immediately vortex the mixture and plate onto pre-warmed IPTG/X-Gal agar plates. Incubate the plate at 37°C overnight.
3. Select a single plaque with a pipette tip and inoculate in 20 mL of LB medium with 200 μL of overnight ER2738 culture in

a 250-mL Erlenmeyer flask. Incubate at 37°C for a minimum of 5 h, shaking at 250 rpm.

4. Transfer the culture to a 50-mL Falcon tube and centrifuge at 4°C at maximum speed for 10 min. Transfer the supernatant containing the phage into a new Falcon tube and add 4 mL of the PEG/NaCl solution to precipitate the phage (*see* **Note 11**). Invert the sample and incubate either on ice for 1–2 h or at 4°C overnight.
5. Pellet the phage by centrifugation at 4°C for 20 min at maximum speed. Discard the supernatant and resuspend the pellet in 1 mL of PBS.
6. Transfer the sample to a 1.5-mL Eppendorf tube and centrifuge at 4°C, 14,000 rpm for 10 min to remove residual cells.
7. Remove the supernatant into a new Eppendorf tube and add 200 μL of the PEG/NaCl solution to reprecipitate the phage. Centrifuge to pellet the phage at 4 °C, 14,000 rpm for 20 min (*see* **Note 12**).
8. Remove the supernatant and resuspend the phage pellet in 495 μL of reaction buffer. Add 5 μL of TCEP (100 mM stock in reaction buffer) and incubate at room temperature, shaking at approximately 200 rpm for 1 h.
9. Add 100 μL of the PEG/NaCl solution and incubate on ice for 1 h. Centrifuge at 4°C, 14,000 rpm for 20 min to pellet the reduced phage.
10. Discard the supernatant and resuspend the phage pellet in 490 μL of PBS. Add 10 μL of BC (1 mM stock in DMF) (Fig. 5). Vortex briefly and incubate at room temperature for 20 min, shaking at ~200 rpm.
11. Add 5 μL of free cysteine (100 mM stock in PBS) and incubate for an additional 30 min at room temperature to quench the reaction.
12. Add 100 μL of PEG/NaCl and incubate on ice for 1 h. Pellet the phage by centrifugation at 4°C, 14,000 rpm for 20 min.
13. Discard the supernatant and resuspend the phage pellet in 100 μL of water. Add 300 μL of recombinant TEV protease (10 μM in TEV cleavage buffer) (Fig. 5). Incubate at 30°C for approximately 16 h.
14. Transfer the sample to a 50 kDa Amicon Ultra-0.5 Centrifugal Filter (Sigma Aldrich, UFC505008) and centrifuge at room temperature, 14,000 rpm for 25 min. The filter separates the phage particles from the cleaved peptide (Fig. 5).
15. Lyophilize the filtrate, which contains the cleaved peptide. Fully redissolve the peptide sample in 30 μL of water.

Centrifuge at room temperature, 14,000 rpm for 10 min to pellet the insoluble debris.

16. Monitor the sample by LC–MS, and injecting 27 μL of the sample (Fig. 5). LC–MS solvent A is 95% water, 5% acetonitrile, 0.1% formic acid and solvent B is 95% acetonitrile, 5% water, 0.1% formic acid. The gradient from 0 to 3 min was 95% A, from 3 to 10 min was 95% B, from 10 to 18 min was 95% B, from 18 to 20 min was 95% A, and from 20 to 25 min was 95% A.
17. Compare the mass before and after the modification to determine the efficiency of cyclization. This method can also be used to analyze other modifications on phage displayed peptides.

4 Notes

1. The tetracycline stock will not be in solution, so before every use vortex thoroughly. A new tetracycline stock should be made once a month.
2. The DNA is extremely fragile and pipetting the solution up and down extensively can shear the insert, leading to low ligation efficiency and transformation efficiency. Never vortex the DNA because this can also cause destruction of the DNA.
3. The restriction digestion enzymes are very sensitive to freeze thaw. The best digestion results are seen when a new aliquot of enzyme is used during the digestion.
4. Make sure to pipette up and down less than 10 times. Extensive pipetting will shear the DNA and result in a low transformation efficiency.
5. Set up around 10–30 samples to get enough vector to be used for the restriction enzyme digestion.
6. Do not amplify the phage for longer than 4 h or this can introduce growth bias into the final library.
7. Before adding the 100% glycerol to the phage library, titer the library to determine the phage concentration. If you want a higher concentration, then reprecipitate the library with the PEG/NaCl solution and resuspend in a smaller volume. If you want a lower concentration, then increase the amount of TBS. Once the phage concentration is what you want, add equal volumes of 100% glycerol and completely resuspend and store at −20°C.
8. When performing phage precipitation, pay attention to the orientation of the Eppendorf tube in the centrifuge. This will

help to locate the phage pellet afterward. The pellet typically appears as a small white dot, which may be faint or barely visible, especially if the phage concentration is below 10^{11} pfu/mL.

9. We observed that preparing the TCEP solution fresh in the reaction buffer helped maintain its reducing activity and consistently resulted in effective disulfide reduction on phage.
10. The phage can stick to the pipette tips so you should pipette up and down multiple times during each dilution step and vortex to ensure accurate transfer. Additionally, a new pipette tip should be used for each dilution to prevent cross-contamination from lower diluted samples to higher diluted samples.
11. The spun down cell pellet can be miniprepped, and the DNA can be sent for sequencing to determine the peptide sequence of the phage.
12. The phage pellet should be large enough to easily see since the total amount of phage will be around 10^{12} pfu in the sample. The phage pellet will be a white circle at the bottom of the Eppendorf tube.

References

1. Smith GP, Petrenko VA (1997) Phage display. Chem Rev 97(2):391–410. https://doi.org/10.1021/cr960065d
2. Cortese R, Monaci P, Luzzago A, Santini C, Bartoli F, Cortese I, Fortugno P, Galfrè G, Nicosia A, Felici F (1996) Selection of biologically active peptides by phage display of random peptide libraries. Curr Opin Biotechnol 7:616–621. https://doi.org/10.1016/S0958-1669(96)80072-3
3. Burritt JB, Bond CW, Doss KW, Jesaitis AJ (1996) Filamentous phage display of oligopeptide libraries. Anal Biochem 238:1–13. https://doi.org/10.1006/abio.1996.0241
4. Cwirla SE, Peters EA, Barrett RW, Dower WJ (1990) Peptides on phage: a vast library of peptides for identifying ligands. Proc Natl Acad Sci U S A 87(16):6378–6382. https://doi.org/10.1073/pnas.87.16.6378
5. Fass D (2012) Disulfide bonding in protein biophysics. Annu Rev Biophys 41:63–79. https://doi.org/10.1146/annurev-biophys-050511-102321
6. Sohrabi C, Foster A, Tavassoli A (2020) Methods for generating and screening libraries of genetically encoded cyclic peptides in drug discovery. Nat Rev Chem 4(2):90–101. https://doi.org/10.1038/s41570-019-0159-2
7. Chen F-J, Pinnette N, Gao J (2024) Strategies for the construction of multicyclic phage display libraries. ChemBioChem 25(9):e202400072. https://doi.org/10.1002/cbic.202400072
8. Chen F-J, Zheng M, Nobile V, Gao J (2022) Fast and cysteine-specific modification of peptides, proteins and bacteriophage using chlorooximes. Chem – Eur J 28(20):e202200058. https://doi.org/10.1002/chem.202200058
9. New England Biolabs (2023) Instruction manual, Ph.D.™ peptide display cloning system. https://www.neb.com/en/-/media/nebus/files/manuals/manuale8101.pdf?rev=2b5c03b454244e469be51c339c3761cc&hash=9E8591E34AF7B0F66323B2432172B0E9&srsltid=AfmBOorxBsOpDq3Uh9d5kShjfzl5ytBcqpt9n2Mr91-nohNjU2ssByWv. Accessed 14 Sept 2025
10. Chen F-J, Pinnette N, Yang F, Gao J (2023) A cysteine-directed proximity-driven crosslinking method for native peptide bicyclization. Angew Chem Int Ed 62(31):e202306813. https://doi.org/10.1002/anie.202306813
11. ThermoFisher Scientific (2025) How to use phenol-chloroform for dna purification. https://www.thermofisher.com/us/en/home/references/protocols/nucleic-acid-purification-and-analysis/dna-extraction-protocols/phenol-chloroform-extraction.html. Accessed 14 Sept 2025
12. Bio Rad (2025) Micro bio-spin chromatography columns. https://www.bio-rad.com/sites/default/files/webroot/web/pdf/lsr/literature/4006051.pdf. Accessed 14 Sept 2025

Check for updates

Chapter 4

Generation of a CDR H3 Randomized Monoclonal Antibody Library by Kunkel Mutagenesis

Jia Xuan Yeoh, Yee Siew Choong and Theam Soon Lim

Abstract

Complementary-determining regions (CDRs) are the primary factor that determines antibody diversity, while CDR H3 plays a central role in antigen binding. Randomization of this loop within a stable framework provides a powerful strategy for generating synthetic antibody libraries. This chapter outlines an approach that is Kunkel mutagenesis based, for constructing a monoclonal antibody library diversified at CDR H3. The method uses uracilated single-stranded DNA templates and degenerate oligonucleotides to introduce targeted variability while suppressing nonrecombinant background through strategically placed stop codons and restriction sites. The resulting repertoire is directly compatible with phage display for downstream selection. This streamlined protocol enables the generation of antibody libraries suitable for applications in affinity maturation, binder discovery, and antibody development.

Keywords Affinity maturation, Monoclonal antibody, Kunkel mutagenesis, Antibody libraries, Phage display

1 Introduction

In vitro antibody discovery platforms, such as phage, yeast, and ribosome display, represent powerful alternatives to traditional animal immunization methods for isolating target-specific antibodies [1, 2]. These technologies offer considerable advantages, including the capacity for high-throughput screening, precise control over selection conditions (e.g., pH, temperature), and the ability to isolate antibodies against challenging antigens, such as toxic molecules or specific conformational epitopes [3]. However, despite the complexity and diversity of initial libraries, primary selections often yield antibody candidates with moderate binding affinities, typically characterized by dissociation constants (KD) exceeding 100 nM [4]. To generate antibodies with enhanced therapeutic or diagnostic utility, sub-nanomolar affinities (pM–low nM range) is often preferred, thus a subsequent process is essential [5].

Huan Peng and Theam Soon Lim (eds.), *Biomolecular Display Technologies*, Methods in Molecular Biology, vol. 3030,
https://doi.org/10.1007/978-1-0716-5249-7_4,

This critical step is known as affinity maturation. Mirroring the natural process that occurs in B lymphocytes during an immune response, in vitro affinity maturation involves the deliberate introduction of genetic variation into antibody-encoding sequences, followed by stringent selection for variants exhibiting improved binding to the target antigen [6]. This iterative cycle of diversification and selection is fundamental to evolving antibodies from initial low-to-moderate affinity binders towards high-affinity molecules with picomolar or even femtomolar dissociation constants [7].

Strategies for introducing genetic diversity through in vitro affinity maturation can be broadly categorized as either random or targeted. Random mutagenesis techniques, such as error-prone PCR or DNA shuffling, introduce mutations across the entire antibody gene. While effective in exploring sequence space, this approach can also inadvertently generate detrimental mutations that compromise antibody stability or expression [8]. In contrast, targeted mutagenesis methods, including site-directed mutagenesis or selective randomization of complementarity-determining regions (CDRs), focus diversity within the paratope-defining CDRs. Since CDRs directly engage the antigen, targeting these regions is more likely to yield affinity improvements while minimizing negative impacts on overall antibody structure and function [9–11]. Although all three CDR loops contribute to antigen recognition, the third complementarity-determining region of the heavy chain (CDR H3) often plays the most critical role in antigen binding due to its exceptional variability in length and amino acid composition [12]. Consequently, CDR H3 is a frequent target for randomization, often incorporating varied lengths to explore a wider range of potential binding conformations [13–16].

Site-directed mutagenesis stands as a cornerstone technology for precisely introducing defined sequence changes during targeted affinity maturation. While early approaches like cassette mutagenesis were utilized, more efficient techniques have been developed [17]. Methods like the QuikChange protocol employ primer-mediated amplification to incorporate mutations, with the parental DNA template subsequently removed [18, 19]. Meanwhile, a highly influential and widely adopted method, which is particularly compatible with phage display systems utilizing M13 bacteriophage, is Kunkel mutagenesis [20–22]. This technique ingeniously leverages a circular, single-stranded DNA template containing uracil residues (dU-ssDNA). A synthetic oligonucleotide carrying the desired mutation is annealed to this template, and in vitro DNA synthesis creates a heteroduplex double-stranded molecule. Upon transformation into a suitable bacterial host, cellular mechanisms preferentially degrade the uracil-containing parental strand, ensuring that the newly synthesized, mutated strand serves as the template for subsequent replication.

However, while Kunkel mutagenesis is highly efficient compared to some earlier methods, it does not yield 100% mutated products [21]. Even with a single primer, a significant proportion (typically around 20%) of clones retain the original, unmutated sequence, and this wild-type background increases when multiple primers targeting distant regions are used (e.g., decreasing to approximately 50% efficiency with three to four primers) [23]. The presence of a substantial wild-type population can critically impede the selection of improved variants, as these clones may dominate the selection process. To overcome this, a common strategy involves constructing an "inactive template" where residues intended for randomization in the library are initially replaced by stop codons (e.g., TAA) or rare arginine codons (e.g., AGA, AGG) [24]. The incorporation of these codons significantly reduces or eliminates the expression of functional protein (such as a pIII fusion in phage display) from the unmutated parental template. Consequently, while the wild-type genotype may persist, its phenotypic representation on the phage surface is severely diminished, effectively excluding it from the binding selection and allowing mutated variants to be preferentially enriched [25].

Building upon the inactive template strategy, this procedure first introduces stop codons into the original template sequence within the regions designated for randomization. This ensures that only templates that have successfully incorporated the mutagenic oligonucleotide and its associated randomized sequence will encode functional protein display, while templates that still retain the original, nonmutated sequence containing stop codons are translationally silent and thus effectively removed from the pool during binding selections. Furthermore, to enhance the efficiency of subsequent selection experiments and improve the likelihood of discovering high-affinity binders, unique restriction endonuclease recognition sites are introduced within the CDR H3 region. This allows for the targeted removal of remaining nonrecombinant or background clones through restriction enzyme digestion prior to selection. It is worth noting that the presence of thymine in the introduced restriction endonuclease recognition sites may also be replaced by uracil during the process, resulting in the resistance of restriction endonuclease digestion [26]. The protocol involves the directed incorporation of mutagenic oligonucleotides into covalently closed circular double-stranded DNA (CCC-dsDNA) using an uracilated single-stranded DNA (dU-ssDNA) template. Following annealing, DNA polymerase extends the primer and followed by ligation by ligase. Introducing this heteroduplex into a *dut*$^+$/*ung*$^-$ *E. coli* strain facilitates the enzymatic degradation of the parental strand that contains uracil, thereby enriching clones bearing the desired mutation (see Fig. 1).

The method reliably yields substantial quantities of mutated DNA suitable for constructing a sizeable library, while allowing

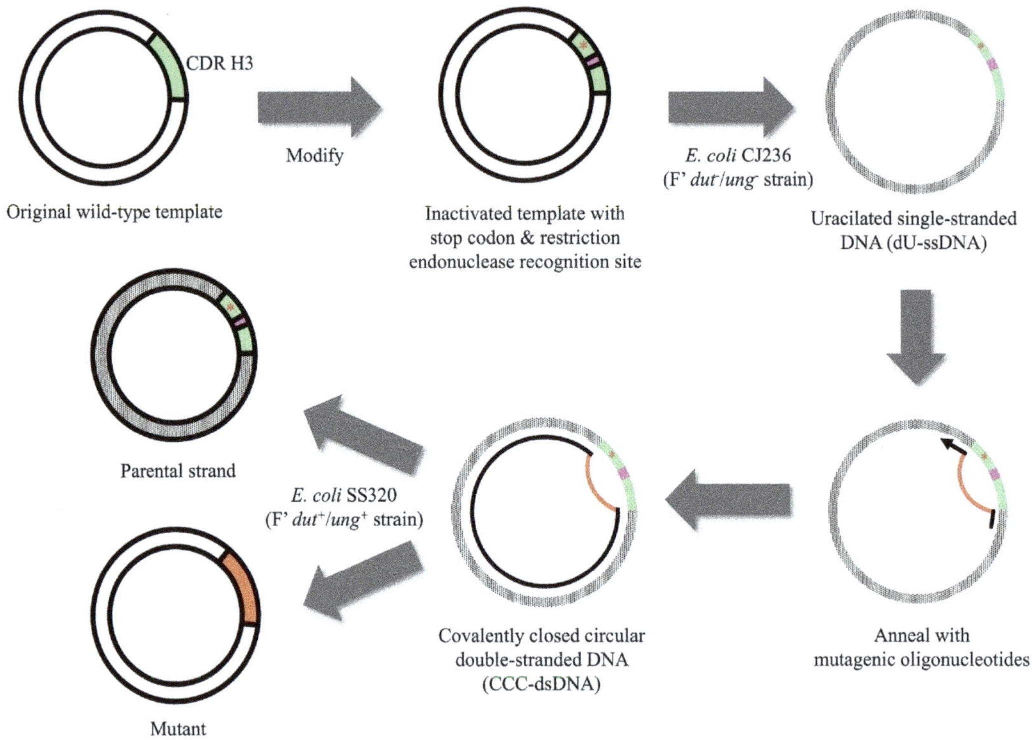

Fig. 1 Kunkel mutagenesis workflow. The DNA template is first modified to include stop codons and restriction endonuclease recognition sites. This modified template is transformed into *E. coli* strain CJ236 via electroporation. Following this, infection with M13K07 helper phage enables the production of uracil-containing single-stranded DNA (dU-ssDNA). Mutagenic, phosphorylated oligonucleotides are then annealed to the ssDNA and serve as primers for synthesizing heteroduplex double-stranded DNA (CCC-dsDNA) using T7 DNA polymerase and T4 DNA ligase. The resulting dsDNA is purified and electroporated into *E. coli* SS320 cells, where the uracil-containing parental strand is selectively degraded. A subsequent restriction endonuclease digestion step removes the leftover original, unmutated template strand. This allows the mutant strand to be retained and converted into the double-stranded, replicative form of the phagemid DNA

simultaneous introduction of mutations across multiple sites or CDRs without reliance on specific restriction enzyme recognition sequences, and enables precise control over the introduced diversity through the use of degenerate codons [23]. This chapter details a robust and efficient protocol based on a modified Kunkel mutagenesis method, optimized for generating diverse antibody libraries specifically targeting CDR H3. Following diversification, biopanning would be employed to select for variants with improved binding characteristics under increasingly stringent conditions. The chapter will only cover the CDR3 mutagenesis protocol to generate a mutant library and not the subsequent panning of the library and affinity determination process.

2 Materials

2.1 Primer Design

Mutagenic Oligos (5′ to 3′; Underlined = Overlapping annealing sites; Bold = Degenerate codons) (*see* **Note 1**):

1. CDR3_NNC-9_Rv: GGTGCCCTGGCCCCA**GNNGNNGNNGNNGNNGNNGNNGNNGNN**GCAATAATACACCGC
2. CDR3_NNC-12_Rv: GGTGCCCTGGCCCCA**GNNGNNGNNGNNGNNGNNGNNGNNGNNGNNGNNGNN**GCAATAATACACCGC

2.2 Preparation of dU-ssDNA Template

1. QIAGEN Qiaprep spin M13 Kit (QIAGEN, Germany): QIAprep spin column, PE buffer, EB buffer.
2. *E. coli* CJ236, genotype: *dut*1, *ung*1,*t hi*-1, *recA*1/pCJ105 (F' *cam*^{r}).
3. 2× YT medium: 16 g tryptone, 10 g yeast extract, and 5 g NaCl in 1 L dH_2O, autoclave and store at room temperature.
4. 2× YT agar: 16 g tryptone, 10 g yeast extract, 5 g NaCl, and 15.5 g agar in 1 L dH_2O, autoclave.
5. 50 mg/mL ampicillin stock solution: 2.5 g ampicillin sodium salt in 50 mL of 50% (v/v) ethanol, filter sterilize and store at −20°C.
6. 30 mg/mL kanamycin stock solution: 1.5 g kanamycin sulfate in 50 mL of dH_2O, filter sterilize and store at −20°C.
7. 40% (w/v) glucose: 40 g D-(+)-glucose in 100 mL of dH_2O, autoclave and store at 4°C.
8. 1 mg/mL Uridine: 1 mg Uridine in 1 mL of dH_2O, filter sterilize and store at −20°C.
9. 0.45 μm nylon filter.
10. 2× YT-amp medium: 2× YT medium, 100 μg/mL ampicillin, and 2% (v/v) glucose.
11. 2× YT-amp/cm medium: 2× YT medium, 100 μg/mL ampicillin, 15 μg/mL chloramphenicol, and 2% (v/v) glucose.
12. 2× YT-amp/cm agar plate: 2× YT agar, 100 μg/mL ampicillin, and 15 μg/mL chloramphenicol.
13. M13K07 helper phage (Invitrogen, USA).
14. PEG/NaCl solution: 200 g polyethylene glycol 6000 (PEG 6000) and 146 g NaCl in 1 L dH_2O, autoclave and store at room temperature.
15. 10× Phosphate buffered saline (PBS), pH 7.4: 8 g NaCl, 0.2 g KCl, 1.44 g $Na_2HPO_4{\cdot}2H_2O$, 0.24 g KH_2PO_4 in 1 L dH_2O, autoclave, and store at room temperature.

16. MP buffer: 3.3 g citric acid monohydrate in 3 mL dH_2O Filter through a 0.2 μm syringe filter.
17. MLB buffer: 1 M sodium perchlorate and 30% (v/v) isopropanol.
18. TAE buffer: 40 mM Tris-acetate and 1.0 mM EDTA, adjust pH to 8.0 and autoclave.
19. TAE/agarose gel: TAE buffer, 1.0% (w/v) agarose.
20. Sterile Petri Dish, 90 mm.
21. MicroPulser™ Electroporator (Bio-Rad, USA).

2.3 Introduction of Degenerate Oligonucleotides and Synthesis of CCC-dsDNA

1. 10× T4 DNA Ligase buffer.
2. T4 polynucleotide kinase.
3. 10× TM buffer: 2 M Tris-HCl and 50 mM $MgCl_2$.
4. 10 mM dNTP mixture.
5. T4 DNA ligase (400 U/μL).
6. T7 DNA polymerase (10 U/μL).
7. QIAquick® PCR Purification kit (QIAGEN, Germany): QIAquick spin column, PB buffer, PE buffer and EB buffer.
8. 10× TAE buffer, pH 8.0: 48.5 g Tris, 11.4 mL glacial acetic acid, and 20 mL 0.5 M EDTA (pH 8.0) in 1 L dH_2O, autoclave and store at room temperature.
9. TAE/agarose gel: 1× TAE buffer, 1.0% (w/v) agarose.

2.4 Conversion to Phage Library Consisting of Mutated CDR H3 Template

1. *E. coli* SS320, genotype: F'[proAB $lacI^qZ$ ΔM15 Tn10 (Tet^R)] araD139 Δ(ara-leu)7696 galE15 galK16 Δ(lac)X74 rpsL (Str^R) hsdR2 (r_K− m_K+) mcrA mcrB1.
2. MicroPulser™ Electroporator (Bio-Rad, USA).
3. SOC medium: 2× YT medium, 2.5 mM KCl, 20 mM $MgSO_4$, and 0.4% (v/v) glucose.
4. 2× YT medium: 16 g tryptone, 10 g yeast extract, and 5 g NaCl in 1 L dH_2O, autoclave and store at room temperature.
5. 2× YT-amp medium: 2× YT medium, 100 μg/mL ampicillin, and 2% (v/v) glucose.
6. 2× YT agar: 16 g tryptone, 10 g yeast extract, 5 g NaCl, and 15.5 g agar in 1 L dH_2O, autoclave.
7. 2× YT-amp agar plate: 2× YT agar and 100 μg/mL ampicillin.
8. Sterile Petri Dish, 90 mm.
9. Nunc™ Square BioAssay Dish, 25 mm (Thermo Scientific, USA).
10. 80% (v/v) glycerol: 40 mL glycerol in 10 mL dH_2O, autoclave and store at room temperature.

2.5 Colony PCR

1. 10× DreamTaq buffer.
2. 10 mM dNTP mixture.
3. DreamTaq DNA Polymerase (Thermo Scientific, USA).
4. Forward primer.
5. Reverse primer.
6. 10× TBE buffer, pH 8.0: 108 g Tris, 55 g boric acid, and 7.4 g EDTA in 1 L dH_2O, autoclave and store at room temperature.
7. TBE/agarose gel: 0.5× TBE buffer, 1.0% (w/v) agarose.

2.6 Phage Library Packaging

1. 2× YT medium: 16 g tryptone, 10 g yeast extract, and 5 g NaCl in 1 L dH_2O, autoclave and store at room temperature.
2. 2× YT agar: 16 g tryptone, 10 g yeast extract, 5 g NaCl, and 15.5 g agar in 1 L dH_2O, autoclave.
3. 50 mg/mL ampicillin stock solution: 2.5 g ampicillin sodium salt in 50 mL of 50% (v/v) ethanol, filter sterilize and store at −20°C.
4. 30 mg/mL kanamycin stock solution: 1.5 g kanamycin sulfate in 50 mL of dH_2O, filter sterilize and store at −20°C.
5. 40% (w/v) glucose: 40 g D-(+)-glucose in 100 mL of dH_2O, autoclave and store at 4°C.
6. 2× YT-amp medium: 2× YT medium, 100 μg/mL ampicillin, and 2% (v/v) glucose.
7. 2× YT-amp/kan medium: 2× YT medium, 100 μg/mL ampicillin, and 50 μg/mL kanamycin.
8. 2× YT-amp agar: 2× YT agar, 100 μg/mL ampicillin, and 2% (v/v) glucose.
9. 2× YT-kan agar: 2× YT agar and 50 μg/mL kanamycin.
10. M13K07 helper phage (Invitrogen, USA).
11. 0.45 μm nylon filter.
12. PEG/NaCl solution: 200 g polyethylene glycol 6000 (PEG 6000) and 146 g NaCl in 1 L dH_2O, autoclave and store at room temperature.
13. 10× Phosphate-buffered saline (PBS), pH 7.4: 8 g NaCl, 0.2 g KCl, 1.44 g $Na_2HPO_4 \cdot 2H_2O$, 0.24 g KH_2PO_4 in 1 L dH_2O, autoclave and store at room temperature.

2.7 Phage Titration

1. 2× YT medium: 16 g tryptone, 10 g yeast extract, and 5 g NaCl in 1 L dH_2O, autoclave and store at room temperature.
2. 2× YT agar: 16 g tryptone, 10 g yeast extract, 5 g NaCl, and 15.5 g agar in 1 L dH_2O, autoclave.
3. 2× YT-amp agar: 2× YT agar, 100 μg/mL ampicillin, and 2% (v/v) glucose.

4. 2× YT-kan agar: 2× YT agar and 50 µg/mL kanamycin.
5. 10× Phosphate-buffered saline (PBS), pH 7.4: 8 g NaCl, 0.2 g KCl, 1.44 g $Na_2HPO_4 \cdot 2H_2O$, 0.24 g KH_2PO_4 in 1 L dH_2O, autoclave and store at room temperature.
6. TGl Electrocompetent Cells (Lucigen, USA), genotype: *supE thi-1* Δ*(lac-proAB)* Δ*(mcrB-hsdSM)5(rK - mK -)* [F' *traD36 proAB lacI^{q}Z* Δ*M15]*.

3 Methods

3.1 Primer Design

Generating a diverse library through site-directed mutagenesis requires the use of degenerate oligonucleotide primers. These primers encode a mixture of amino acid sequences at the target positions designated for randomization, allowing for the exploration of sequence space within specific regions, such as the CDRs. NNN degeneracy (where N represents any of the four nucleotides: A, C, G, or T) was commonly employed, as it theoretically covers all 64 possible codons [8]. However, a significant drawback of NNN is the inherent inclusion of three stop codons, which can lead to a high frequency of nonfunctional clones in the resulting library, complicating screening and selection efforts [27]. To avoid this issue, alternative reduced codon sets have been developed and are widely utilized. Examples include NNK (N = A/C/G/T, K = G/T), NNS (N = A/C/G/T, S = C/G), and NNB (N = A/C/G/T, B=C/G/T). These sets minimize the frequency of stop codons while still encoding all 20 standard amino acids, offering a more favorable balance between diversity and the proportion of functional sequences [28].

Effective primer design for Kunkel mutagenesis requires careful consideration of several technical parameters to ensure efficient annealing and extension. The degenerate region encoding the randomized positions must be flanked by sequences that are reverse complementary to the packaged strand of template DNA. A minimum length of approximately 15 complementary bases both upstream and downstream of the randomized segment is crucial to ensure stable and specific annealing of the primer to the uracilated template strand, thereby accurately initiating DNA synthesis at the desired location (see Fig. 2). Practical limitations in oligonucleotide synthesis efficiency generally restrict the overall length of the primer to approximately 100 base pairs [25].

3.2 Preparation of dU-ssDNA Template

Template is prepared by using a modified QIAGEN QIAprep spin M13 kit protocol.

1. Transform the phagemid vector carrying the template sequence to be mutated into competent *E. coli* CJ236 (or analogous *dut-/ung-* strain). Thaw 50 µL of CJ236

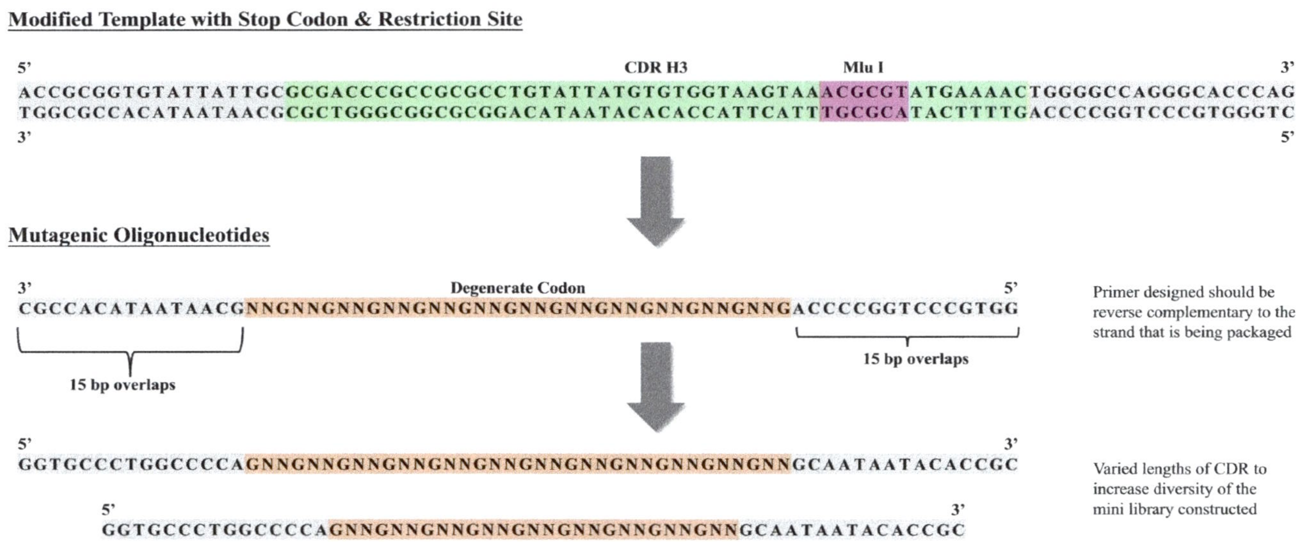

Fig. 2 Design of mutagenic oligonucleotides. Modified DNA template sequence incorporating a stop codon and Mlu I restriction site downstream of the CDR H3. Mutagenic oligonucleotides are designed to introduce randomized codons (NNC) into the CDR H3 region, with 15 base pairs overlaps flanking both upstream and downstream region to enable proper annealing. They are also designed to be reverse complementary to the packaging strand. Moreover, variations in the length degenerate codons support the generation of CDRs of differing lengths, further enhancing diversity.

electrocompetent cells on ice for 2 min, mix with 1 μg of plasmid DNA.

2. Transfer the mixture to a prechilled 0.1 cm electroporation cuvette. Electroporate at 1.7 kV using an electroporator.
3. Immediately recover the electroporated mixture with 1 mL of prewarmed 2× YT medium and transfer the suspension to a 1.5 mL microcentrifuge tube. Incubate the cell suspensions at 37°C and 800 rpm for 30 min.
4. Plate the recovered cells on 2× YT agar plate supplemented with appropriate antibiotics (e.g., ampicillin and chloramphenicol) to select for the vector and incubate overnight at 37°C.
5. Pick a single colony of *E. coli* CJ236 containing the phagemid vector and inoculate 5 mL 2× YT medium supplemented with appropriate antibiotics and grow overnight at 37°C and 200 rpm.
6. Inoculate 2 mL of overnight culture into 200 mL 2× YT medium supplemented with appropriate antibiotics at 37°C and 200 rpm until OD_{600} reaches ~0.5. Infect with M13KO7 (10^{10} cfu/mL) and incubate at 37°C and 200 rpm for 1 h.
7. Transfer cultures to 50 mL Falcon tubes and pellet the cells by centrifugation at 3200×*g* at 25°C for 15 min.
8. Discard supernatant, gently resuspend pellet and equally distribute into 500 mL conical shake flasks with 100 mL of 2× YT medium supplemented with appropriate antibiotics and kanamycin (50 μg/mL) to select for bacteria coinfected with helper phage M13KO7. Uridine (0.25 μg/mL) is also supplemented. Culture for approximately 22 h at 25°C, 200 rpm.
9. To harvest the phage, transfer cultures to 50 mL Falcon tubes and centrifuge at 7000×*g* at for 10 min. Transfer supernatants to a new tube and repeat centrifugation again.
10. Filter the clarified phage-containing supernatant with 0.45 μ m nylon filter.
11. Transfer filtrate to a new tube containing 20% final volume of PEG/NaCl and incubate supernatant on ice for 1 h to precipitate phage.
12. Centrifuge precipitated phage at 8000×*g* for 15 min at room temperature and discard supernatant. Briefly spin again at 2000×*g* for 2 min and aspirate the remaining supernatant with care.
13. Resuspend phage pellets with 16 mL of 1× PBS by using a pipette, filter resuspended phage through a 0.45 μm nylon filter.

14. Repeat the PEG/NaCl precipitation (see Steps 11 and 12). After the second precipitation, resuspend the final phage pellet in 1 mL of 1× PBS by using a pipette.
15. Clarify the phage by centrifugation at 13,000 rpm for 10 min using a bench top microcentrifuge at room temperature to remove any residual cell debris. Repeat centrifugation until no bacteria pellet is observed.
16. To isolate the ssDNA, transfer supernatant to a new tube, add 10 μL of MP buffer (1:100 dilution), vortex briefly to mix and incubate at room temperature for 10 min. A visible cloudiness indicates successful DNA precipitation.
17. Load the sample onto a QIAprep spin column in a 2 mL collection tube. Centrifuge at 13,000 rpm for 1 min and discard the flow-through.
18. Add 700 μL MLB buffer to the column. Centrifuge at 13,000 rpm for 1 min and discard the flow-through.
19. Add another 700 μL MLB buffer and incubate at room temperature for at least 1 min. Centrifuge at 13,000 rpm for 1 min and discard the flow-through.
20. Add 700 μL buffer PE, centrifuge for 1 min at 13,000 rpm, discard the flow-through, and repeat step once more.
21. Centrifuge the empty column at 13,000 rpm for 1 min to remove residual PE buffer.
22. Transfer the QIAprep spin column to a 1.5 mL microcentrifuge tube. Add prewarmed 100 μL EB buffer to the center of the column membrane. Incubate at room temperature for 10 min and elute by centrifuging at 13,000 rpm for 1 min.
23. Quantify the amount of recovered dU-ssDNA using a nanodrop at absorbance at 260 nm (A_{260} = 1.0 for 33 ng/μL of dU-ssDNA).
24. Analyze the dU-ssDNA by running a small aliquot on a TAE/agarose gel. The DNA should appear as a predominant single band.

3.3 Introduction of Degenerate Oligonucleotides and Synthesis of CCC-dsDNA

To enable ligation during complementary strand synthesis, the degenerate oligonucleotides must carry a 5′-phosphate group [25]. These can either be ordered prephosphorylated from commercial suppliers or can be phosphorylated enzymatically later in-house [29].

1. To phosphorylate the degenerate oligonucleotide, combine 0.6 μg oligonucleotide with 2 μL 10× T4 DNA Ligase buffer and autoclaved dH_2O to a total volume of 20 μL in a 1.5 mL microcentrifuge tube.
2. Add 20 U T4 polynucleotide kinase (T4 PNK) to the mixture and incubate at 37°C for 1 h. Place the mixture on ice and proceed directly to the annealing step.

3. Mix the phosphorylated oligonucleotide with 20 μg of dU-ssDNA template at a molar ratio of 3:1. Add 25 μL 10× TM buffer and top up the total volume to 250 μL with autoclaved dH_2O.
4. Divide the mixture into PCR tubes evenly and heat to 90°C for 2 min, then gradually cool to 25°C at a rate of 1°C/min using a thermocycler or dry block to allow for controlled annealing.
5. To the 250 μL annealing mixture, add 17 μL 10× T4 DNA Ligase buffer, 25 μL 10 mM dNTP mix, 5 μL T4 DNA ligase (400 U/μL), and 3 μL T7 DNA polymerase (10 U/μL).
6. Mix and incubate the reaction at 20°C for at least 3 h, followed by a 20 min incubation at 65°C to heat inactivate the ligase. During this step, the heteroduplexed DNA is converted to covalently, closed, circular DNA (CCC-dsDNA) via strand extension and ligation.
7. Use QIAquick PCR Purification kit to purify and desalt the synthesized CCC-dsDNA by adding 1.5 mL of PB buffer and mix thoroughly.
8. Apply the mixture to a QIAquick spin column in a 2 mL collection tube. Centrifuge at 13,000 rpm for 1 min and discard the flow-through.
9. Add 750 μL PE buffer, centrifuge for 1 min at 13,000 rpm, discard the flow-through, and repeat step once more.
10. Centrifuge the empty column at 13,000 rpm for 1 min to remove residual PE buffer.
11. Transfer the QIAquick spin column to a fresh 1.5 mL microcentrifuge tube and elute by adding 31 μL of prewarmed EB buffer to the center of the column membrane. Incubate at room temperature for 10 min and elute by centrifuging at 13,000 rpm for 1 min.
12. Measure the amount of CCC-dsDNA recovered using a nanodrop at absorbance at 260 nm (A_{260} = 1.0 for 50 ng/μL of CCC-dsDNA). The purified product can be used immediately for transformation by electroporation or stored frozen at −20°C for future use.
13. Analyze the CCC-dsDNA by running a small aliquot on a TAE/agarose gel. CCC-dsDNA typically appears as multiple bands with distinct electrophoretic mobilities. The fastest-migrating band corresponds to the desired CCC-dsDNA, which is fully extended and ligated, and exhibits high mutation frequency and transformation efficiency. A slower-migrating upper band reflects strand-displacement products from aberrant T7 polymerase activity and has low transformation efficiency. Occasionally, a third band of intermediate mobility may

be observed, representing unligated yet extended dsDNA. This can result from incomplete phosphorylation or suboptimal ligase activity.

3.4 Conversion to Phage Library Consisting of Mutated CDR H3 Template

To generate a functional phage display library, the covalently closed circular double-stranded DNA (CCC-dsDNA) must be introduced into *E. coli* cells harboring the F' episome, enabling subsequent M13 phage replication [25]. The *E. coli* strain SS320 is well-suited for this purpose due to its high electroporation efficiency and robust phage production capabilities [30]. It is important to note that SS320 is not an amber suppressor strain, so the antibody sequence must not have an amber stop in between the antibody sequence and pIII gene sequence in the phagemid.

3.4.1 Library Conversion

1. Thaw 50 µL of SS320 electrocompetent cells on ice for 2 min. Add 1 µg of CCC-dsDNA to the thawed cells. The number of electroporations required depends on the desired library size and complexity of the degenerate oligonucleotides. To achieve a diversity range of 10^9–10^{10}, approximately 10–20 electroporations may be pooled, depending on transformation efficiency.
2. Transfer the mixture to a prechilled 0.1 cm electroporation cuvette. Electroporate at 1.7 kV using an electroporator.
3. Immediately recover the electroporated mixture with 1 mL of prewarmed SOC medium and transfer the suspension to a 1.5 mL microcentrifuge tube. Incubate the cell suspensions at 37°C and 800 rpm for 30 min.
4. Pool the cell suspension according to the oligonucleotide variant used. To determine the transformation efficiency, dilute 10 µL of pooled cells in 90 µL 2× YT-amp and plate out on 2× YT-amp agar plates in 90 mm petri dish.
5. Plate out the remainder of the pooled cell suspension on BioAssay Dishes with 2× YT-amp agar. Incubate all plates overnight at 37°C.
6. Scrape the colonies on the BioAssay Dish with 2× YT-amp.
7. Estimate the library diversity by titrating an aliquot of the scraped library suspension (see Sect. 3.4.1).
8. Prepare glycerol stocks of the library for long-term storage (see Sect. 3.4.2).
9. To confirm the presence of CDR H3 mutations, perform colony PCR on randomly picked colonies from the 90 mm petri dish (see Sect. 3.5).

3.4.2 Library Size Estimation

1. Take 10 µL of cells from the scraped library suspension and perform a ten-fold serial dilution series down to 10^{-13}.
2. Spot 10 µL from each dilution on the 2× YT-amp agar plate and incubate overnight at 37°C.

3. Count the total library size using the following formula:

$$Library\ size = \frac{number\ of\ colonies \times\ \ dilution\ factor}{total\ volume}$$

3.4.3 Preparation of Bacteria Library Stock

1. Pellet the scraped library suspension by centrifugation at 4500×*g* for 10 min.
2. Resuspend cell the pellet with appropriate amount of 2× YT-amp and add 80% (v/v) sterile glycerol to the cells suspension to make a 20% glycerol library stock (*see* **Note 2**).
3. Aliquot 1 mL of the final library suspension into 2 mL cryogenic vial and keep in −80°C until use.

3.5 Colony PCR

1. Randomly select single colonies and resuspend each in 10 μL of autoclaved dH_2O.
2. Prepare the PCR reaction using 2 μL of colony suspension as the DNA template. In the reaction mixture, add 200 μM dNTPs, 0.5 μM each of forward and reverse primers, 1× DreamTaq buffer and 0.5 U DreamTaq DNA Polymerase. Top up the total reaction volume to 20 μL with autoclaved dH_2O.
3. Run the PCR with the following thermal cycling conditions: initial denaturation at 95°C for 5 min, 20 cycles of amplification with denaturation at 95°C for 30 s, annealing at 55°C for 30 s, elongation at 72°C for 2 min and finally, elongation at 72°C for 5 min.
4. Analyze the amplified PCR products by gel electrophoresis on 0.5% TBE/agarose at 120 V for 50 min.
5. Select colonies with amplicons of the expected size and send them for sequencing.
6. Use IMGT/V-QUEST (www.imgt.org/IMGT_vquest/vquest) to analyze the sequencing results for V, D, J gene usage and identify introduced mutations (*see* **Note 3**).

3.6 Phage Library Packaging

1. Thaw a tube of glycerol stock for the library and inoculate it into 500 mL of 2× YT-amp. Incubate at 37°C with shaking at 200 rpm until the culture reaches an OD_{600} of approximately 0.5.
2. Infect 250 mL of the culture with M13KO7 helper phage, maintaining the multiplicity of infection (MOI) of 1:20. Incubate the infected culture statically at 37°C for 30 min.
3. Centrifuge the culture at 3500×*g* for 10 min and discard the supernatant (*see* **Note 4**).

4. Resuspend the pellet in 300 mL 2× YT-amp/kan. Incubate overnight at 30°C with shaking at 200 rpm.
5. Pellet down the culture at 7000×*g* for 15 min.
6. Carefully transfer the phage-containing supernatant to fresh 50 mL Falcon tubes containing 20% volume of PEG/NaCl solution to 80% volume of supernatant. Mix well and incubate on ice for 1 h to precipitate phage (*see* **Note 5**).
7. Centrifuge the mixture at 8000×*g* for 30 min at 4°C. Discard the supernatant and resuspend the phage pellet in 16 mL of 1× PBS.
8. Filter the resuspension through a 0.45 µm nylon filter to remove bacterial debris.
9. Add an additional 20% volume of PEG/NaCl solution (4 mL for 16 mL suspension), mix well and incubate on ice for at least 20 min.
10. Centrifuge the mixture at 8000×*g* for 30 min at 4°C. Discard the supernatant, short spin briefly and carefully removes any remaining PEG/NaCl solution by pipetting.
11. Resuspend the final phage pellet in 2 mL of 1× PBS.
12. Clarify the suspension by centrifugation at 13,000 rpm for 10 min using a bench top microcentrifuge at room temperature to eliminate remaining residual cell debris. Repeat centrifugation if needed until no visible pellet remains.
13. Take 10 µL of the final phage suspension to determine the titer of the packaged library (see Sect. 3.7).
14. Store the library at 4°C until further use (*see* **Note 6**).

3.7 Phage Titration

1. Dilute 10 µL of phage library in 90 µL of 1× PBS and perform a ten-fold serial dilution.
2. To each dilution, add 100 µL of *E. coli* TG1 cells grown to an OD_{600} of approximately 0.5.
3. Spot 10 µL each of the infected cells onto both 2× YT-amp agar plate and 2× YT-kan agar plate. Incubate the plates overnight at 37°C (*see* **Note 7**).
4. Calculate the phage titer using the formula:

$$\text{Phage titer (cfu/mL)} = \frac{\text{Number of colonies} \quad \times \text{Dilution factor}}{\text{Total volume spotted}}$$

5. The library can now be packaged for panning to identify higher affinity mutants.

4 Notes

1. Overlapping annealing sites of mutagenic oligos may differ based on the original antibody template sequence.
2. The glycerol stocks of library are prepared to have a starting OD_{600} of approximately 0.1 when the tube of stock is thawed into 500 mL of 2× YT-amp during library packaging.
3. Deep sequencing can be employed to comprehensively assess the diversity of the antibody library repertoire.
4. Cells should be pelleted and the glucose-containing medium discarded, as residual glucose can repress expression of the pIII fusion protein.
5. The efficiency of phage particle precipitation using PEG/NaCl solution can be improved by extending the incubation on ice to 2 h.
6. Store prepared phage library at 4°C for no more than 4 weeks. To avoid degradation of displayed antibodies, fresh phage preparations are recommended before downstream applications. If the phagemid has an amber stop at the C-terminal end of the antibody sequence, an additional step of phage infection with an amber suppressor strain would be necessary before panning.
7. Colony counts on ampicillin plates should be at least twice those on kanamycin plates, indicating lower levels of helper phage produced than the phage library. These counts also provide a preliminary estimate of library size before biopanning.

Acknowledgments

The authors would like to acknowledge the support of Malaysian Ministry for Higher Education through the Fundamental Research Grant Scheme (FRGS/1/2024/STG01/USM/02/10).

References

1. Valldorf B, Hinz SC, Russo G, Pekar L, Mohr L, Klemm J, Doerner A, Krah S, Hust M, Zielonka S (2022) Antibody display technologies: selecting the cream of the crop. Biol Chem 403(5-6):455–477
2. Hairul Bahara NH, Tye GJ, Choong YS, Ong EB, Ismail A, Lim TS (2013) Phage display antibodies for diagnostic applications. Biologicals 41(4):209–216
3. Bradbury ARM, Sidhu S, Dübel S, McCafferty J (2011) Beyond natural antibodies: the power of in vitro display technologies. Nat Biotechnol 29(3):245–254
4. Langreder N, Schäckermann D, Unkauf T, Schubert M, Frenzel A, Bertoglio F, Hust M (2023) Antibody affinity and stability maturation by error-prone PCR. Methods Mol Biol 2702:395–410

5. Steinwand M, Droste P, Frenzel A, Hust M, Dübel S, Schirrmann T (2014) The influence of antibody fragment format on phage display based affinity maturation of IgG. mAbs 6(1):204–218
6. Doria-Rose NA, Joyce MG (2015) Strategies to guide the antibody affinity maturation process. Curr Opin Virol 11:137–147
7. Lo K-M, Leger O, Hock B (2014) Antibody engineering. Microbiol Spectr 2(1):319–343
8. Lim CC, Choong YS, Lim TS (2019) Cognizance of molecular methods for the generation of mutagenic phage display antibody libraries for affinity maturation. Int J Mol Sci 20(8):1861
9. de Wildt RMT, Mundy CR, Gorick BD, Tomlinson IM (2000) Antibody arrays for high-throughput screening of antibody–antigen interactions. Nat Biotechnol 18(9):989–994
10. Pini A, Viti F, Santucci A, Caremolla B, Zardi L, Neri P, Neri D (1998) Design and use of a phage display library: human antibodies with subnanomolar affinity against a marker of angiogenesis eluted from a two-dimensional gel. J Biol Chem 273(34):21769–21776
11. Frenzel A, Schirrmann T, Hust M (2016) Phage display-derived human antibodies in clinical development and therapy. mAbs 8(7):1177–1194
12. Chiu ML, Goulet DR, Teplyakov A, Gilliland GL (2019) Antibody structure and function: the basis for engineering therapeutics. Antibodies (Basel) 8(4):55
13. Mason DM, Friedensohn S, Weber CR, Jordi C, Wagner B, Meng SM, Ehling RA, Bonati L, Dahinden J, Gainza P, Correia BE, Reddy ST (2021) Optimization of therapeutic antibodies by predicting antigen specificity from antibody sequence via deep learning. Nat Biomed Eng 5(6):600–612
14. Grzeschik J, Könning D, Hinz SC, Krah S, Schröter C, Empting M, Kolmar H, Zielonka S (2018) Generation of semi-synthetic shark IgNAR single-domain antibody libraries. In: Hust M, Lim TS (eds) Phage display: methods and protocols. Springer, New York, pp 147–167
15. Chen X, Gentili M, Hacohen N, Regev A (2021) A cell-free nanobody engineering platform rapidly generates SARS-CoV-2 neutralizing nanobodies. Nat Commun 12(1):5506
16. Sevy AM, Chen M-T, Castor M, Sylvia T, Krishnamurthy H, Ishchenko A, Hsieh C-M (2020) Structure-and sequence-based design of synthetic single-domain antibody libraries. PEDS 33:gzaa028
17. Wells JA, Estell DA (1988) Subtilisin—an enzyme designed to be engineered. Trends Biochem Sci 13(8):291–297
18. Vandeyar MA, Weiner MP, Hutton CJ, Batt CA (1988) A simple and rapid method for the selection of oligodeoxynucleotide-directed mutants. Gene 65(1):129–133
19. Sugimoto M, Esaki N, Tanaka H, Soda K (1989) A simple and efficient method for the oligonucleotide-directed mutagenesis using plasmid DNA template and phosphorothioate-modified nucleotide. Anal Biochem 179(2):309–311
20. Kunkel TA (1985) Rapid and efficient site-specific mutagenesis without phenotypic selection. Proc Natl Acad Sci U S A 82(2):488–492
21. Kunkel TA, Roberts JD, Zakour RA (1987) Rapid and efficient site-specific mutagenesis without phenotypic selection. Methods Enzymol 154:367–382
22. Scholle MD, Kehoe JW, Kay BK (2005) Efficient construction of a large collection of phage-displayed combinatorial peptide libraries. Comb Chem High Throughput Screen 8(6):545–551
23. Sidhu SS, Weiss GA (2004) Constructing phage display libraries by oligonucleotide-directed mutagenesis. In: Clackson T, Lowman HB (eds) Phage display. Oxford University Press, Oxford, pp 27–41
24. Sidhu SS, Geyer CR (2015) Phage display in biotechnology and drug discovery. CRC Press, Boca Raton
25. Frei JC, Lai JR (2016) Protein and antibody engineering by phage display. Methods Enzymol 580:45–87
26. Huang R, Fang P, Kay BK (2012) Improvements to the kunkel mutagenesis protocol for constructing primary and secondary phage-display libraries. Methods 58(1):10–17
27. Siloto RMP, Weselake RJ (2012) Site saturation mutagenesis: methods and applications in protein engineering. Biocatal Agric Biotechnol 1(3):181–189
28. Nov Y (2012) When second best is good enough: another probabilistic look at saturation mutagenesis. Appl Environ Microbiol 78(1):258–262
29. Tonikian R, Zhang Y, Boone C, Sidhu SS (2007) Identifying specificity profiles for peptide recognition modules from phage-displayed peptide libraries. Nat Protoc 2(6):1368–1386
30. Sidhu SS, Lowman HB, Cunningham BC, Wells JA (2000) Phage display for selection of novel binding peptides. In: Thorner J, Emr SD, Abelson JN (eds) Methods in enzymology, vol 328. Academic Press, Cambridge, pp 333–335

Part II

Display System Optimization

Check for updates

Chapter 5

Yeast Display of Single-Chain Fc Fragments with Modulated Binding of Effector Molecules

Katharina Stadlbauer, Cecilia Wick, Julia Gobl, Wolfgang Wallner, Annika de Sousa Linhares, Jochen Stritzker and Gordana Wozniak-Knopp

Abstract

Yeast display platform has proven instrumental for directed evolution of diverse proteins towards altered binding specificity, affinity, or improved biophysical properties. Particularly in antibody display, this method has delivered variants that are featured today as integral parts of approved therapeutic agents. While broadly used for discovery of binding agents, yeast display has also been applied for optimization of properties of Fc fragment. Among the bispecific antibody formats, which come in a variety of different molecular architectures, the single-chain Fc is a less explored alternative. This format offers novel opportunities for positioning of binding sites in a multispecific molecule, however, necessitates special design due to its unique features such as linker. We tested the amenability of yeast system for the efficient presentation of the single-chain IgG Fc and characterized the displayed fragments for binding of structural markers and Fc gamma receptors. Taken together, this chapter sets the base for successful use of yeast display in isolation of single-chain Fc variants with tailored ligand-binding properties.

Keywords Single-chain Fc, Fc-gamma receptor, Copy number, Directed evolution, Yeast display

1 Introduction

1.1 Directed Evolution of Fc Fragments for Altered Ligand Recognition

Antibodies are traditionally seen as composed of the antigen-binding variable region, and effector-function mediating Fc region. While the discovery and optimization of antigen-binding regions has traditionally harvested the power of molecular display techniques, the engineering of the Fc region towards a particular binding function for improved or novel functionalities via directed evolution is more novel and intensely pursued by the antibody research community not longer than for the past two decades. Nevertheless, this approach made a difference for human health as it delivered molecules that are currently increasingly present as parts of newly approved therapeutic antibodies. In the Fc engineering, three large groups of properties are being addressed: (i) interaction with the Fc ligand molecules,

Huan Peng and Theam Soon Lim (eds.), *Biomolecular Display Technologies*, Methods in Molecular Biology, vol. 3030,
https://doi.org/10.1007/978-1-0716-5249-7_5,

mostly those present on the surface of the effector cells, to steer the reactivity of the Fc with a certain ligand and the corresponding activity of the affected cell type, or protein cascade in the case of complement activation, (ii) interaction with the neonatal Fc receptor (FcRn), leading towards extended half-life in vivo, and (iii) increased Fc stability (Fig. 1).

The interaction of the Fc fragment with ligand molecules on effector cells can elicit both positive and negative signaling, resulting in either activation or inhibition of the responding cell groups. For IgG, currently the only antibody class present in the approved therapeutic antibodies, both kinds of receptors share overlapping binding sites, located on the N-terminal loops of the IgG C_H2 domain and additionally involving hinge region of the antibody [1]. Interestingly, the IgG subclasses interact differently with the IgG effector ligands and elicit various responses of the effector cells, which also dictates the choice of antibody isotype to optimize its biological function. While IgG1-Fc, the isotype traditionally used in clinical antibodies, shows strong reactivity with agonistic receptor FcγRI and weak reactivity with FcγRIIa and FcγRIIIa, and can hence induce potent cellular activity such as phagocytosis or antibody-dependent cellular cytotoxicity, the IgG2- and IgG4-Fcs interact with these ligands with lower affinity, leading to less pronounced cellular functions. For each of the isotypes, the interaction with the inhibitory receptor FcγRIIb is at least for an order of magnitude lower than

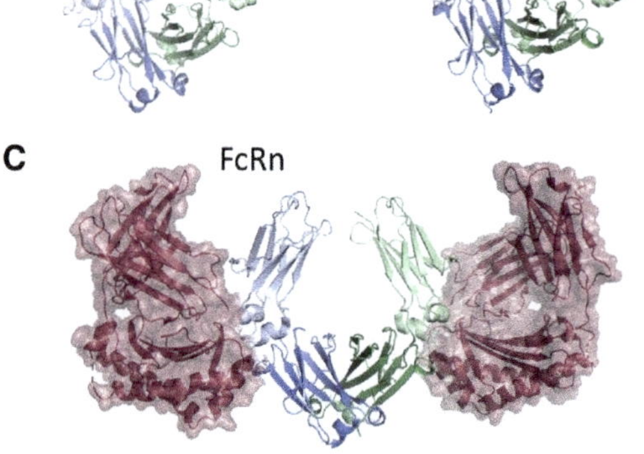

Fig. 1 Fc fragment (light blue and light green: C_H2 domains, deep blue and deep green: C_H3 domains) complexed with the ligands conveying its biological activity, shown in purple with surfaced cartoon presentation. (**A**) FcγRIIIa (CD16), PDB: 1E4K. (**B**) C1q complement component, PDB: 6FCZ. (**C**) neonatal Fc receptor (FcRn), PDB: 7Q15. The figure was prepared using PyMOL (Schrödinger LLC)

can be measured for its activating analogue FcγRIIa [2]. Antibody variants with enhanced effector functions, owing to a more potent interaction with activating Fcγ receptors and decreased inhibitory receptors, have been isolated using yeast library screenings [3], and indeed presently benefit patients as they importantly contribute to the beneficial properties of several recently approved antibody therapeutics, such as margetuximab [4]. To conclude, modification of the Fc fragment sequence leading to an improved interaction with activating Fc receptors is a valuable strategy for design of therapeutic antibodies with superior biological activity. At the same time, boosting of the IgG-Fc binding to activating receptors by modification of N-linked glycan pattern towards low content of proximal fucose is also a valuable strategy for improving the mode of action based on antibody-dependent cytotoxicity driven by several clinically applied antibodies, such as seen in obinutuzumab, mogamulizumab, and benralizumab [5]. Recent reports list approximately the same numbers of INN-labeled antibodies where augmented interactions with Fc gamma receptors have been achieved over fucose reduction or amino acid substitutions (14 vs. 16) [6].

Interestingly, the molecular evolution of the Fc fragment via display and selection is powerful enough to functionalize even aglycosylated Fc fragments for novel or enhanced effector functions. For example, mutated Fc fragments that enable binding to FcγRI have been isolated using bacterial display and flow cytometry-guided selections, and such binders incited antibody-dependent cytotoxicity (ADCC) by monocyte-derived dendritic cells [7, 8]. Unglycosylated Fc variants exhibiting stronger reactivity with FcγRIII and simultaneously showing less F/V158 allele bias than clinical grade IgG1 antibodies were isolated with a similar system [9]. Even Fc fragments with 1000-fold potentiated ability to interact with FcγRIIa, and with 25-fold lower affinity towards the inhibitory allele FcγRIIb, were designed using a bacterial expression system displaying a complete IgG, and such antibodies mediated potent macrophage phagocytosis of the relevant antigen-positive tumor cells [10].

Moreover, also the obliteration of effector functions has proved advantageous for certain antibodies. Fc fragments with reduced binding to Fcγ receptors were applied to avoid the unwanted inflammatory responses to therapeutic antibodies, and complete elimination of effector functions is still a property pursued by many recent studies [6]. Another situation where inert Fc proves beneficial are antiviral agents where the internalization via Fc receptors can lead to antibody-dependent enhancement (ADE) mechanisms, a serious safety concern. Several promising novel antiviral antibodies developed to counter SARS-CoV-2 infection such as etesevimab, tixagevimab, and cilgavimab [11, 12] feature Fc fragments rendered inert using point mutations discovered by rational engineering.

In this context, also the antibody complement-activating activity was engineered through molecular display techniques, although the documented efforts oriented into this direction are fewer than the engineering of the effector functions, probably due to a lower number of indications that exploit complement activation as a therapeutic mode of action. Bacterial Fc display was instrumental in isolating variants that could mediate complement-dependent cellular cytotoxicity when combined with variable domains of anti-CD20 antibody rituximab, with only two-fold to five-fold lower potency of the original antibody [13].

The interaction of Fc fragment with FcRn is essential for the favorable long half-life in vivo of several types of antibodies. The lower affinity of IgG3 towards FcRn is also the likely reason why the increased use of this isotype in therapeutic agents is first expected after the recent engineering achievements, oriented towards increased FcRn engagement, enhanced stability and aggregation resistance [14, 15]. Even for the best interaction partner IgG1 the enhanced interaction with FcRn has proven instrumental for therapeutic use: Fc mutants isolated using directed evolution approach with phage display are today a hallmark of approved therapeutic nirsevimab, directed against the respiratory syncytial virus [16]. The Fc version M252Y/S254T/T256E (YTE) isolated via phage display and screening reacts more potently with FcRn, which makes it a long-acting antibody [17, 18], and is one of the important factors why nirsevimab presents a solution for anti-RSV immunotherapy after six decades of quest for a suitable medication. When the variant is equipped with further mutations (H433K/N434F), providing long-lasting binding to FcRn [19], such Fc fragment can efficiently prevent binding of other IgGs by competition [20]. This caused up to 50% reduction in antibody levels in healthy individuals, and led to approval of the IgG Fc fragment modified in this way, efgartigimod, for treatment of myasthenia gravis and immune thrombocytopenia [21]. Additionally, this medication is in advanced phases of clinical testing for several other autoimmune conditions where the antibodies are the causative agents of the disease pathology, such as pemphigus vulgaris, foliaceus, and chronic inflammatory demyelinating polyneuropathy. A further development of YTE-variant was its application in the monomeric Fc, which served as a scaffold for mutagenesis to eventually enable the selection of variants providing IgG1-like half-life in vivo in mouse experiments, when fused with a Fab and a single-chain Fc fragment, thus allowing bispecific antigen binding while ensuring monovalent antigen interaction for each binding partner [22].

1.2 Asymmetric Fc Fragments and Single-Chain Fc

To conclude, the quest for molecules opening novel therapeutic options via directed evolution is often based on formats different from a classical homodimeric bivalent IgG. The rise of the bispecific antibodies led to increasing numbers of approvals in the past two decades, reflecting their unique functioning in certain biological situations, such as mediating effector-to-target cell interactions, linking two different ligands or epitopes on one cell, or acting to transfer biological activity over cellular of tissue compartments [23]. This has also significantly increased the recognition of their diverse formats as decisive for their successful differentiation. Breaking the traditional symmetry of the Fc was a crucial feature for the forthcoming of bispecific antibodies, based on the linkages of the binding entities to heterologous half-Fcs, heterodimerized, for example, via selective steric compatibility or electrostatic steering. To accelerate the transition of binding agents from their discovery platforms to expression and screening in soluble format, several ingenuine methods for display of alternative variants of Fc fragments, often heterodimerized already when displayed in biological platforms for selection and screening, have been documented. Very soon after the discovery of knobs-into-holes strategy [24], phage display was used to isolate heterodimeric Fc variants with increased stability [25]. Later, yeast platform yielded improved electrostatic steering-based asymmetric Fc fragments optimized for expression yield, with variants featuring mutated residues that were unexpected and could not be designed by rational mutagenesis methods [26]. Apart from improved biophysical properties, yeast display was instrumental in isolating heterodimeric mutated Fc fragments that contain de novo created antigen binding sites within structural elements [27]. Monovalent Fc-based antigen-binding clones of similar format can indeed prove of advantage in certain biological situations, for example, enhanced biodistribution of brain-delivered enzyme substitutes as compared with Fc fragments with bivalent binding of molecular shuttling protein CD98 [28].

One example where asymmetric structure of the displayed Fc can be beneficial for affinity selections for ligand binding is the engineering for improved FcγR binding as these molecules require an Fc dimer for interaction but contact both half-Fcs in one to one stoichiometry, and different residues of both half-Fcs are involved into this interaction to a different extent. Interestingly, for the Fc fragments with enhanced interaction with FcγRIII, mutated identically in both Fc halves, it was shown that not all mutated residues contribute equally to the improvement of receptor binding [29]. Using extensive mutagenesis and screening, an Fc that introduces substitutions in each Fc half asymmetrically was discovered that can mediate more potent ADCC than IgG1 [30] by interacting with FcγRI 1000-fold more potently than the wild-type IgG1 and at the same time showing no difference in affinity towards the inhibitory receptor FcγRIIb. This differential recognition was not seen either in the original homodimeric DLE mutant or in the corresponding heterodimeric half-wild type Fc. In strong contrast with the symmetrically mutated DLE variant (S239D/A330L/I332E), destabilized for about 20°C when both Fc halves were mutated, the asymmetrical Fc variant was less impaired in its thermostability, for only 6°C.

Among the plethora of asymmetrical antibody formats available, the strategy of joining heterologous Fc monomers with a linker in a single-chain Fc (scFc) has until now been less explored. Only recently, the first antibody drug with scFc, tarlatamab, which simultaneously targets DLL3 antigen on tumor cells and CD3 on T cells, was approved [31]. In this antibody, the scFc is joined with a bispecific T-cell engager (BiTE) for its in vivo half-life extension, and the molecule represents the first BiTE approved for treatment of solid tumors. Several other scFc-containing drugs are in preclinical development at the moment, promising novel therapeutic options in situations where small molecular size paired with monovalent binding mode is decisive for optimal activity, such as in molecular Trojan horse-mediated brain delivery [32].

Topologically, bispecific or multispecific reagents containing a single-chain Fc fragment, binding fragments containing antigen-binding sites can be linked to either or both N- and C-termini, avoiding the formation of heterogeneously paired species that may result from the coexpression of multiple chains.

With the increasing realization value of gene therapies, tissue-specific targeting for Adeno-associated virus (AAV) vectors is a major limiting factor, and bispecific antibodies have proven highly efficient for redirection to specific complex signatures of target receptors [33, 34]. Bispecific formats containing linker-bound-single-chain Fcs offer several advantages when used for anchoring the attached antigen-binding fragments onto the surface of virus or virus-like particles. As the covalent bonding dictates the correct chain pairing, a large proportion of correctly formed heterodimer is formed, which is important as the polishing purification methods are not amenable here. On the other hand, an arrayed constellation of the target-receptor binding entities is ensured with covalent bonding.

Apart of supporting construction of bispecific antibodies and enabling enhanced effector ligand molecules due to novel architectures achieved by asymmetrical mutagenesis, single chain-Fc fragments are also optimally suited for construction of monomeric fusion proteins with protein drugs such as enzymes and hormones [35]. While the first clinical candidates in this class with markedly improved half-life in comparison to drug alone were dimers, monomeric Fc fusions (with monomeric drug and dimeric Fc fragment) promise enhanced biological activity and better options of noninvasive delivery [36]. Currently, three of the total 17 approved Fc-fusion proteins feature such format [37].

1.3 Linker

In the scFc proteins described until now the composition of linker mostly follows the most commonly used one in the design of antibody scFv fragments, the repeats of G_4S sequence. The reason for this is its expected high flexibility, low propensity to aggregation and protease resistance. At the same time, the neutral character of glycine and serine should contribute to retaining the binding properties of the Fc fragment towards its diverse ligands more predictable. The exact number of GS-rich repeats, however, differs in the reports. In the study of the hGH-scFc fusions, constructs with between 8 and 14 repeats were compared for the expression level and the percentage of monomer, and it was found that the increasing number of linker repeats up to 12 or 13 had a positive influence on the yield of the recombinant protein, and that the variant with 13 repeats showed the lowest level of impurities upon the expression [35]. In the future, alternatives in the linker sequence design can also prove to be of advantage when trying to increase the solubility of the molecule, as shown in the past for the linkers connecting variable domains of the antibodies [38], or when trying to ensure that the linker works as a spacer between protein domains [39].

1.4 Expression and Purification of scFc Fragments

The optimization of display conditions is steered by a prerequisite of the format of the yeast-displayed protein being one that can be well expressed and possibly well folded also when produced in the soluble form. For this purpose, we produced the wild-type scFcs of IgG1 and IgG2 in mammalian cells and purified them with Protein A-based affinity chromatography. The results were compared with those obtained with constructs where the immunogen ovalbumin (OVA) was fused N-terminally with the construct. For the expression, the mammalian cell-based pTT/HEK293-6E system was used. The yields after Protein A purification amounted to several tens of mg per L expression supernatant, and apart from a dominant monomer peak the preparations contained higher molecular weight species, corresponding to dimers and multimers of the protein (Fig. 2A). Interestingly, the amount of these aggregates was lower for

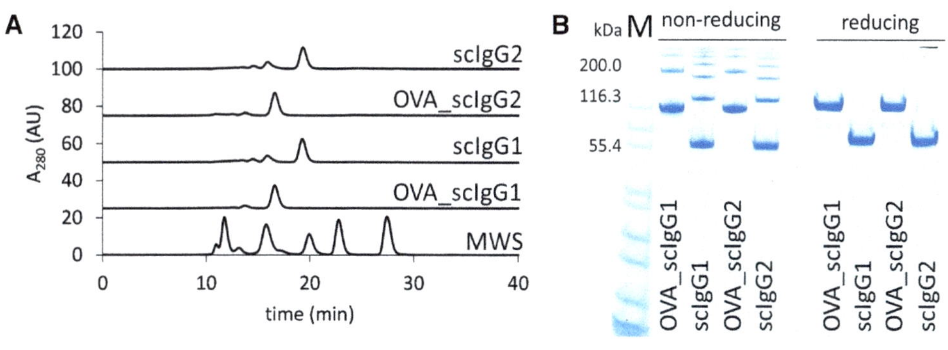

Fig. 2 (**A**) Size exclusion chromatography in native conditions revealing the profile of single chain Fc fragments of IgG1 and IgG2 and their fusions with ovalbumin (OVA) after Protein A-based purification. MWS: molecular weight standard with proteins of 670, 158, 44, 17, and 1.35 kDa. (**B**) Coomassie-stained SDS-PAGE gel with 2 μg of each of the proteins resolved, either in nonreduced or reduced sample (M is Mark12 protein ladder, Thermo Fisher Scientific)

the OVA-fused scFcs. The analysis with SDS-PAGE has confirmed that the multimers are formed owing to cysteine mispairing, as only monomer bands were visible upon reduction and heating of the protein preparation (Fig. 2B).

1.5 Visualization of Linker-Connected Fc Using In Silico Methods

The emergence of multimeric structures in scFc preparations is most likely to be led back to the possible mispairing of the cysteine residues present in the hinge region. We were, therefore, interested if the molecular dynamics-derived information on the studied fragment could further shed light on this topic. We applied crystal structures of the Fc fragments and the G_4S unit for linker assembly of the primordial scFc structure and established that there should be no strain of linker imposed over the length of 10 G_4S repeats. We constructed the scFc models using homology modeling [40] or artificial intelligence-based tool AlphaFold3 [41] (Fig. 3A), and it was interesting to see that even the models derived with the same method strongly differ in the position of residues pertaining to the Fc hinge and linker sequence (Fig. 3B). We used the homology-derived model to perform molecular dynamics simulations over 50 ns using WebGRO for Macromolecular Simulations (https://simlab.uams.edu/) [42]. We then compared the root mean square fluctuation (RMSF) of the atoms in individual amino acid residues for homodimeric Fc and scFc

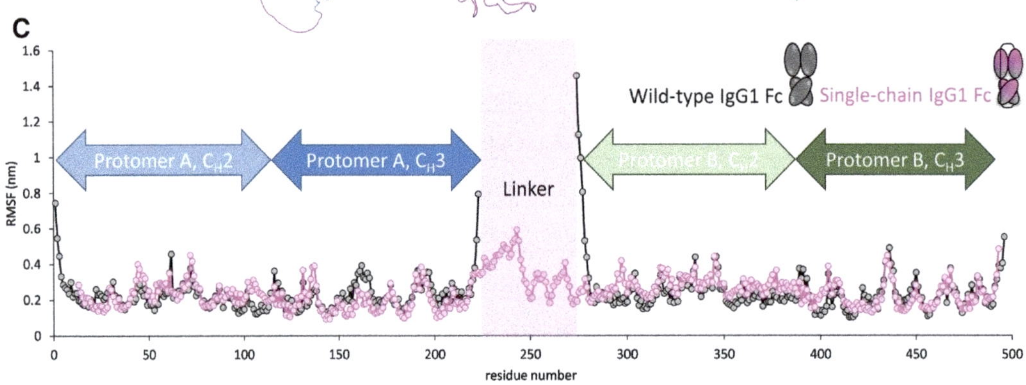

Fig. 3 (**A**) Models of single chain Fc, left: schematic showing C_H2 domain of Protomer A in light blue, C_H3 of protomer A in deep blue, linker in magenta, C_H2 domain of Protomer B in light green and C_H3 domain of Protomer B in deep green, center: AlphaFold 3-derived scFc model, right: Swiss Model-derived scFc model. (**B**) Overlays of five AlphaFold3-derived models of scFc. (**C**) RMSF data derived from molecular dynamics simulation of a homodimeric Fc and an scFc with indicated molecular regions

(Fig. 3C). There were no conspicuous differences between the RMSF of the atoms of two structures, except for the amino acid residues at the C-terminus of protomer A and N-terminus of protomer B, which were more flexible in the case of homodimer. The residues in the linker region showed most flexibility in the sc IgG1 Fc sequence.

1.6 Yeast Surface Display of the Single-Chain Fc

Yeast surface display has been instrumental in applying methods of directed evolution to engineer beneficial properties such as superior activity or stability into a vast repertoire of very diverse proteins. The advantageous features of this display system include eukaryotic folding apparatus, the ability of N-linked glycosylation, and the compatibility with fluorescence-activated cell sorting. The multiparametric analysis characteristic for this method allows the normalization of inspected signal, for example antigen binding strength, to the number of binding sites expressed per cell, which are usually measured via an antipeptide tag antibody, such as HA-tag or FLAG-tag [43, 44]. Owing to increasing popularity of yeast display in the last decade, the methods for highly efficient transformation have been developed, which are conducive to simple creation of very large libraries. A second beneficial feature of yeast display in *Saccharomyces cerevisiae* is certainly the simple but efficient library construction, as the gap-driven homologous recombination in this yeast species requires only 25 base pairs of homology for sealing the DNA strands, with only about 1% illegitimate recombination [45]. Moreover, this mechanism extends to the assembly of up to 25 DNA fragments with the expression vector [46].

In the investigation of feasibility of yeast display for scFc fragments, we aimed to optimize the conditions for the expression of scFc fragment on the yeast surface and compared the expression parameters for yeast-displayed wild-type IgG1 Fc and sc IgG1 Fc fragments. We also evaluated the binding properties towards typical Fc ligands that could be informative for the evaluation of integrity of the displayed fragment. For this purpose, we have chosen an anti-N-terminal tag antibody anti-Xpress, whose binding is not dependent on the structural properties of the displayed construct, and should, therefore, be indicative of the number of displayed copies; a peptide-derived anti-hinge antibody; an anti-C_H2 antibody, whose binding depends on the proper conformation of the domain; FcγRI (CD64), which would only bind to dimerized Fc when glycosylated; protein A, the reactivity of which is dependent on conformation of both C_H2 and C_H3 domains, and a polyclonal anti-IgG1 antibody (Fig. 4A). Although the level of display of scFc, judged by median fluorescence intensity, amounted only to about 30% of that achieved with a homodimeric Fc fragment, staining with other markers was about 60%–70% of the control, indicating good suitability for display (Fig. 4B). The relative values did not differ between the cultures that were induced at the temperature of 20°C, and those induced at 37°C,

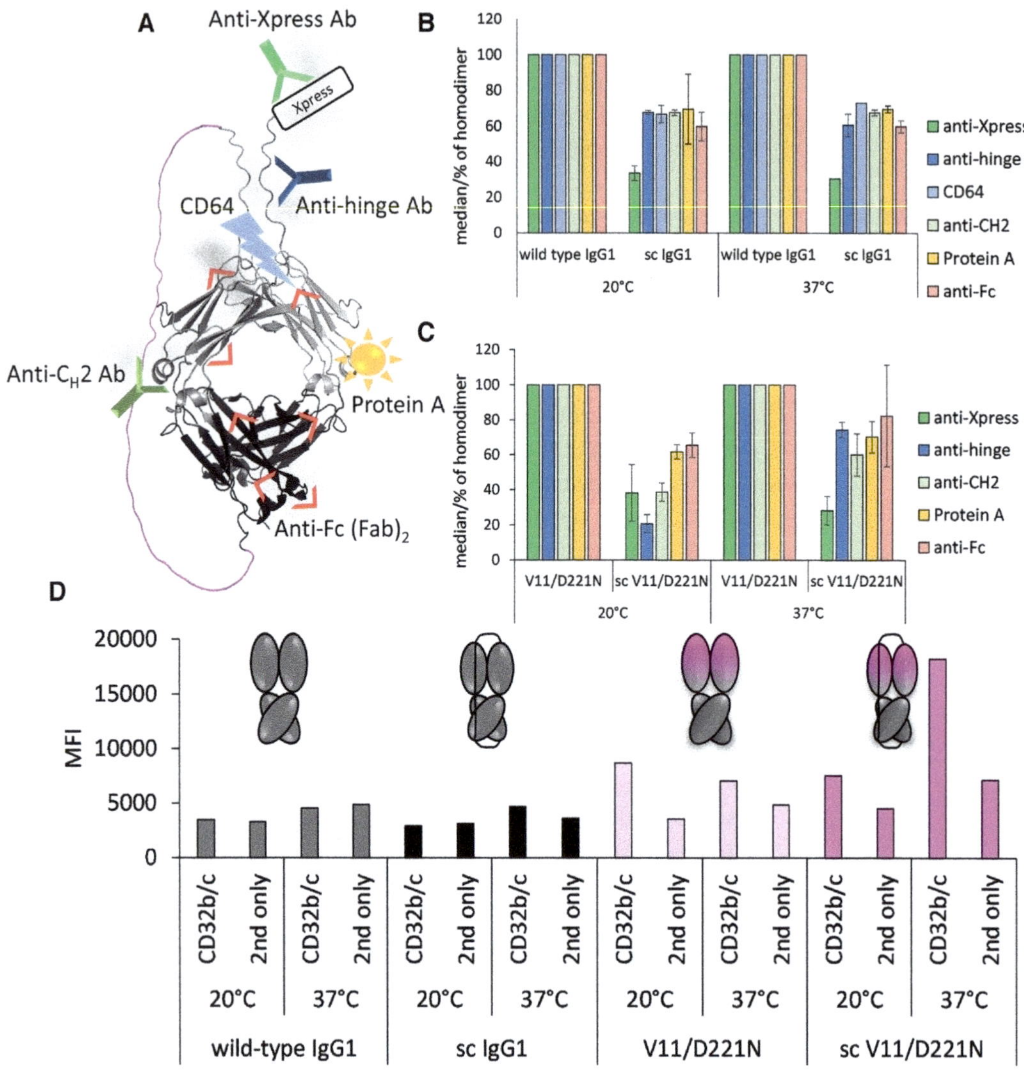

Fig. 4 (**A**) Cartoon diagram of an scFc with C_H2 domains in light and C_H3 domains in dark gray with linker in magenta and indicated ligands anti-Xpress antibody, anti-hinge antibody, FcγRI, anti-CH2 antibody, protein A and polyclonal anti-Fc serum. (**B**) Comparison of median fluorescence for ligand binding to yeast-displayed sc IgG1 Fc in ratio to homodimeric IgG1 Fc, when the cells were induced at 20°C or at 37°C. (**C**) Comparison of median fluorescence for ligand binding to yeast-displayed sc IgG1 V11/D221N mutant Fc in ratio to homodimeric V11/D221N, when the cells were induced at 20°C or at 37°C. (**D**) Interaction of engineered wild-type IgG1 Fc and V11/D221N in homodimeric or sc format with FcγRIIb/c (CD32b/c), when the cells were induced at 20°C or at 37°C (2nd only: staining with secondary reagent only)

where higher protease activity, but also stress imposed on folding and secretory machinery could negatively affect the level of display of a difficult-to-fold protein. The reason for this can be that only a single Xpress tag is available per scFc construct, while there are two in the homodimeric Fc translated from a single expression cassette.

Further, we were also interested in characterizing the amenability for display for designed Fc and scFc fragments, optimized for preferential interaction with certain effector ligand binding molecules. For this purpose, we have first chosen the well characterized Fc variant V11/D221N [47, 48], which is engineered to interact preferentially with FcγRIIb (CD32b) ligand, but is refractory to Fcγ RIIa (CD32a) and other activating ligands (Fig. 4C). The outcome of staining with several markers has confirmed a high level of display and positive reactivity with all conformation-dependent indicators used. In comparison with V11/D221N homodimer, the fluorescent intensity indicating the level of display was again at about 30%, while the structure-dependent ligands produced over 50% of the signal when induced at 37°C. To discover if we can visualize the stronger CD32b binding in yeast system, we induced both unmutated and mutated IgG1 variants and could confirm positive staining for V11/D221N, which was most intense for the sc variant when induced at stress temperature (Fig. 4D).

We were further interested in determining the precise number of displayed Fc or scFc copies per cell. In addition to the variants described above, we have characterized an asymmetrical scFc, the "asym mAb-1" [30] that is engineered for strong binding to both alleles of the activating FcRγIIIa (CD16a). While the expression of homodimeric wild-type Fc or V11/D221N homodimer was about 50,000 copies per yeast cell, about 5000–10,000 copies were measured for all three scFc variants, regardless of the temperature conditions of the induction (Fig. 5).

Regarding this discrepancy in the display level, we compared the ability of yeast-displayed IgG1 Fc, sc IgG1 Fc, and sc asym mAb-1 to interact with CD16a 158 V allele. Reportedly, the interaction of asym mAb-1 should be enhanced for about 1000 times judging from K_D as determined in surface plasmon resonance experiments by passing soluble receptor molecules over immobilized antibody variants [30]. Due to the low display level, the maximal fluorescence produced by the asym mAb-1 displaying yeast was indeed much lower than measured for the homodimeric IgG1 Fc and sc IgG1 Fc displaying cells; however, the EC_{50} was calculated to be 2 nM vs. 85 and 150 nM, confirming improved antigen affinity (Fig. 6A). The titration of asym mAb-1 displayed on yeast cells with both alleles of CD16a revealed similar activity, in line with reported data [30] (Fig. 6B). These findings are valuable for design of antigen selection experiments with scFc constructs and indicate that it is crucial to use a low antigen concentration, or alternatively kinetic competition-based selection procedures, to successfully isolate strong antigen-binding clones.

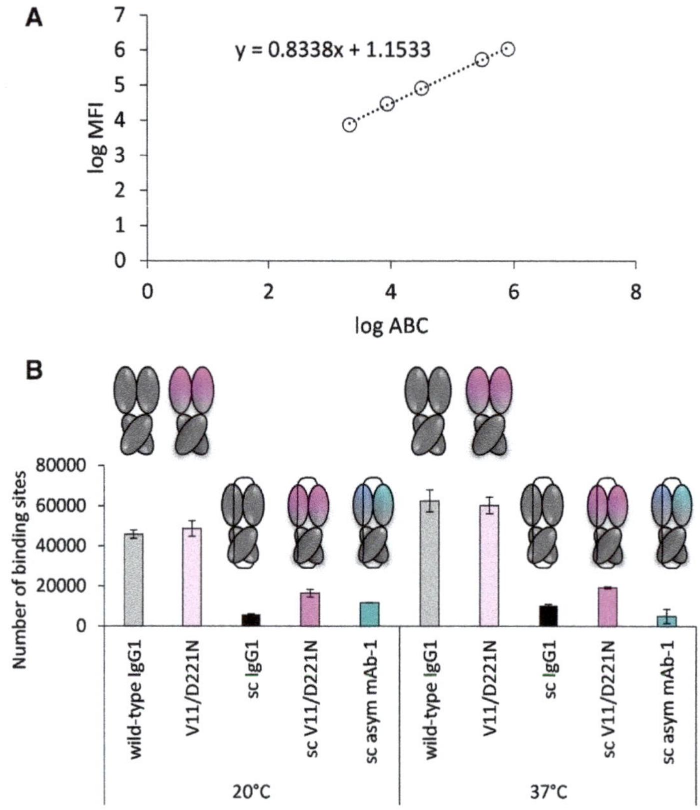

Fig. 5 Determining the number of Fc fragments displayed per yeast cell. (**A**) Calibration curve derived from standard populations of QIFIKIT beads. (**B**) Calculated number of displayed fragments for homodimeric IgG1 Fc and homodimeric V11/D221N mutant, and sc IgG1, V11/D221N and asym mAb-1 Fc fragments after the cells were induced at 20°C or at 37°C

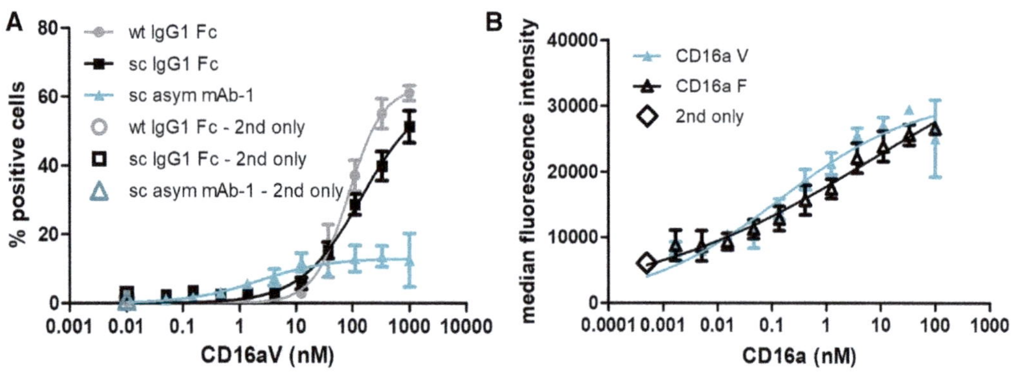

Fig. 6 (**A**) Titration of yeast-displayed homodimeric IgG1 Fc, sc IgG1 Fc, and asym mAb-1 with CD16a (FcγRIIIa) V158 allele. (**B**) Comparison of binding of yeast-displayed asym mAb-1 to CD16a (FcγRIIIa) V and F 158 alleles. Figure has been prepared with Prism5

2 Materials

2.1 Reagents

1. Oligonucleotide primers (sequences are specified in Table 1)
2. MyTaq™ Red Mix
3. EZ-Link™ Sulfo-NHS-LC-LC-Biotin
4. Anti-Xpress antibody (46-05-28, Thermo Fisher Scientific) (all antibody working dilutions are specified in Table 2)
5. Anti-C_H2 antibody-FITC conjugate (MCA647F, Bio-RAD)
6. Protein A-biotin (203195, Calbiochem)
7. CD64 (FcγRI) (his-tagged) (10256-H08H, Sino Biological)
8. CD32b/c (FcγRIIb/c) (his-tagged) (1875-CD, R&D Systems)
9. CD16a (FcγRIIIa), V158 allele (his-tagged) (10389-H27H1, Sino Biological)
10. CD16a (FcγRIIIa), F158 allele (his-tagged) (10389-H08H, Sino Biological)

Table 1
Primers for amplification and sequencing of scFc expression cassette

Primer	Sequence
T7 promotor	taatacgact cactataggg
Pydl reverse	gtcgattttg ttacatctac ac

Table 2
Reagents for detection and characterization of yeast-displayed scFcs

Compound	Dilution
Anti-Xpress antibody	1 μg/mL
Anti-hinge antibody	1 μg/mL
CD64	1 μg/mL
Protein A-biotin	10 μg/mL
Anti-C_H2-FITC antibody	1 μg/mL
Anti-his-antibody, Alexa Fluor 488 conjugate	5 μg/mL
Anti-his-antibody, Alexa Fluor 647 conjugate	2 μg/mL
Anti-mouse Fab-FITC	1 μg/mL
Anti-mouse Fc-PE	0.5 μg/mL
Streptavidin-Alexa Fluor 647 conjugate	0.5 μg/mL

11. Anti-human γ chain-PE conjugate (P-8047, Sigma-Aldrich)
12. Anti-pentahis antibody Alexa Fluor-488 conjugate (35310, QIAgen)
13. Anti-pentahis antibody Alexa Fluor-647 conjugate (35370, QIAgen)
14. Goat anti-mouse IgG (H+L) cross-adsorbed secondary antibody-PE conjugate (405307, BioLegend)
15. Anti-mouse Fc $(Fab)_2$ fragment-FITC conjugate (F-2653, Sigma-Aldrich)
16. Streptavidin-Alexa Fluor-647 conjugate
17. Propidium iodide (working dilution in Table 3)
18. TO-PRO-3 (working dilution in Table 3)
19. Bacterial strain *E. coli* TOP10 (*F- mcrA (mrr-hsdRMS-mcrBC) 80lacZ M15 lacX74 recA1 ara 139 (ara-leu)7697 galU galK rpsL (StrR) endA1 nupG*)
20. Yeast strain *S. cerevisiae* EBY100 (*MAT*a *GAL1-AGA1::URA3 ura3-52 trp1 leu2Δ1 his3Δ200 pep4::HIS2 prb1_1.6R can1 GAL*) (ATCC® MYA4941™)

2.2 Solutions and Buffers

1. 50% PEG3350
2. 1 M Li-acetate solution
3. salmon sperm DNA 2 mg/mL salmon sperm DNA diluted in TE buffer (10 mM Tris, 1 mM EDTA, pH 8.0)
4. 500 mM EDTA, pH 8.0
5. Buffer for yeast media Potassium phosphate buffer, 1 M, pH 6.0
6. 10× DO supplements (-Leu/-Trp) 15.6 g/L DO supplements (-Leu/-Trp)
7. 100× leucine solution 10 g/L leucine
8. Phosphate-buffered saline (PBS) 137 mM NaCl, 2.7 mM KCl, 10 mM Na_2HPO_4, 2 mM KH_2PO_4
9. FACS staining solution 2% BSA in PBS
10. Freezing buffer 30% glycerol

Table 3
Viability probes for yeast cells

Compound	Dilution	Excitation	Emission detected
Propidium iodide	1 μg/mL	493 nm	Red (636 nm)
TO-PRO-3	1 μM	642 nm	Far red (664 nm)

2.3 Media

1. YPD 20 g/L peptone, 10 g/L yeast extract, and 2% glucose
2. SD-CAA 1% CAA solution with 1.34% YNB with ammonium sulphate, 100 mM KH_2PO_4/K_2HPO_4 buffer, pH 6.0, 2% glucose
3. SG/R-CAA 1% CAA solution with 1.34% YNB with ammonium sulphate, 100 mM KH_2PO_4/K_2HPO_4 buffer, pH 6.0, 2% galactose, 1% raffinose
4. YPD solid media 1.5% agar with 20 g/L peptone, 10 g/L yeast extract, and 2% glucose
5. SD-Leu solid media 1.5% agar with 1× DO supplements (-Leu/-Trp), 1.34% YNB with ammonium sulphate, 100 mM KH_2PO4/K_2HPO_4 buffer, 2% glucose, and 0.1 mg/mL leucine
6. LB medium 1.5% agar with 10 g/L peptone, 5 g/L yeast extract, and 10 g/L NaCl
7. 100× pen-strep solution 100,000 U/mL penicillin and 10 mg/mL streptomycin
8. 1000× ampicillin solution 100 mg/mL ampicillin solution

2.4 Kits

1. Gel and DNA purification kit
2. Plasmid isolation kit (for mini- or midi-preparation)
3. Zymoprep II kit
4. QIFIKIT

2.5 Equipment

1. 96-well microtiter plates
2. 1.5-mL microcentrifuge tubes
3. 1.0-mL cryotubes
4. 15- and 50-mL conical tubes
5. 125-, 500-, 1000-, and 2000-mL Erlenmeyer flasks
6. 90-mm Petri dishes
7. Pipettes from P10 to P1000 range with respective tips and multichannel pipettes
8. Rotating wheel
9. −80°C refrigerator
10. Incubator with shaking platform that can be heated to 20°C, 30°C, and 37°C
11. Heat blocks or water baths
12. FACS analysis apparatus

3 Methods

3.1 Transformation and Culturing of *S. cerevisiae* Displaying scFc

For transformation into *S. cerevisiae*, scFc expression sequence was cloned into pYD1 vector, amplified in *E. coli* TOP10 and the plasmids were isolated using minipreparation. To avoid potential undesired recombination events, nonhomologous sequences were used for the two IgG Fc protomers (*see* **Note 1**). We observed that the relatively large expression sequence, even if dehomologized, can lead to the secondary products in the PCR, and therefore, identified pairs of pYD1-vector specific primers that produced clean specific amplicons suitable for sequencing without preparative gel purification (Table 1), when used in a PCR reaction with MyTaq Red with the program in Table 4. Either *E. coli* or yeast colony lysate can be used as a template.

1. Start an overnight culture of *S. cerevisiae* EBY100 in 10 mL YPD, on an orbital shaker at 30°C.
2. Next day, determine the OD_{600} of the culture and dilute to 500 mL of OD_{600} of 0.4 in YPD medium.
3. Incubate the yeast culture on an orbital shaker at 30°C for about 5 h, until it reaches an OD_{600} between two and three.
4. Distribute the culture to 50-mL-conical tubes.
5. Pellet the yeast by centrifugation at 1000×*g*, 5 min, at room temperature.
6. Wash pellets with 25 mL distilled water per tube.
7. Collect the cells by centrifugation at 1000×*g*, 5 min, at room temperature.
8. Resuspend each pellet with 3 mL 200 mM Li-acetate solution and let shake at 30°C for 15 min.
9. Collect the cells by centrifugation at 1000×*g*, 5 min, at room temperature. Discard the Li-acetate solution.
10. Resuspend the cells in the remains of the Li-acetate solution.

Table 4
PCR program for amplification of scFc expression cassette

Step	Temperature (°C)	Time (s)	Cycle
Initial denaturation	95	30	
Denaturation	95	20	
Annealing	55	20	
Extension	72	60	Back to denaturation, 35×
Final extension	72	300	

11. Add to each tube 2.4 mL 50% PEG3350, 360 µL 1 M Li-acetate, 500 µL heat-shocked (5 min at 95°C) salmon sperm DNA and plasmid DNA in a volume that should not exceed 340 µL. Let shake at 30°C for 30 min.
12. Incubate at 42°C in a water bath for 45 min. Invert the tubes every 10 min.
13. Pellet the yeast and remove the transformation solution.
14. Add 5 mL YPD medium to each pellet and incubate with shaking at 30°C for 30 min.
15. Collect the cells by centrifugation at 1000×*g*, 5 min, at room temperature. Inoculate into 500 mL SD-CAA medium with pen/strep.
16. Plate the aliquots to SD-Trp plates to isolate single colonies. Incubate at 30°C for at least 3 days. About 1×10^6 colonies/µg vector used for transformation are expected.
17. Inoculate the yeast clones from a single colony or yeast libraries (at least 20-fold excess of the number of independent library members) into SD-CAA with pen/strep at an OD_{600} of 0.2.
18. Let grow at 30°C overnight, with shaking, to an OD_{600} of at least five.
19. Collect the cells by centrifugation at 1000×*g*, 5 min at room temperature.
20. Remove the supernatant.
21. Resuspend the cells in SG/R-CAA medium.
22. Alternatively, yeast can be induced by transferring an aliquot of SD-CAA grown culture into SG/R-CAA; however, the volume should not exceed 5% of the total culture volume (*see* **Note 2**).
23. The remaining cells can be frozen by centrifuging them at 1000×*g*, 5 min at 4°C, resuspending them in an equal volume of freezing buffer and placing to −80°C.
24. Incubate the yeast cultures with shaking at 20°C for 48 h or at 37°C overnight, when stress induction conditions should be used.

3.2 Basic Display Parameters: Staining with Fc Ligands

Several ligands of the Fc can be instrumental in determining the display level and the integrity of the displayed molecules. The binding of a tag-specific antibody, such as anti-Xpress recognizing the Xpress tag present in the pYD1-vector, is not dependent on the structural features of the displayed protein and therefore a valuable tool for determining the display level. The reactivity with Fc receptors is indicative of the integrity of the C_H2 domain; due to the highest affinity, preferably CD64 is used for staining of IgG1-based constructs. Along the same lines, the binding of the conformation-dependent anti-C_H2 antibody confirms proper folding of this domain. Strong staining with Protein A is encouraging as it hints at the possibility of using the upscalable affinity purification method based on this ligand if the displayed proteins are later to be isolated in soluble form.

The scFc constructs can be expressed in-frame with C-terminal tags; c-myc and a his-tag are present in the pYD1 vector. However, as several Fc ligands, including the receptor molecules, are commercially available as his-tagged proteins, expressing the scFcs without the C-terminal tag allows the use of these ligands with straightforward detection with an anti-his antibody. This can be helpful before the protocol for biotinylation or other labeling methods are established (*see* **Note 3**).

1. Determine the OD_{600} of induced yeast cultures.
2. Resuspend the cells at an OD_{600} of one, corresponding to 1×10^7 cells/mL, in FACS staining solution.
3. Incubate the cell suspension with agitation on a shaking platform or on a rotating wheel for 30 min at room temperature.
4. Distribute the cells in 100-μL-aliquots to the wells of a 96-U-shaped-well microtiter plate.
5. Collect the cells with centrifugation at 1000×*g*, 5 min at room temperature, and remove the blocking solution.
6. Resuspend the cells in FACS staining solution with primary antibody at a concentration as stated in Table 2.
7. Incubate on a shaking platform for 1 h at room temperature.
8. Collect the cells by centrifugation the cells at 1000×*g*, 5 min at 4°C. From this point on, washing steps should be performed with cold solutions, and the incubations should follow on ice to reduce dissociation of the ligand from the yeast-displayed Fc.
9. Wash cell pellet briefly in ice-cold PBS and centrifuge at 1000×*g*, 5 min at 4°C.
10. Resuspend the cells in ice-cold FACS staining solution of fluorescently labeled secondary detection reagent or directly labeled tag-specific antibody.
11. Incubate for 30 min on ice, protected from light.
12. Collect the cells at 1000×*g*, 5 min at 4°C and remove the staining solution.
13. Wash cell pellet briefly in 100 μL ice-cold PBS and centrifuge at 1000×*g*, 5 min at 4°C.
14. Resuspend the cells in 200 μL ice-cold PBS and keep on ice until the fluorescence measurement.

3.3 Determining the Number of Displayed scFc Proteins on the Surface of Yeast Cells

Surface expression levels are determined using the QIFIKIT (Agilent K0078) employing flow cytometry. Five populations of calibration beads with different numbers of mouse mAb molecules are used as a calibration standard.

1. For the blocking of yeast cells, follow Steps 1–3 of the protocol 3.2.
2. Label 10^6 yeast cells with a saturating concentration of 1 μg/mL of the anti-Xpress antibody in FACS staining solution in 100 μL volume with shaking for 30 min at RT.
3. Collect the cells by centrifugation at 1000×*g*, 5 min at 4°C.
4. Wash cell pellet briefly in 100 μL ice-cold PBS and centrifuge at 1000×*g*, 5 min at 4°C.
5. Stain beads and cells with secondary goat anti-mouse Fc $F(ab')_2$-FITC conjugate, provided with the kit, at 1:50 dilution in 100 μL of FACS staining solution in volume for 30 min, on ice, protected from light.
6. Collect the beads and cells by centrifugation at 1000×*g*, 5 min at 4°C.
7. Resuspend the cells and beads in 200 μL ice-cold PBS.
8. Determine the mean fluorescence intensity (MFI) values by flow cytometry.
9. Plot the MFI values for the standard bead populations against the number of antibody molecules per bead (on a log/log scale). Fit the values with linear regression and establish a standard curve.
10. Using this equation, convert the MFI values of yeast cells samples to the number of antibody binding sites per cell (*see* **Note 4**).

3.4 Viability Staining

Determining the viability of the yeast cells in the induced cultures is crucial in the design of sorting campaigns. Stress-induced yeast cultures displaying scFcs contain only a low percentage of dead cells, comparable to the clones displaying homodimeric IgG1 Fc without a linker (Fig. 7). For the cells displaying CD32b-binding mutant V11/D211N, the results were similar. The nonviable cells cannot contribute to the propagation and enrichment of antigen-binding clones, yet these are the ones that frequently show strong fluorescence with secondary reagents labeled with fluorophores. To avoid selecting such cells, a gate where all members of the population with high irrelevant fluorescence are excluded can be applied. Including the viability probe in the staining procedure for sorting sample can actually impair the viability of the cells, especially upon a longer exposition, because most of these are toxic compounds. When setting up the experiment, yeast heated to 95°C for 5 min can be used as a positive control (*see* **Note 5**).

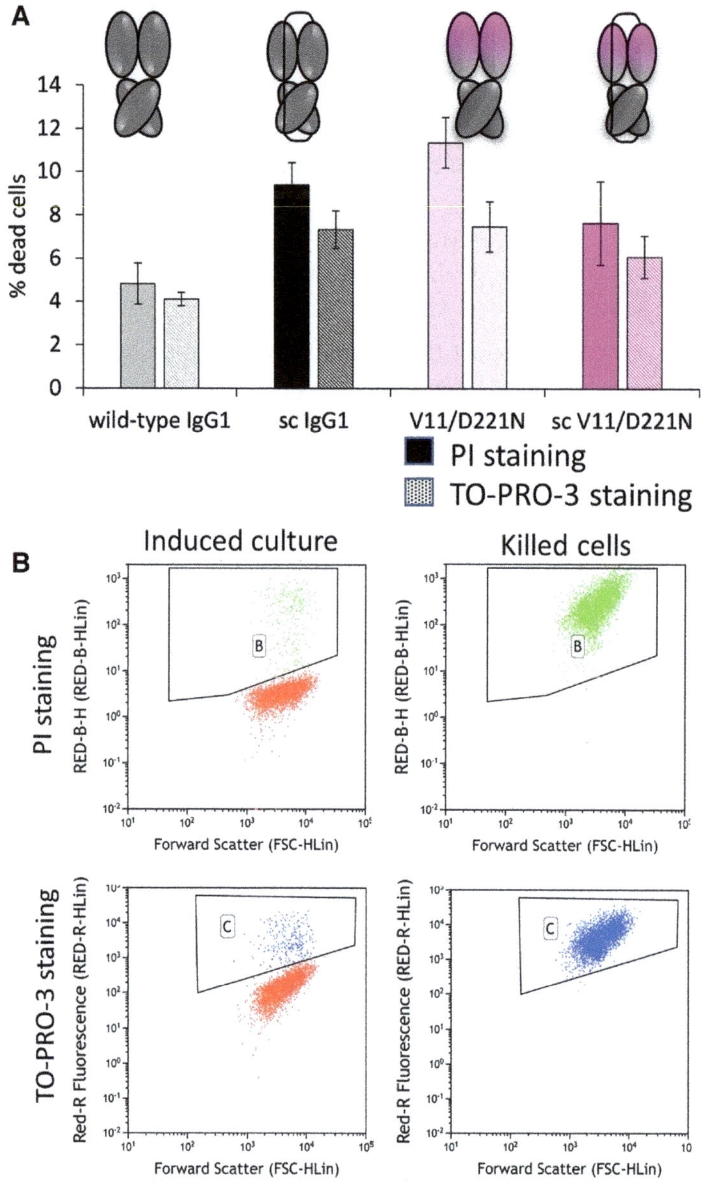

Fig. 7 (**A**) Percent of dead cells determined with PI or TO-PRO-3 in cultures displaying different homodimeric and sc Fc fragments when induced at 37°C. (**B**) Representative dot plot analysis showing the gating of dead cells and the outcome of the measurement of the positive control for staining, for PI and TO-PRO-3 protocol

1. Dilute the sample to 10^7 cells/mL in FACS staining solution.
2. Incubate at room temperature for 30 min with shaking.
3. Distribute 100-μL-aliquots of the blocked cells to the wells of a 96-U-shaped well plate.
4. Centrifuge the cells at 1000×*g*, 5 min at room temperature.

5. Add 100 µL of viability probe, diluted in PBS according to Table 3.
6. Incubate at room temperature for 30 min, protected from light.
7. Centrifuge the sample at 1000×*g* for 5 min at 4°C and remove the supernatant.
8. Resuspend the cells in 200 µL ice-cold PBS and place on ice until the FACS measurement.

3.5 Single-Chain Fc Variants with Biased Fc Receptor Recognition

When designing the expression protocols for performing display experiments with Fc mutants, one must keep in mind that thermal destabilization due to the mutagenesis can affect the integrity of the displayed Fc when expressed at a higher temperature. Such an example is the homodimeric DLE-mutant with improved binding to CD16a, where the midpoint of transition for C_H2 domain is 20°C lower than what can be measured for the wild-type Fc, at about 50°C. Considering a typical additional decrease of about 10°C due to no-mammalian glycosylation, it is obvious that the thermal denaturation of the protein already progresses at 37°C, causing the low integrity of the displayed mutant. Before testing the yeast-displayed sc Fc variants for the ability or bias in ligand interaction, it is recommendable to consider the data on their biophysical properties when expressed as soluble proteins, for example thermostability determined with differential scanning calorimetry or a similar method.

1. Prepare a dilution series of the Fcγ receptor of interest in FACS staining solution in a nonprotein binding plate. Start concentration and the dilution factor should be determined according to the expected affinity of the mutant; for a pilot experiment, starting concentrations of 1–5 µM and three-fold to four-fold dilution steps are usually used.
2. Follow Steps 1–5 of the protocol 3.2 for the blocking of yeast cells.
3. Add 100 µL of the solution containing the Fc ligand and incubate at room temperature for 1 h.
4. Place the microtiter plate with stained cells on ice and add 200 µL of ice-cold PBS.
5. Incubate on ice for 10 min.
6. Centrifuge the cells at 1000×*g*, 5 min at 4°C.
7. Remove the supernatant and place the plate on ice.
8. Resuspend the cells in 100 µL fluorescently labeled secondary reagent diluted in ice-cold FACS staining solution.
9. Incubate on ice for 30 min, protected from light.
10. Remove the supernatant and resuspend the cells in 200 µL ice-cold PBS.

11. Keep the plate on ice until the FACS analysis.
12. Record the fluorescence values and calculate EC_{50} by applying nonlinear regression analysis for MFI against the concentration of the Fcγ receptor. Useful programs for the calculation are Prism or Sigma Plot.

4 Notes

1. Dehomologization of the protomer-encoding sequence can be performed by several online tools, such as https://www.ebi.ac.uk/jdispatcher/st/emboss_backtranseq, which will back-translate the protein sequence using the codon table of choice. Determining the percent of homology is the next step in optimizing the sequence. The use of natively occurring nucleotide sequence for one of the protomers is a good option as otherwise than in synthetic genes, the codons encoding the same amino acid do not repeat, again reducing the likelihood of recombination.
2. Keeping the concentration of glucose below 0.1% is relevant upon the induction as glucose acts as a strong suppressor of *GAL1,10*-promotor which is driving the display in pYD1-based systems.
3. Fcγ receptors are available from several sources as his-tagged or biotinylated proteins, allowing simple detection. If biotinylation is carried out in-house, binding tests should be performed to confirm the activity of the receptor. In general, biotinylation with relatively low biotin to protein molar ratios, such as 5:1, leads to labeled functional receptor.
4. It is expected that the MFI values of the stained samples largely exceed the MFI of the samples stained with the secondary reagent only and the latter is, therefore, negligible. However, in case the number of binding sites is low, the estimation is more accurate if the MFI of this control sample is subtracted from the test samples, and the MFI of the control uncoupled bead population from the MFI of standard beads used for construction of the calibration curve.
5. For the positive control of yeast cell viability staining, cells can be heated to 95°C for 5 min. For this purpose, the aliquot of induced cultured should be washed briefly in PBS and resuspended in PBS alone, without addition of any protein, which might denature and render the sample unsuitable for FACS analysis.

Acknowledgments

Financial support from the Austrian Research Promotion Agency (FFG) and the Federal Ministry for Innovation, Mobility and Infrastructure in frame of the program "Expedition Zukunft Wissenschaft" is gratefully acknowledged. The FACS equipment was kindly provided by the Connective Base GmbH, and the project was supported by the BOKU Core Facility Biomolecular & Cellular Analysis.

References

1. Shields RL, Namenuk AK, Hong K et al. (2001) High resolution mapping of the binding site on human IgG1 for FcγRI, FcγRII, FcγRIII, and FcRn and design of IgG1 variants with improved binding to the FcγR. J Biol Chem 276:6591–6604. https://doi.org/10.1074/jbc.M009483200
2. Bruhns P, Iannascoli B, England P, Mancardi DA, Fernandez N, Jorieux S, Daëron M (2009) Specificity and affinity of human Fcγ receptors and their polymorphic variants for human IgG subclasses. Blood 113:3716–3725. https://doi.org/10.1182/blood-2008-09-179754
3. Stavenhagen JB, Gorlatov S, Tuaillon N, Rankin CT, Li H, Burke S, Huang L, Johnson S, Bonvini E, Koenig S (2007) Fc optimization of therapeutic antibodies enhances their ability to kill tumor cells *in vitro* and controls tumor expansion *in vivo* via low-affinity activating Fcγ receptors. Cancer Res 67:8882–8890. https://doi.org/10.1158/0008-5472.CAN-07-0696
4. Markham A (2021) Margetuximab: first approval. Drugs 81:599–604. https://doi.org/10.1007/s40265-021-01485-2
5. Wilkinson I, Hale G (2022) Systematic analysis of the varied designs of 819 therapeutic antibodies and Fc fusion proteins assigned international nonproprietary names. Mabs 14:1–15. https://doi.org/10.1080/19420862.2022.2123299
6. Hale G, De Vos J, Davy AD, Sandra K, Wilkinson I (2024) Systematic analysis of Fc mutations designed to reduce binding to Fc-gamma receptors. Mabs 16:1–15. https://doi.org/10.1080/19420862.2024.2402701
7. Jung ST, Reddy ST, Kang TH, Borrok MJ, Sandlie I, Tucker PW, Georgiou G (2010) Aglycosylated IgG variants expressed in bacteria that selectively bind FcγRI potentiate tumor cell killing by monocyte-dendritic cells. Proc Natl Acad Sci U S A 107:604–609. https://doi.org/10.1073/pnas.0908590107
8. Jung ST, Kang TH, Kim Dil (2014) Engineering an aglycosylated Fc variant for enhanced FcγRI engagement and pH-dependent human FcRn binding. Biotechnol Bioprocess Eng 19:780–789. https://doi.org/10.1007/s12257-013-0432-z
9. Jo M, Kwon HS, Lee KH, Lee JC, Jung ST (2018) Engineered aglycosylated full-length IgG Fc variants exhibiting improved Fcγ RIIIa binding and tumor cell clearance. Mabs 10:278–289. https://doi.org/10.1080/19420862.2017.1402995
10. Jung ST, Kelton W, Kang TH, Ng DTW, Andersen JT, Sandlie I, Sarkar CA, Georgiou G (2013) Effective phagocytosis of low Her2 tumor cell lines with engineered, aglycosylated igg displaying high FcγRIIa affinity and selectivity. ACS Chem Biol 8:368–375. https://doi.org/10.1021/cb300455f
11. Shi R, Shan C, Duan X et al. (2020) A human neutralizing antibody targets the receptor-binding site of SARS-CoV-2. Nature 584:120–124. https://doi.org/10.1038/s41586-020-2381-y
12. Loo YM, McTamney PM, Arends RH et al. (2022) The SARS-CoV-2 monoclonal antibody combination, AZD7442, is protective in nonhuman primates and has an extended half-life in humans. Sci Transl Med 14:1–14. https://doi.org/10.1126/scitranslmed.abl8124
13. Lee CH, Romain G, Yan W et al. (2017) IgG Fc domains that bind C1q but not effector Fc3 receptors delineate the importance of complement-mediated effector functions. Nat Immunol 18:889–898. https://doi.org/10.1038/ni.3770
14. Saito S, Namisaki H, Hiraishi K, Takahashi N, Iida S (2019) A stable engineered human IgG3 antibody with decreased aggregation during antibody expression and low pH stress. Protein Sci 28:900–909. https://doi.org/10.1002/PRO.3598
15. Chu TH, Patz EF, Ackerman ME (2021) Coming together at the hinges: therapeutic prospects of IgG3. Mabs 13:1–15. https://doi.org/10.1080/19420862.2021.1882028
16. Keam SJ (2023) Nirsevimab: first approval. Drugs 83:181–187. https://doi.org/10.1007/s40265-022-01829-6

17. Acqua WFD, Woods RM, Ward ES, Palaszynski SR, Patel NK, Brewah YA, Wu H, Kiener PA, Langermann S (2002) Increasing the affinity of a human IgG1 for the neonatal Fc receptor: biological consequences. J Immunol 169:5171–5180. https://doi.org/10.4049/jimmunol.169.9.5171
18. Dall'Acqua WF, Kiener PA, Wu H (2006) Properties of human IgG1s engineered for enhanced binding to the neonatal Fc receptor (FcRn). J Biol Chem 281:23514–23524. https://doi.org/10.1074/jbc.M604292200
19. Vaccaro C, Zhou J, Ober RJ, Ward ES (2005) Engineering the Fc region of immunoglobulin G to modulate *in vivo* antibody levels. Nat Biotechnol 23(10):1283–1288. https://doi.org/10.1038/nbt1143
20. Ulrichts P, Guglietta A, Dreier T et al. (2018) Neonatal Fc receptor antagonist efgartigimod safely and sustainably reduces IgGs in humans. J Clin Invest 128:4372–4386. https://doi.org/10.1172/JCI97911
21. Heo YA (2022) Efgartigimod: first approval. Drugs 82:341–348. https://doi.org/10.1007/S40265-022-01678-3
22. Shan L, Dyk NVan, Haskins N et al. (2021) *In vivo* pharmacokinetic enhancement of monomeric Fc and monovalent bispecific designs through structural guidance. Commun Biol 4:1–11. https://doi.org/10.1038/s42003-021-02565-5
23. Labrijn AF, Janmaat ML, Reichert JM, Parren PWHI (2019) Bispecific antibodies: a mechanistic review of the pipeline. Nat Rev Drug Discov 18:585–608. https://doi.org/10.1038/s41573-019-0028-1
24. Ridgway JBB, Presta LG, Carter P (1996) "Knobs-into-holes" engineering of antibody CH3 domains for heavy chain heterodimerization. Protein Eng 9:617–621. https://doi.org/10.1016/1380-2933(96)80685-3
25. Atwell S, Ridgway JBB, Wells JA, Carter P (1997) Stable heterodimers from remodeling the domain interface of a homodimer using a phage display library. J Mol Biol 270:26–35. https://doi.org/10.1006/JMBI.1997.1116
26. Choi HJ, Kim YJ, Choi DK, Kim YS (2015) Engineering of immunoglobulin Fc heterodimers using yeast surface-displayed combinatorial Fc library screening. PLoS One 10:e0145349. https://doi.org/10.1371/JOURNAL.PONE.0145349
27. Benedetti F, Stadlmayr G, Stadlbauer K, Rüker F, Wozniak-Knopp G (2023) Selection of high-affinity heterodimeric antigen-binding Fc fragments from a large yeast display library. Methods Mol Biol 2681:131–159. https://doi.org/10.1007/978-1-0716-3279-6_9
28. Chew KS, Wells RC, Moshkforoush A et al. (2023) CD98hc is a target for brain delivery of biotherapeutics. Nat Commun 14:1–17. https://doi.org/10.1038/s41467-023-40681-4
29. Lazar GA, Dang W, Karki S et al. (2006) Engineered antibody Fc variants with enhanced effector function. Proc Natl Acad Sci U S A 103:4005–4010. https://doi.org/10.1073/pnas.0508123103
30. Mimoto F, Igawa T, Kuramochi T, Katada H, Kadono S, Kamikawa T, Shida-Kawazoe M, Hattori K (2013) Novel asymmetrically engineered antibody Fc variant with superior FcγR binding affinity and specificity compared with afucosylated Fc variant. Mabs 5:229–236. https://doi.org/10.4161/MABS.23452
31. Dhillon S (2024) Tarlatamab: first approval. Drugs 84:995–1003. https://doi.org/10.1007/s40265-024-02070-z
32. Morrison JI, Metzendorf NG, Rofo F, Petrovic A, Hultqvist G (2023) A single-chain fragment constant design enables easy production of a monovalent blood–brain barrier transporter and provides an improved brain uptake at elevated doses. J Neurochem 165:413–425. https://doi.org/10.1111/JNC.15768
33. Oslund RC, Holland PM, Lesley SA, Fadeyi OO (2024) Therapeutic potential of cis-targeting bispecific antibodies. Cell Chem Biol 31:1473–1489. https://doi.org/10.1016/J.CHEMBIOL.2024.07.004
34. Mazor Y, Sachsenmeier KF, Yang C, Hansen A, Filderman J, Mulgrew K, Wu H, Dall'Acqua WF (2017) Enhanced tumor-targeting selectivity by modulating bispecific antibody binding affinity and format valence. Sci Rep 7:1–11. https://doi.org/10.1038/srep40098
35. Zhou L, Wang HY, Tong S, Okamoto CT, Shen WC, Zaro JL (2017) Single chain Fc-dimer-human growth hormone fusion protein for improved drug delivery. Biomaterials 117:24–31. https://doi.org/10.1016/J.BIOMATERIALS.2016.11.051
36. Dumont JA, Low SC, Peters RT, Bitonti AJ (2006) Monomeric Fc fusions: impact on pharmacokinetic and biological activity of protein therapeutics. BioDrugs 20:151–160. https://doi.org/10.2165/00063030-200620030-00002
37. Binder U, Skerra A (2024) Strategies for extending the half-life of biotherapeutics: successes and complications. Expert Opin Biol Ther 25:93–118. https://doi.org/10.1080/14712598.2024.2436094
38. Hennecke F, Krebber C, Plückthun A (1998) Non-repetitive single-chain Fv linkers selected by selectively infective phage (SIP) technology. Protein Eng Des Sel 11:405–410. https://doi.org/10.1093/PROTEIN/11.5.405
39. Hultqvist G, Syvänen S, Fang XT, Lannfelt L, Sehlin D (2017) Bivalent brain shuttle increases antibody uptake by monovalent binding to the transferrin receptor. Theranostics 7:308–318. https://doi.org/10.7150/thno.17155
40. Waterhouse A, Bertoni M, Bienert S et al. (2018) SWISS-MODEL: homology modelling of protein structures and complexes. Nucleic Acids Res

46:W296–W303. https://doi.org/10.1093/NAR/GKY427
41. Abramson J, Adler J, Dunger J et al. (2024) Accurate structure prediction of biomolecular interactions with AlphaFold 3. Nature 630(8016):493–500. https://doi.org/10.1038/s41586-024-07487-w
42. Lindahl E, Bjelkmar P, Larsson P, Cuendet MA, Hess B (2010) Implementation of the CHARMM force field in GROMACS: analysis of protein stability effects from correction maps, virtual interaction sites, and water models. J Chem Theory Comput 6:459–466. https://doi.org/10.1021/CT900549R
43. Boder ET, Wittrup KD (1997) Yeast surface display for screening combinatorial polypeptide libraries. Nat Biotechnol 15:553–557. https://doi.org/10.1038/nbt0697-553
44. Chao G, Lau WL, Hackel BJ, Sazinsky SL, Lippow SM, Wittrup KD (2006) Isolating and engineering human antibodies using yeast surface display. Nat Protoc 1:755–768. https://doi.org/10.1038/nprot.2006.94
45. Raymond CK, Powder TA, Sexson SL (1999) General method for plasmid construction using homologous recombination. Biotechniques 26:134–141. https://doi.org/10.2144/99261RR02
46. Gibson DG, Benders GA, Axelrod KC, Zaveri J, Algire MA, Moodie M, Montague MG, Venter JC, Smith HO, Hutchison CA (2008) One-step assembly in yeast of 25 overlapping DNA fragments to form a complete synthetic *Mycoplasma genitalium* genome. Proc Natl Acad Sci U S A 105:20404–20409. https://doi.org/10.1073/pnas.0811011106
47. Knorr DA, Dahan R, Ravetch JV (2018) Toxicity of an Fc-engineered anti-CD40 antibody is abrogated by intratumoral injection and results in durable antitumor immunity. Proc Natl Acad Sci USA 115:11048–11053. https://doi.org/10.1073/pnas.1810566115
48. Blundell PA, Le NPL, Allen J, Watanabe Y, Pleass RJ (2017) Engineering the fragment crystallizable (Fc) region of human IgG1 multimers and monomers to fine-tune interactions with sialic acid-dependent receptors. J Biol Chem 292:12994–13007. https://doi.org/10.1074/jbc.M117.795047

Check for updates

Chapter 6

A Simple and Rapid Method for Preparing VHH Antibody-Template DNA Conjugates for Loop-Mediated Isothermal Amplification (LAMP) Method from cDNA Display

Junpei Yamashita and Naoto Nemoto

Abstract

Generally, in vitro display technology serves as a fundamental method for performing in vitro selection by linking genotypes to phenotypes. This study introduces a rapid and simple method for preparing VHH antibody-template DNA conjugate suitable for the LAMP method (Loop-mediated isothermal amplification), known for its rapid and highly sensitive detection, using cDNA display, an in vitro display technology.

Keywords cDNA display, Immune PCR, VHH, Antibody-DNA conjugate, Isothermal PCR, Loop-mediated isothermal amplification (LAMP)

1 Introduction

Immuno-PCR is a technology with an exceptionally promising concept, combining the high recognition specificity characteristic of antibodies with the high-sensitivity detection characteristic of PCR [1]. However, attaching a single strand of DNA for PCR detection to an antibody presented a technical challenge. Specifically, attaching just one strand of succinimide-modified DNA to the lysine residue of an antibody is extremely difficult stoichiometrically. Consequently, various methods using genotype-phenotype linking molecules have been proposed. Representative examples include both a method using phage display [2] and a method attaching DNA to antibody [3]. Additionally, we have developed a method to realize immuno-PCR using in vitro display technology based on a cell-free translation system [4]. A particular strength of this approach is that using single-domain antibodies like VHH antibodies as the displayed molecules allows for the rapid and simple synthesis of molecules with a one-to-one correspondence between VHH antibodies and nucleic acids using the cell-free translation system. We demonstrated this

Huan Peng and Theam Soon Lim (eds.), *Biomolecular Display Technologies*, Methods in Molecular Biology, vol. 3030,
https://doi.org/10.1007/978-1-0716-5249-7_6,

detection method and named it cDNA display mediated immune-PCR (cD-IPCR) [5]. A major advantage of this method is that it allows for simpler and faster synthesis of molecules for immuno-PCR compared to conventional methods, provided that suitable VHH antibodies are already available. However, detection requires a PCR machine, making it difficult to use outside of a laboratory setting. Therefore, we focused on isothermal PCR methods, which enable DNA amplification anywhere with a constant-temperature device. Among these, the LAMP method is known for its high reproducibility and detection sensitivity [6, 7].

However, designing six primers is necessary, and finding the optimal DNA amplification conditions using these primers often requires considerable time and effort. Consequently, designing these six primers sets for each VHH antibody targeting different antigens to perform cD-IPCR was considered highly inefficient. A major feature of cDNA display is the ability to readily link a puromycin linker to mRNA using photo-crosslinking [8, 9]. The cnvK used here crosslinks a pyrimidine base of mRNA at over 95% efficiency within seconds at 366 nm, but reversibly cleaves upon irradiation at 312 nm (Fig. 1A) [10]. Utilizing this property, mRNA-VHH antibody conjugates are first created as mRNA displays by irradiating with 366 nm light after hybridization between mRNA and puromycin-linker. Subsequently, after translation reaction, 312 nm light irradiation is applied to separate the VHH antibody-linker conjugate from the mRNA. Next, the LAMP-specific DNA and this VHH antibody-linker conjugate are linked by 312 nm light

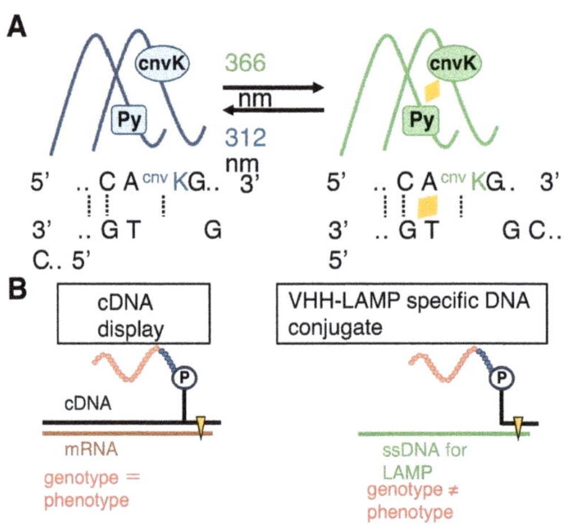

Fig. 1 (**A**) Schematic illustration of photo-crosslinking and cleavage of a pyrimidine base with cnvK. (**B**) Schematic representation of cDNA display and VHH-LAMP specific DNA conjugate. cDNA display: The polypeptide (VHH) is covalently linked to its coding cDNA through puromycin. VHH-LAMP specific DNA conjugate: The polypeptide is covalently linked to an arbitrary nucleic acid-in this case, an ssDNA for LAMP-through puromycin. Because the DNA sequence is independent of the polypeptide sequence, this approach avoids the sequence constraints inherent to cDNA display

irradiation. This enables the simple and rapid synthesis of the VHH antibody-LAMP-specific DNA conjugate using a cell-free translation system (Fig. 1B). However, the LAMP method does have its challenges, which must be overcome if the desired results are to be achieved. We believe that one of its key areas of application is the use of this technology in nucleic acid therapeutics, whereby DNA or RNA is linked to VHH to streamline experimental procedures through the synthesis of VHH-nucleic acid conjugates.

2 Materials

All reagents should be of molecular biology grade to avoid contamination of ribonuclease. If indicated, prepare all solutions with Nuclease-free ultrapure distilled water (UPDW). Except of cnvK linker, all template DNA and primers were ordered from a DNA supplier (Eurofins Genomics, Japan).

2.1 Design of the cnvK Linker

1. DNA oligomer for cnvK linker composed of the following sequence: 5'- Cyanine5 -AAGAATTTCCA- (cnvK) -GCCGCCCCCGTCC- (Spacer 18) × 2 -CC- puromycin -3'. This oligomer can be obtained from a DNA supplier (Hokkaido System Science, Japan).

2.2 Synthesis of Single-Stranded (ss) DNA Template for LAMP Method

2.2.1 Design of dsDNA Template for LAMP Method

1. Double-stranded (ds) DNA template for LAMP method (shown in Fig. 2): 5'- AGCCGTAGCC CTGTATGCCC GAGAGTGCCTGTGAGGGCGACGCAGACGCC GTTGCCTGTAGCATAGAAGATCCGTGCGGC GGCGGGCCGGTGGGTTTCTGCTTCTTGGGT TTGGGAGGCCCGCCGCCCTCGCCGTCTTCT CCGGGCACGGACTGCACTCCTCCGATGGAG TGAAACTGGAACTGTCTGATGAGCGTGGGG TCAAAGTTGCACATGGGCAGTCCGCTGGCC TCGGAGAGCATGACGGCGATGGAGTTGGGG TTGATCCACGGGGGGCGGCGTGGAAATTCT TCCCTATAGT GAGTCGTATT AATTTCGCGG GATC -3'.

2.2.2 Transcription of dsDNA Template for LAMP Method

1. dsDNA template for LAMP method (Sect. 2.2.1).
2. T7 RiboMax™ Express Large Scale RNA Production System (Promega).
3. Heat block "Cool Stat 5200 (anatech, Japan)."
4. RQ1 RNase-Free DNase (Promega, U.S.A.).

DNA sequences of LAMP method for ssDNA synthesis

Base (nt)	Explanation
11 ~ 28	F3 primer
54 ~ 70	F2 region
75 ~ 86	LF region
92 ~ 115	F1c region
155 ~ 176	B1c region
177 ~ 196	LB region
202 ~ 221	B2 region
239 ~ 256	B3 region
268 ~ 291	Hybridization region of cnvK Linker
292 ~ 311	T7 promoter

AGCCGTAGCC CTGTATGCCC GAGAGTGCCT GTGAGGGCGA CGCAGACGCC
GTTGCCTGTA GCATAGAAGA TCCGTGCGGC GGCGGGCCGG TGGGTTTCTG
CTTCTTGGGT TTGGGAGGCC CGCCGCCCTC GCCGTCTTCT CCGGGCACGG
ACTGCACTCC TCCGATGGAG TGAAACTGGA ACTGTCTGAT GAGCGTGGGG
TCAAAGTTGC ACATGGGCAG TCCGCTGGCC TCGGAGAGCA TGACGGCGAT
GGAGTTGGGG TTGATCCACG GGGGGCGGCG TGGAAATTCT TCCCTATAGT
GAGTCGTATT AATTTCGCGG GATC

Fig. 2 DNA sequences of dsDNA template for LAMP method

5. RNase Inhibitor (Thermo Fisher Scientific, U.S.A.).
6. RNAClean XP (BECKMAN COULTER).
7. Magnetic separator.
8. NanoDrop 1000, Micro volume spectrophotometer (Thermo Fisher Scientific, U.S.A.).

2.2.3 Reverse Transcription of RNA Template for LAMP Method

1. RNA template for LAMP method (Sect. 2.2.2).
2. High Efficient Reverse Transcription Kit (e.g., ReverTra Ace).
3. 10 mM dNTPs Mixture (Promega, U.S.A.).
4. Reverse transcription primer: 5'-CTGTATGCCCGAGAGTGC-3'.
5. RNase Inhibitor (Thermo Fisher Scientific, U.S.A.).
6. Thermal cycler "Biometra TRIO T3 Thermocycler (Analytik Jena, Germany)."

2.2.4 RNase H Treatment for ssDNA Template of LAMP Method

1. Reverse transcription products (Sect. 2.2.3).
2. RNase H (TaKaRa, Japan).
3. 5× ReverTra Buffer (TOYOBO, Japan).

4. NucleoSpin® Gel and PCR Clean-up (TaKaRa, Japan).
5. NanoDrop 1000, Micro volume spectrophotometer (Thermo Fisher Scientific).

2.3 LAMP Method

1. ssDNA for LAMP method (Sect. 2.2.4) (*see* **Note 1**).
2. Bst DNA Polymerase (NIPPON GENE, Japan).
3. 10× Bst Reaction Buffer (NIPPON GENE, Japan).
4. 10 mM dNTPs Mixture (Promega, U.S.A.).
5. F3 Primer: 5'- CTGTATGCCCGAGAGTGC -3'.
6. Forward Inner Primer (FIP) (F1c-F2): 5'- CCCAAACCCAAGAAGCAGAAACCC-GTTGCCTGTAGCATAGAAGA -3' (*see* **Note 2**).
7. Loop Forward primer (LF): 5'- CCCGCCGCCGCA -3'.
8. B3 Primer: 5'- AACTCCATCGCCGTCATG -3'.
9. Backward Inner Primer (BIP) (B1c-B2): 5'- CACTCCTCCGATGGAGTGAAAC-TGCCCATGTGCAACTTTG -3' (*see* **Note 2**).
10. Loop Backward Primer (LB): 5'- TGGAACTGTCTGATGAGCGT -3'.
11. 5 M Betaine solution (FUJIFILM Wako, Japan).
12. 99.9% DMSO (Sigma-Aldrich, Japan).
13. Heat block "Cool Stat 5200 (anatech, Japan)."
14. 2% Agarose gel.
15. Gelgreen Nucleic Acid Gel Stain, 10000× in DMSO (COSMO BIO, Japan).
16. Ez-Capture MG AE-9300Z bioluminescence and fluorescence imaging system (ATTO, Japan).

2.4 Synthesis of mRNA Display

2.4.1 Transcription of VHH-Encoding DNA

1. dsDNA template encoding a VHH for mRNA display (Shown in Fig. 3): 5'- GATCCCGCGA AATTAATACG ACTCACTATA GGGAGACCACAACGGTTTCCCTCTAGAAAT AATTTTGTTTAACTTTAAGAAGGAGATATA CCAATGGAAGTTCAATTAGTAGAAAGTGGA GGTGGCCTGGCACAGCCTGGTGGATCTCTT CGTCTGAGCTGTCTGGCTTCGGGCTTCGCG GTTGGCACGTCTCCGATGTTCTGGTACCGC CAGGCTCCGGGTCAAGAACGTGAGTTTGTG GCACGTATTTCCAGTGGGTTCGGCGCCGGT TTCACCCAGTATGCTGAAAGCGTAAAAGGC CGCTTTACTATCTCTCGTGACAAAAACAAG

Base (nt)	Explanation
14 ~ 33	T7 promoter
34 ~ 80	T7 for PURE
81 ~ 85	RBS (Ribosome Binding Site)
94 ~ 96	Start codon
97 ~ 468	VHH coding region
469 ~ 480	GGGS
481 ~ 507	HA tag
508 ~ 516	GGS
534 ~ 541	Hybridization region of cnvK Linker
520 ~ 541	cnvK New Y tag

GATCCCGCGA AATTAATACG ACTCACTATA GGGAGACCAC AACGGTTTCC
CTCTAGAAAT AATTTTGTTT AACTTTAAGA AGGAGATATA CCAATGGAAG
TTCAATTAGT AGAAAGTGGA GGTGGCCTGG CACAGCCTGG TGGATCTCTT
CGTCTGAGCT GTCTGGCTTC GGGCTTCGCG GTTGGCACGT CTCCGATGTT
CTGGTACCGC CAGGCTCCGG GTCAAGAACG TGAGTTTGTG GCACGTATTT
CCAGTGGGTT CGGCGCCGGT TTCACCCAGT ATGCTGAAAG CGTAAAAGGC
CGCTTTACTA TCTCTCGTGA CAAAAACAAG AATACCGTTT TCCTGCAGAT
GAACTCCCTG AAACCGGAAG ATACTGCGGT CTACTACTGC AACGCACACA
CGCAAGTTGT GACCGGTCTG AAAGCTTATG ACTACTGGGG CCAGGGTACT
CAGGTAACCG TTAGCTCTGG GGGAGGCAGC TACCCATACG ACGTTCCAGA
CTACGCAGGC GGAAGCTCTA GGACGGGGGG CGGCGTGGAA A

Fig. 3 Full-length of VHH-coding dsDNA

AATACCGTTTTCCTGCAGATGAACTCCCTG
AAACCGGAAGATACTGCGGTCTACTACTGC
AACGCACACACGCAAGTTGTGACCGGTCTG
AAAGCTTATGACTACTGGGGCCAGGGTACT
CAGGTAACCGTTAGCTCTGGGGGAGGCAGC
TACCCATACGACGTTCCAGACTACGCAGGC
GGAAGCTCTA GGACGGGGGG CGGCGTGGAA A -3'.

2. T7 RiboMax™ Express Large Scale RNA Production System (Promega, U.S.A.).
3. RQ1 RNase-Free DNase (Promega, U.S.A.).
4. Heat block "Cool Stat 5200 (anatech, Japan)."
5. RNAClean XP (BECKMAN COULTER, U.S.A.).
6. Magnetic separator.
7. NanoDrop 1000, Micro volume spectrophotometer (Thermo Fisher Scientific, U.S.A.).

2.4.2 Photo-Crosslinking of cnvK Linker and RNA

1. 10 mM Tris-HCl, pH 7.5.
2. 500 mM NaCl.
3. 0.01% Tween-20 (Sigma-Aldrich, Japan).
4. 10 mM ethylenediaminetetraacetic acid (EDTA).
5. mRNA (transcript of full-construct DNA coding VHH).
6. cnvK linker (Sect. 2.1).
7. Thermal cycler "Biometra TRIO T3 Thermocycler (Analytik Jena, Germany)."
8. UV Crosslinker "CL-1000 Ultraviolet Crosslinker (Funakoshi, Japan)."
9. Gel electrophoresis apparatus.
10. 5× Tris-Borate-EDTA (TBE) running buffer, pH 8.3.
11. 4% polyacrylamide gel containing 8 M urea.
12. SYBR Gold Nucleic Acid Gel Stain (Thermo Fisher Scientific, U.S.A.).
13. Typhoon FLA 9500 fluorescence scanner (Cytiva, Sweden).

2.4.3 Synthesis of mRNA Display by Cell-Free Translation

1. Cell-free translation kit (e.g., PUREflex series).
2. mRNA-puromycin linker conjugate (photo-crosslinking product).
3. 3 M KCl (FUJIFILM Wako, Japan).
4. 1 M $MgCl_2$(FUJIFILM Wako, Japan).
5. 0.5 M ethylenediaminetetraacetic acid (EDTA), pH 8.0.
6. Heat block "Cool Stat 5200 (anatech, Japan)."
7. Micro Bio Spin columns filled with Bio-Gel P-6 (Bio-Rad, USA).
8. 10 mM Tris-HCl (pH 7.5) (FUJIFILM Wako, Japan).

2.5 Synthesis of VHH-LAMP Specific DNA

2.5.1 Degradation of mRNA and Photo-Crosslinking Cleavage (Preparation of Linker-VHH Conjugate)

1. Buffer-exchanged mRNA display.
2. RNase H (TaKaRa, Japan).
3. RNase T1 (Thermo Fisher Scientific).
4. 10× NE Buffer 2 (New England Biorabs, USA).
5. Heat block "Cool Stat 5200 (anatech, Japan)."
6. UV transilluminator "CI-210B (BIO CRAFT, Japan)."

2.5.2 Photo-Crosslinking of Linker-VHH Conjugate and ssDNA (Preparation of VHH-LAMP Specific DNA)

1. Linker-VHH conjugate.
2. ssDNA template for LAMP method.
3. 10 mM Tris-HCl, pH 7.5.
4. 500 mM NaCl.
5. Tween-20.
6. 10 mM ethylenediaminetetraacetic acid (EDTA).
7. Thermal cycler "Biometra TRIO T3 Thermocycler (Analytik Jena, Germany)."
8. UV Crosslinker "CL-1000 Ultraviolet Crosslinker (Funakoshi, Japan)."
9. Micro Bio Spin columns filled with Bio-Gel P-6 (Bio-Rad, USA).
10. 10 mM Tris-HCl (pH 7.5).
11. 10× PBS Buffer (NIPPON GENE, Japan).
12. Anti HA Antibody Beads (FUJIFILM Wako Chemicals, U.S.A.).
13. Bovine Serum Albumin (BSA).
14. Sheared Salmon Sperm, DNA.
15. Thermo block rotator.
16. Gel electrophoresis apparatus (SDS-PAGE).
17. 10× SDS running buffer (NIPPON JENE, Japan).
18. 4% stacking gel containing 8 M urea.
19. 6% separating gel containing 8 M urea.
20. Typhoon FLA 9500 fluorescence scanner (Cytiva, Sweden).

3 Methods

A schematic representation of VHH-LAMP specific DNA formation is shown in Fig. 4. (1) The VHH-coding dsDNA is transcribed into mRNA (Sect. 3.5.1). (2) An mRNA is photo-crosslinking with puromycin linker (Sect. 3.5.2). (3) The crosslinked product is in vitro translated (Sect. 3.5.3). (4) mRNA is degraded (Sect. 3.6.1) (*see* **Note 3**). (5) The crosslink of cnvK was cleaved by UV irradiation at 312 nm, yielding the linker–VHH conjugate (Sect. 3.6.2). (6) A ssDNA for LAMP is photo-crosslinked with linker-VHH conjugate (Sect. 3.6.3).

3.1 Design of the cnvK Linker

1. Modify the 5' terminus with a Cyanine 5 (Cy5) fluorescent label (*see* **Note 4**).
2. Modify the 3' terminus with a puromycin.

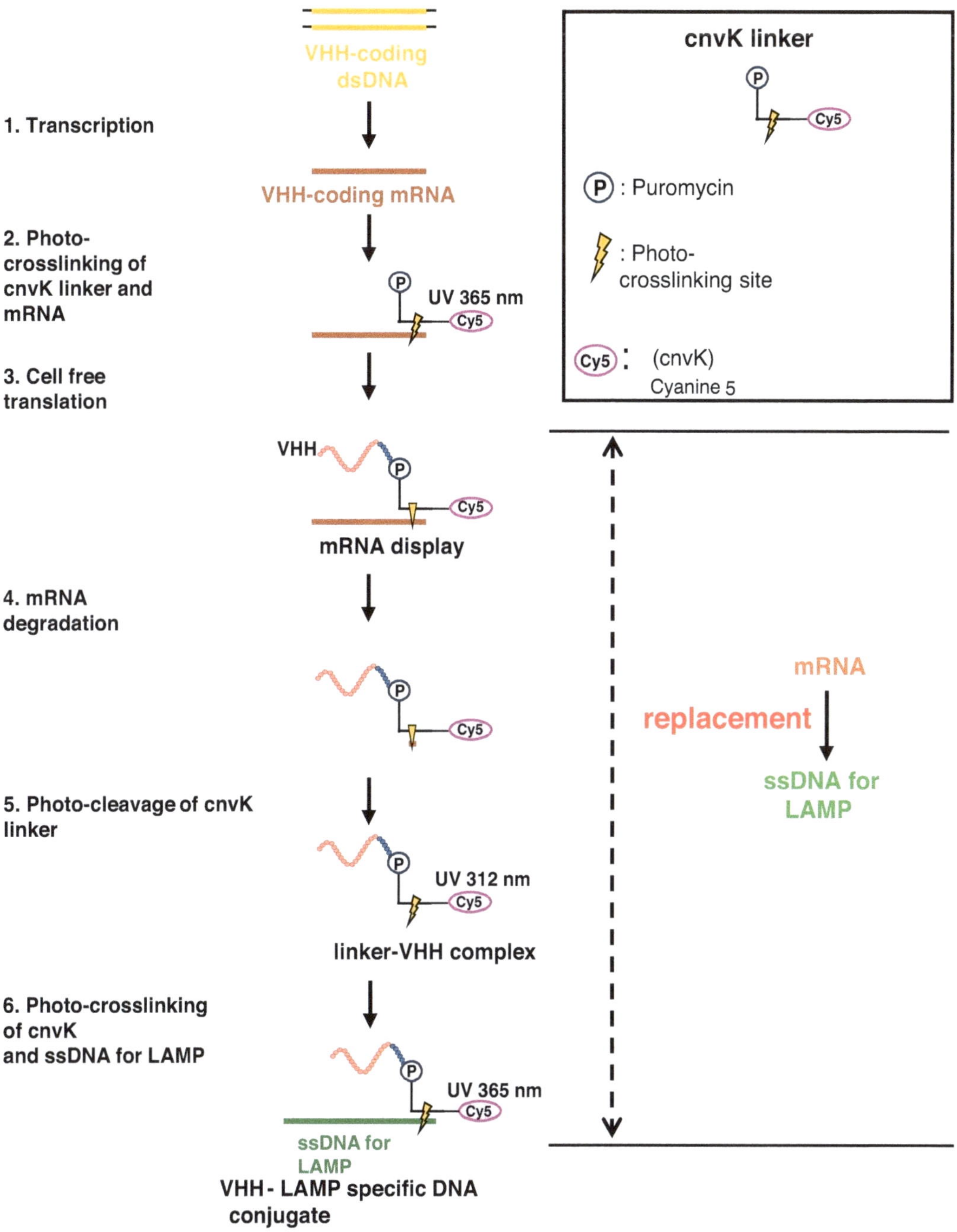

Fig. 4 Schematic representation of VHH-LAMP specific DNA molecules

3.2 Synthesis of ssDNA Template for LAMP Method

3.2.1 Design of dsDNA Template for LAMP Method

1. Synthesize dsDNA for LAMP method by ordering a DNA synthesis supplier as in Fig. 2.
2. *See* **Note 5** for more information.

3.2.2 Transcription of dsDNA Template for LAMP Method

1. Prepare the transcription reaction solution as follows: mix 5 μL of RiboMax™ Express T7 2× buffer, 50 ng of the template DNA for LAMP method from Sect. 3.2.1, 1 μL of Enzyme Mix T7 express, 0.5 μL of RNase Inhibitor, and add nuclease-free water up to 10 μL.
2. Incubate at 37°C for 30 min on a heat block (*see* **Note 6**).
3. Add 1 μL of RQ1 RNase-free DNase (1 U/μL) and incubate at 37°C for 15 min on a heat block.
4. Purify the transcript (mRNA) with RNAClean XP.
5. Determine its concentration by absorbance at 260 nm using a spectrophotometer.
6. Store the mRNA at −80°C until use.

3.2.3 Reverse Transcription of RNA Template for LAMP Method

1. Prepare the reverse transcription reaction solution as follows: mix 4 μL of 5× ReverTra buffer, 3 μg of the template RNA from Sect. 3.2.2, 2 μL of 10 mM dNTPs Mixture, 1.2 μL of 50 μM reverse transcription primer, and add nuclease-free water up to 19 μL.
2. Heat the mixture at 65°C for 3 min followed by lowering the temperature to 55°C at a rate of 0.1°C/s and incubate for 1 min. The temperature was then cool down to 45°C at a rate of 0.01°C/s and incubated for 1 min and subsequently lowered to 25°C at a rate of 0.1 °C/s. (*see* **Note 7**).
3. Add 1 μL of ReverTra Ace® (100 U/μL) and incubate at 50°C for 30 min on a heat block.
4. Incubate the mixture at 95°C for 3 min on a heat block to inactivate the enzyme.

3.2.4 RNase H Treatment for ssDNA Template of LAMP Method

1. Prepare the RNase H treatment solution as follows: mix all reverse transcription products from Sect. 3.2.3, 1 μL of 5× ReverTra buffer, 0.25 μL of RNase H (20~60 U/μL), and add nuclease-free water up to 25 μL.
2. Incubate the mixture at 37°C for 20 min on a heat block.
3. Purify the RNase H treatment product (ssDNA) with NucleoSpin® Gel and PCR Clean-up (*see* **Note 8**).
4. Determine its concentration by absorbance at 260 nm using a spectrophotometer.
5. Store the ssDNA at −25°C until use.

3.3 LAMP Method

1. Prepare the LAMP method solution as follows: mix 2.5 μL of 10× Beast Reaction buffer, 1 μL of Bst DNA Polymerase (8 U/μL), 3.5 μL of 10 mM dNTPs Mixture, 5 μL of Primer Mixture (containing 40 pmol of FIP, BIP, 10 pmol of F3, B3 primer, 20 pmol of LF, LB primer), 8.0 μL of 5 M Betaine solution,

1.5 μL of DMSO, 1.0 μL of 1 nM template DNA, and add nuclease-free water up to 25 μL (*see* **Note 9**).

2. Incubate the mixture at 65°C for 60 min on a heat block.
3. Analyze the amplification for LAMP method on a 2% agarose gel electrophoresis by staining with the Gelgreen Nucleic Acid Gel Stain and visualized by the bioluminescence and fluorescence imaging system (*see* **Note 10**).

3.4 Design of VHH-Coding DNA for cDNA Display

1. Synthesize VHH-coding DNA template by ordering a DNA synthesis supplier as in Fig. 3.
2. *See* **Note 11** for more information.

3.5 Synthesis of mRNA Display

3.5.1 Transcription of VHH-Coding DNA

1. Prepare the transcription reaction solution as follows: mix 2 μL of RiboMax™ Express T7 2× buffer, 100 ng of the template VHH DNA from Sect. 3.4, 1 μL of Enzyme Mix T7 express, and add nuclease-free water up to 10 μL.
2. Incubate at 37°C for 30 min on a heat block (*see* **Note 6**).
3. Add 1 μL of RQ1 RNase-free DNase and incubate at 37°C for 15 min on a heat block.
4. Purify the transcript (mRNA) with RNAClean XP.
5. Determine its concentration by absorbance at 260 nm using a spectrophotometer.
6. Store the mRNA at −80°C until use.

3.5.2 Photo-Crosslinking of cnvK Linker and mRNA

1. Prepare the photo-crosslinking reaction solution as follows: mix 2 μL of 5× Annealing Buffer (500 mM NaCl, 50 mM Tris–HCl (pH7.5), 0.01% Tween-20, 50 mM EDTA), 15 pmol of cnvK linker, 15 pmol of VHH mRNA prepared in Sect. 3.5.1, and nuclease-free water up to 10 μL (*see* **Note 12**).
2. Heat the mixture at 90°C for 1 min followed by lowering the temperature to 70°C at a rate of 1.0°C/s and incubate for 1 min. The temperature was then cool down to 50°C at a rate of 0.01°C/s and incubated for 1 min and subsequently lowered to 25°C at a rate of 0.1°C/s.
3. Irradiate the mixture with UV light at 365 nm for about 2 min using a UV crosslinker (*see* **Note 13**).
4. Analyze the ligated product on a denaturing 4% polyacrylamide gel containing 8 M urea by imaging the Cy5 using a fluorescence scanner and subsequently stained with the SYBR Gold nucleic acid gel stain and visualized by the fluorescence scanner (*see* **Note 14**).
5. Store the ligated sample at −80°C until use.

3.5.3 Synthesis of mRNA Display by Cell-Free Translation

1. Prepare the translation mixture as follows: mix 10 pmol of photo-crosslinking product from Sect. 3.5.2, 12.5 μL of PUREfrex 1.0 Solution I, 1.25 μL of PUREfrex 1.0 Solution II, 2.5 μL of PUREfrex 1.0 Solution III, and nuclease-free water up to 25 μL.
2. Incubate the mixture at 37°C for 15 min on a heat block.
3. Add 12 μL of 3 M KCl and 3 μL of 1 M $MgCl_2$ to translation sample.
4. Incubate at 37°C for 60 min (*see* **Note 15**).
5. Add 9 μL of 0.5 M EDTA solution.
6. Incubate at 37°C for 10 min.
7. Exchange the buffer into 10 mM Tris-HCl (pH 7.5) using Micro Bio Spin columns.

3.6 Synthesis of VHH-LAMP Specific DNA Conjugate

3.6.1 mRNA Degradation and Photo-Crosslinking Cleavage (preparation of linker-VHH conjugate)

1. Prepare the translation mixture as follows: mix all of translation products from Sect. 3.5.3, 5.3 μL of 10× Ne Buffer 2, 0.5 μL of RNase H (1000 U/μL), 0.5 μL of RNase T1 (1000 U/μL), nuclease-free water up to 53 μL (*see* **Note 16**).
2. Incubate at 30°C for 20 min.
3. Irradiate the mixture with UV light at 312 nm for about 4 min using a UV transilluminator (*see* **Note 17**).

3.6.2 Photo-Crosslinking of Linker-VHH Conjugate and ssDNA (preparation of VHH-LAMP Specific DNA conjugate)

1. Prepare the photo-crosslinking reaction solution as follows: mix all linker-VHH conjugate products from Sect. 3.6.1, 10 pmol of ssDNA for LAMP method, 5× Annealing Buffer, nuclease-free water up to 75 μL (*see* **Note 18**).
2. Incubate the mixture at 70°C for 1 min followed by cooling to 50°C at a rate of 0.01°C/s and incubate for 1 min. The temperature was then cool down to 25°C at a rate of 0.1°C/s.
3. Irradiate the mixture with UV light at 365 nm for about 2 min using a UV crosslinker.
4. Exchange the buffer into 1× PBS Buffer using Micro Bio Spin columns.

3.6.3 HA-Tag Affinity Purification of VHH-LAMP Specific DNA Conjugate

1. Take 40 μL of Anti HA Antibody beads (*see* **Note 19**) into a tube and centrifuge the beads slurry at 8000×*g* for 30 s at 4°C.
2. Incubate for 1–2 min on ice and then remove the supernatant.
3. Add 200 μL of blocking buffer (500 μg/mL Sheared Salmon Sperm DNA, 3% (w/v) BSA, 0.05% (v/v) Tween-20,

1× PBS) and mix by thermo block rotator for 1 h at 4°C (*see* **Note 20**).

4. Centrifuge the beads slurry at 8000×*g* for 30 s at 4°C and remove the supernatant.
5. Add 500 μL of PBS and mix by vortex mixer and then centrifuge the beads slurry at 8000×*g* for 30 s at 4°C and remove the supernatant. This step was performed twice.
6. Add 200 μL of VHH-LAMP specific DNA conjugate into washed beads.
7. Mix by thermo block rotator for 2 h at 4°C.
8. Centrifuge the beads slurry at 8000×*g* for 30 s at 4°C and remove the supernatant.
9. Wash beads as described in Step 5.
10. Resuspend the beads in 100 μL of 4× SDS running buffer and boil at 95°C in heat block for 3 min (*see* **Note 21**).
11. Centrifuge the beads slurry at 8000×*g* for 30 s at 25°C and collect the supernatant containing purified VHH-LAMP specific DNA conjugate molecules (Fig. 5).

4 Notes

1. Although dsDNA is generally used as the template for LAMP, we found that single-stranded DNA (ssDNA) facilitates primer annealing and generally provides higher amplification efficiency than dsDNA. Therefore, we used single-stranded DNA (ssDNA) as the template for the LAMP. In addition, ssDNA shorter than approximately 150 bases

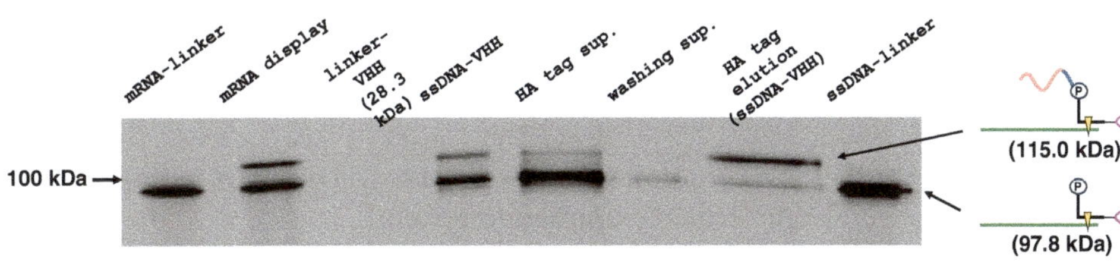

Fig. 5 Confirmation of VHH-LAMP specific DNA conjugate. mRNA-linker (see Sect. 3.5.2, lane 1) was translated to mRNA display (lane 2, upper band. Note that the lower band corresponds to the mRNA-linker that was not conjugated to a peptide), and mRNA degradation (preparation of linker-VHH conjugate), in lane 3). After photo-crosslinking with linker-VHH conjugate and ssDNA for LAMP, VHH-LAMP specific DNA conjugate (crude) was formed (lane 4). Further purification with anti HA beads (supernatant was analyzed in lane 5, and wash supernatant was analyzed in lane 6) yielded pure VHH-LAMP specific DNA conjugate (lane 7). Samples were analyzed by SDS-PAGE containing 8 M urea, and fluorescence of Cyanine5 attached to the puromycin linker (see Sect. 2.1) was visualized with gel imager

can be readily obtained by chemical synthesis from a DNA supplier.

2. We recommend using HPLC-purified FIP and BIP primers to ensure high purity and consistent LAMP performance.
3. Efficient UV (312 nm) absorption by cnvK requires that no RNA residues remain in close proximity to the cnvK unit. Moreover, if the mRNA stays hybridized to the linker, it interferes with the annealing of the ssDNA probe and consequently inhibits photo-crosslinking. To avoid this issue, the mRNA is degraded before initiating the reaction.
4. For the fluorescent labeling of the linker, dyes that do not significant absorb UV light at 300–400 nm, such as Cy5. Please contact Epsilon Molecular Engineering, Inc. (Japan) to request the synthesis of a puromycin linker.
5. If you want to use other LAMP template DNA, please change "LAMP sequence" part. The DNA construct can be directly synthesized as an artificial gene on a plasmid or overlap extension PCR from several fragments.
6. Optimization of the template DNA amount and reaction time is required to minimize the by-products during the transcription reaction.
7. Annealing of the RNA and the reverse transcription primer improves synthesis efficiency.
8. Any standard nucleic acid purification method, for example ethanol precipitation, can be used for purification.
9. Amplification enhancers, such as betaine and DMSO, require optimization depending on the sequence and experimental conditions.
10. Any type of gel-staining reagent can be used.
11. This sequence was codon-optimized for PUREfrex; therefore, when using this construct in other cell-free translation systems, codon usage must be reoptimized accordingly. In addition, please ensure that there is no stop codon before cnvK NewYtag region.
12. The amount of mRNA needs to be optimized depending on the cell-free translation system.
13. After annealing the linker to the mRNA, UV irradiation was performed immediately.
14. Binding efficiency can be estimated by analyzing the band intensity ratios of bound and unbound mRNA.
15. Using the improved version PUREfrex 2.0, a reaction time of 40 min is sufficient.

16. By using not only RNase H but also RNase T1, the mRNA is fragmented, which improves the efficiency of subsequent ssDNA annealing.
17. Heat the photo-crosslinking sample in a PCR tube at 65°C for 1 min by the thermal cycler. Furthermore, warm the surface of the transilluminator for preheating. This step is essential for achieving efficient photo-crosslinking cleavage of the cnvK. After the heating, place the PCR tube directly on UV lamp of the transilluminator.
18. The amount of ssDNA to be added depends on the translation efficiency.
19. To minimize nonspecific binding of ssDNA, purification using the HA tag was chosen. However, with appropriate optimization of the purification conditions, other purification, such as His tag, could also be used.
20. To prevent unbound ssDNA from binding nonspecifically to the anti-HA beads, a blocking step should be required.
21. Elution with SDS carries a high risk of protein denaturation; therefore, alternative elution strategies should be employed depending on the intended downstream application.

Acknowledgments

This work was supported in part by KAKENHI, Japan (17K19471, and 21H05025 to N.N.). We thank Prof. Masatoshi Yamaguchi and Prof. Miho Suzuki for valuable scientific discussion.

References

1. Sano T, Smith CL, Cantor CR (1992) Immuno-PCR: very sensitive antigen detection by means of specific antibody-DNA conjugates. Science 258(5079):120–122
2. Guo YC, Zhou YF, Zhang XE, Zhang ZP, Qiao YM, Bi LJ, Wen JK, Liang MF, Zhang JB (2006) Phage display mediated immuno-PCR. Nucleic Acids Res 34(8):e62
3. van Buggenum JAGL, Gerlach JP, Eising S, Schoonen L, van Eijl RA, Tanis SE, Hogeweg M, Hubner NC, van Hest JC, Bonger KM, Mulder KW (2016) A covalent and cleavable antibody-DNA conjugation strategy for sensitive protein detection via immuno-PCR. Sci Rep 6: 22675
4. Anzai H, Terai T, Jayathilake C, Suzuki T, Nemoto N (2019) A novel immuno-PCR method using cDNA display. Anal Biochem 578:1–6
5. Jayathilake C, Nemoto N (2021) cDNA display-mediated immuno-PCR (cD-IPCR): an ultrasensitive immunoassay for biomolecular detection. Methods Mol Biol 2261:307–321
6. Notomi T, Okayama H, Masubuchi H, Yonekawa T, Watanabe K, Amino N, Hase T (2000) Loop-mediated isothermal amplification of DNA. Nucl Acids Res 28:e63
7. Yoshino M, Watari H, Kojima T, Ikedo M (2006) Sensitive and rapid detection of koi herpesvirus by LAMP method. Fish Pathol 41(1):19–27
8. Yamaguchi J, Naimuddin M, Biyani M, Sasaki T, Machida M, Kubo T, Funatsu T, Husimi Y, Nemoto N (2009) cDNA display: a novel screening method for functional disulfide-rich peptides by solid-phase synthesis and stabilization of mRNA-protein fusions. Nucleic Acids Res 37(16):e108

9. Mochizuki Y, Suzuki T, Fujimoto K, Nemoto N (2015) A versatile puromycin-linker using cnvK for mRNA/cDNA display by a novel. J Biotechnol 212:174–180
10. Yoshimura Y, Fujimoto K (2008) Ultrafast reversible photo-cross-linking reaction: toward in situ DNA manipulation. Org Lett 10(15):3227–3230

Chapter 7

M13 Bacteriophage pVIII Protein: Display Strategies, Chemical Modification, and Antibacterial Activity Investigations

Xuanliang Wang, Zongyuan Fan, Ziyue Huang, Zishan Wang, Zhijie Hu, Dairong Li and Huan Peng

Abstract

The excessive and inappropriate use of antibiotics has driven the proliferation of antibiotic-resistant bacterial strains, posing significant challenges to conventional antimicrobial therapies. Endowed with remarkable engineering versatility, the M13 bacteriophage has emerged as a versatile platform for the development of novel antimicrobial strategies. In this chapter, we focused on the major coat protein pVIII of the M13 phage, utilizing genetic engineering and chemical modification approaches to engineer pVIII mutants with tailored surface charge properties. Through comparative analysis of the antibacterial efficacy of phage variants with distinct surface charges, we systematically assessed the influence of positive and negative charge densities on bactericidal activity, aiming to advance the development of innovative antimicrobial therapies.

Keywords M13 bacteriophage, Phage display, Chemical modification, Antibacterial activity

1 Introduction

Although antibiotics have revolutionized the treatment of bacterial infections, their overuse and inappropriate administration have fueled an increasingly severe antimicrobial resistance (AMR) crisis. AMR is spreading globally at an alarming rate, posing a paramount threat to public health [1]. More critically, the pipeline for new antibiotic development has significantly stagnated in recent years, resulting in progressively dwindling therapeutic alternatives in clinical practice. Thus, there is an urgent need to develop alternative therapeutic strategies based on novel mechanisms to mitigate the challenges arising

The authors "Xuanliang Wang" and "Zongyuan Fan" contribute equally.

Huan Peng and Theam Soon Lim (eds.), *Biomolecular Display Technologies*, Methods in Molecular Biology, vol. 3030,
https://doi.org/10.1007/978-1-0716-5249-7_7,

from the diminishing efficacy of conventional antimicrobial agents [2]. Phages are natural predators of bacteria and were widely used for pathogens control before the discovery of antibiotics. However, utilizing wild-type lytic phages for bacterial infection treatment face challenges such as uncontrolled released of lysate. More recently, the nonlytic M13 phage has attract more and more interest from researchers due to the unique filamentous structure and ease for capsid protein modification. The properties of the capsid protein, especially the pVIII protein, significantly influence the function or activity of the phage particles. Two primary strategies: phage display and chemical modification, has well developed for engineering the pVIII proteins [3].

Phage display is a powerful tool leveraging gene fusion to present target peptides or protein fragments on bacteriophages, typically involving molecular cloning to insert exogenous peptide-encoding DNA sequences into phage capsid protein genes [4–6]. In contrast, chemical modification enables covalent conjugation of exogenous moieties (e.g., positively charged arginine or polyethyleneimine) to side-chain functional groups of proteins, including lysine's ε-amino group, glutamic acid/aspartic acid's carboxyl groups, and cysteine's sulfhydryl group [7, 8]. Incorporating positively charged ligands can augment phage surface positive charge density to strengthen bacterial cell membrane interactions and enhance direct bactericidal activity.

In this chapter, we used the M13 bacteriophage as a model system to engineer pVIII protein mutants with tailored surface charge profiles via a combination of genetic modification and chemical functionalization approaches. The experimental workflow encompassed site-directed mutagenesis, transformation and expression, phage amplification and preservation, as well as structural characterization. Ultimately, the minimum inhibitory concentration (MIC) of each phage variant was determined via the plate count method to systematically analyze the correlation between surface charge distribution and bactericidal efficacy. The findings of this work are anticipated to lay theoretical and experimental groundwork for the development of highly efficient and specific phage-based antimicrobial agents, thereby contributing to mitigating the growing AMR crisis.

2 Materials

2.1 Primer Design and PCR

1. P520 [2× Phanta Flash Master Mix (Dye Plus)]: A premixed PCR reagent containing Phanta Flash ultrahigh fidelity DNA polymerase, dNTPs, optimized buffer, and electrophoresis dye. Keep at −20°C. Before utilizing, thaw it on ice first. Directly add 25 μL of P520 to a 50 μL PCR reaction volume.
2. Upstream and downstream primers.

3. Template DNA.
4. ddH_2O.

2.2 Electrophoresis

1. Agarose
2. 1× TAE buffer
3. 10,000× nucleic acid dye
4. 1 kb DNA Ladder

2.3 Materials for Gel Product Recovery

1. Gel DNA Precipitation Buffer (Buffer GDP)
2. Gel Wash Buffer (Buffer GW)
3. Elution Buffer

2.4 Transformation

1. *E. coli* competent cells: Culture *E. coli* in LB medium to an OD600 ≈ 0.4–0.6. Cool on ice, then centrifuge at 4000 rpm for 10 min at 4°C. Resuspend cells in ice-cold 0.1 M $CaCl_2$ and incubate on ice for 30 min. Centrifuge again, resuspend in $CaCl_2$ solution containing 15% glycerol, aliquot 50 μL/tube, and rapidly freeze at −80°C.
2. LB (without antibiotics): Take 10 g of trypticase peptone, 5 g of yeast extract, and 10 g of sodium chloride. Substances are dissolved in 950 mL deionized water. To achieve a pH of 7.0, utilize sodium hydroxide for adjustment and subsequently dilute the solution to 1 L. Heat the autoclave to a temperature of 121°C and maintain it for a duration of 15 min. Then, keep it cool and store it at room temperature.
3. Solid LB: Add 15 g agar/L to prepared LB (without antibiotics). After sterilization, cool to 50°C. Incorporate Kanamycin (50 μg/mL) and IPTG (1 mM). Pour into plates. Store at 4°C. Warm to room temperature before use.
4. Liquid LB: Prepare 1 L as described above for LB. After sterilization, cool to 50°C. Add filter-sterilized Kanamycin stock solution (50 mg/mL) to a final concentration of 50 μg/mL and IPTG stock solution (1 M) to a final concentration of 1 mM.

2.5 Phage Purification

1. IPTG (1:1000 final concentration): Weigh 2.38 g IPTG powder and dissolve in 10 mL deionized water to prepare a 1 M stock solution. Sterilize by filtration through a 0.22 μm membrane, aliquot, and store at −20°C. Dilute 1:1000 in culture medium prior to use.
2. PEG/NaCl Solution: Weigh 200 g PEG-8000 and 146.1 g NaCl, dissolve in 800 mL deionized water with stirring. Add water to 1 L, then autoclave at 121°C or filter through a 0.22 μ m membrane. Store at room temperature.
3. PBS Buffer: Prepare 8 g NaCl, 0.2 g KCl, 1.44 g Na_2HPO_4, and 0.24 g KH_2PO_4. Dissolve in 800 mL deionized water. Adjust

pH to 7.4 with HCl. Dilute to 1 L with water. Autoclave at 121°C. Store at room temperature.

2.6 MIC Assay

1. Antibiotic-Free Mueller-Hinton (MH) Agar Plates: Weigh 38 g MH agar powder and dissolve in 1 L deionized water. Heat and boil for 1 min to dissolve. Autoclave at 121°C for 15 min, cool to 50°C, pour into Petri dishes (20 mL per dish), and store at 4°C after solidification.
2. MH Broth: Weigh 21 g of MH broth powder and dissolve in 1 L of deionized water. Heat to dissolve. Autoclave at 121°C for 15 min and store at room temperature.

3 Methods

3.1 PCR

1. Thaw reagents: Slowly thaw 2× Phanta Flash Master Mix (Dye Plus), upstream primer, downstream primer, template DNA, and ddH_2O on ice. Gently mix after thawing and promptly return unused portions to −20°C storage.
2. Prepare the PCR reaction mixture (using a 50 μL reaction as an example) (Table 1): P520 [2× Phanta Flash Master Mix (Dye Plus)] is a novel high-fidelity rapid PCR premix utilizing directionally evolved Phanta Flash Super-Fidelity DNA Polymerase (*see* **Note 1**).
3. Add all components to the PCR tube. Gently pipette or briefly centrifuge until the liquid settles at the bottom. Thoroughly mix the reaction mixture.
4. Set the PCR instrument reaction program: Select an appropriate reaction program based on the primer Tm values and template characteristics, then save it (Table 2).

Table 1
PCR system

Reagent	Volume (μL)
PCR master mix	50
2× mix buffer (p520)	25
F primer	2
R primer	2
DNA template	4
ddH_2O	17

Table 2
PCR reaction protocol settings

Step	Temperature	Time	Description
Predenaturation	98°C	30 s	Thoroughly denature template DNA
Denaturation	98°C	10 s	Denaturation step for each cycle
Annealing	Set based on primer Tm	5 s	Primer annealing to template
Extension	72°C	4–5 s/kb	For M13 phage plasmid (8048 bp), set to approximately 45 s
Cycles	28–35 cycles		
Final extension	72°C	1 min	Ensure complete extension of all products
Hold	4°C	Indefinite	Maintain sample stability after reaction completion

3.2 Electrophoresis

1. Prepare a 1% agarose gel: Weigh 0.3 g of agarose and add it to 30 mL of 1× TAE buffer. Mix thoroughly, then put it into a microwave oven. Heat it up until the agarose is completely dissolved (*see* **Note 2**). Rinse the bottom of the conical flask with cold water and allow to cool slightly to approximately 60°C. Add 10,000× nucleic acid dye. Pour the solution into the gel tank with the comb in place and allow to solidify at room temperature for approximately 20–30 min.
2. Preparation of electrophoresis buffer: Pour 1× TAE electrophoresis buffer into the electrophoresis tank, ensuring the liquid level covers the gel surface by 2–3 mm.
3. Add 3 μL of 1 kb DNA Ladder for loading preparation.
4. Using a pipette, draw 5 μL of PCR product and slowly inject it into the sample well of the gel.
5. Set voltage to approximately 100 V, current to 30 mA, and electrophoresis time to 20 min. Alternatively, stop when a marker band reaches the 2/3 point of the gel.
6. After electrophoresis, remove the gel and visualize under UV transilluminator (Fig. 1).

3.3 Gel Product Recovery

1. Cut target DNA band: Visualize the electrophoresis gel under UV light and locate the target DNA band. Using a gel cutter, cut close to the edge of the target band. Transfer the excised gel fragment into a preweighed 1.5 mL centrifuge tube and record its weight.
2. Dissolve gel fragment: Add three volumes of Buffer GDP based on the gel fragment weight. Incubate at 50°C in a water bath for 10 min, gently shaking or to vortex every 2–3 min until complete gel dissolution.

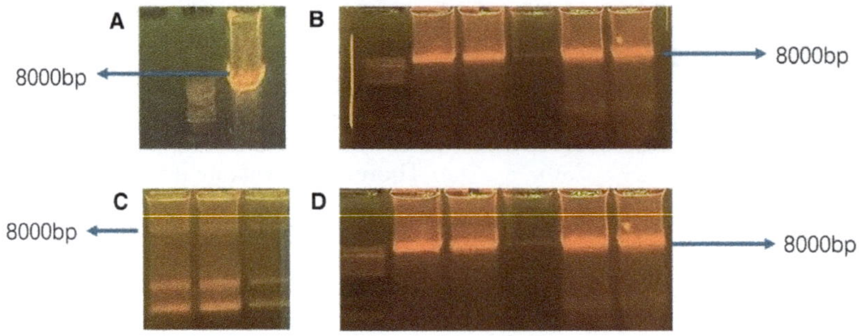

Fig. 1 Observing electrophoresis gel products under an ultraviolet transilluminator. (**A**) The electrophoresis band for 24 25-R; (**B**) The electrophoresis band for 25-R; (**C**) The electrophoresis band for 25 26-R; (**D**) The electrophoresis band for 25 26 27-R

3. DNA binding: Transfer the dissolved gel solution to a spin column (placed within a collection tube). Centrifuge at ≥ 12,000 rpm for 1 min. Discard the eluate, retaining the spin column within the same collection tube.
4. Wash: Add Buffer GW along the walls of the column to thoroughly rinse residual salts adhering to the tube walls. Add 500 μ L of wash buffer, centrifuge at ≥12,000 rpm for 1 min, and repeat twice. Discard the supernatant and place the column in the recovery tube. Centrifuge at ≥12,000 rpm for 2 min.
5. DNA Elution: Insert the column into a sterile 1.5 mL centrifuge tube. Prewarm the Elution Buffer to 55°C (*see* **Note 3**). Slowly add 20–30 μL of buffer to the center of the column, as close to the column base as feasible. Incubate for 2 min. Centrifuge at a speed of 12,000 rpm for a duration of 1 min. Discard the column. To ensure the preservation of DNA, it is recommended to store it at a temperature of −20°C.

3.4 Transformation

1. Remove the competent cells from the −80°C freezer and thaw on ice for approximately 10–15 min until completely thawed.
2. On ice, add 5 μL of the previously extracted DNA solution to 50 μL of thawed competent cells and mix gently (*see* **Note 4**).
3. Incubate the mixed cells on ice for 30 min to promote DNA-cell membrane binding.
4. Immerse the bottom 1/2 to 2/3 of the reaction tube in a 42°C water bath for 90 s of heat shock. Immediately return the tube to ice and cool for a duration of 2–3 min.
5. Add 500–800 μL antibiotic-free LB to each tube. Incubate on a shaker at 37°C and 200 rpm for 45 min to allow cells to express the resistance gene.

6. Centrifuge at the speed of 5000 rpm for 1 min to collect cells. Discard the supernatant, reserving approximately 100 μL of the suspension for plating.
7. Spread the cell suspension evenly onto preprepared LB solid medium plates.
8. Turn the plates upside down and let them sit at a temperature of 37°C for a duration of 12–16 h. Monitor the growth of the colonies on the next day and select in single colonies for further experiments. Take the chosen colonies and carefully transfer them using a pipette tip into 300 μL of LB liquid medium. The sample should be incubated at a temperature of 37°C with a rotation speed of 200 rpm for a duration of 6–8 h prior to being sent for sequencing by the company.

3.5 Phage Purification

1. After infecting competent *E. coli* with phage, incubate at 37°C on a shaking incubator until the culture reaches an $OD_{600} \approx 0.5$ (*see* **Note 5**). Add IPTG to a final concentration of 1:1000, then transfer to 30°C and continue shaking overnight to induce phage expression and release.
2. The following day, extract the culture, subject it to centrifugation at a temperature of 4°C and a speed of 5000 g for 10 min, and gather the supernatant (*see* **Note 6**). Add 1/5 of the supernatant's volume and add it to a PEG/NaCl solution. Mix thoroughly and place in a 4°C refrigerator on ice for at least 4 h (*see* **Note 7**).
3. Following the ice bath, centrifuge at a temperature of 4°C and a speed of 10,000 g for a duration of 15 min. A white flocculent precipitate will form at the bottom or sides of the tube, representing the phages. Carefully remove the supernatant. Resuspend the phage in PBS buffer at 1/10 the volume of the original bacterial suspension (e.g., 20 mL for 200 mL original) (*see* **Note 8**).
4. Take 1/5 volume of PEG/NaCl solution and add it to the resuspended phage solution. Then, incubate the sample on ice at a temperature of 4°C for a duration of 2–3 h, and subsequently perform a centrifugation process at a speed of 10,000 g for a time span of 15 min. Remove the supernatant and resuspend the phage in a smaller volume of PBS (*see* **Note 9**) to increase concentration.
5. Aliquot the final high-concentration phage suspension and refrigerate at −80°C for subsequent use.

3.6 Determination of Minimum Inhibitory Concentration (MIC)

1. To prepare the bacterial stock, streak the target strain onto MH agar plates that are free of antibiotics, and then incubate them at a temperature of 37°C for a duration of 18–24 h.

Select three to five morphologically consistent colonies and inoculate into 5 mL MH broth. The culture should be maintained at a temperature of 37°C while being shaken continuously for a duration of 18–24 h. To obtain an OD_{450} value of 0.01, measure it using a spectrophotometer and then dilute the culture with MH broth accordingly.

2. Prepare the 96-well plate:
   Column 1: Each well should be filled with 100 μL of phage stock solution.
   For columns 2–11: Add a volume of 50 μL of MH broth to each well.
   Column 12: Each well should be supplemented with 100 μL of MH broth, which will serve as the negative control.
3. Dilute the phage gradient. Transfer 50 μL from each well of Column 1 to the corresponding well in Column 2, mixing by pipetting up and down four to six times. Repeat this step down to Column 10. Finally, discard 50 μL from Column 10 (*see* **Note 10**).
4. Vortex the diluted bacterial suspension (OD_{450} = 0.01) to mix thoroughly. Add 50 μL of bacterial suspension to each well in columns 1–11 (final volume 150 μL). Column 12 serves as the negative control and remains uninoculated.
5. Seal the 96-well plate with a sealing membrane to prevent evaporation. Measure the OD_{600} value at 0 h using a spectrophotometer. Incubate at 37°C for 16–24 h. Subsequently, measure the OD_{600} value at 24 h.
6. MIC determination: Subtract the OD_{600} value at 0 h from the OD_{600} value at 24 h. Identify wells with a difference <0.1; the corresponding phage concentration is the minimum inhibitory concentration (MIC).

4 Notes

1. P520 exhibits a low mismatch rate (1/81 that of standard Taq enzymes) and high amplification speed (4–5 s/kb). P520 is premixed with DNA polymerase, dNTPs, optimized buffer, and electrophoresis dye, enabling direct use for PCR amplification and product electrophoresis analysis. Its amplification products feature blunt ends, suitable for subsequent cloning operations.
2. Mix thoroughly till the liquid becomes clear and free of particles.
3. Since the M13 plasmid is 8048 bp long, resulting in a recovered fragment >3 kb, prewarming the elution buffer to 55°C enhances recovery efficiency.

4. Gently tap the bottom of the tube to mix, avoiding vigorous mixing.
5. OD_{600} Measurement: Take an appropriate amount of sample from the bacterial culture medium. Ensure thorough mixing to prevent measurement errors caused by cell sedimentation; Blank Calibration: Fill a cuvette with an equal volume of culture medium (uninoculated with bacteria). Place it in the spectrophotometer and perform a "zero" calibration at 600 nm wavelength to establish the baseline. Sample Measurement: Add the mixed bacterial culture to a clean cuvette, ensuring no water droplets or fingerprints on the outer surface. Insert into the spectrophotometer and read the absorbance value at 600 nm, which is the OD_{600} value.

$$\text{virions/mL} = (A_{269} - A_{320}) \times 6 \times 10^{16} / (\textit{number of bases/virion})$$

where: A_{269} is the absorbance at 269 nm; A_{320} is the absorbance at 320 nm (background correction); *number of bases/virion* is the base count of the phage genome; M13 typically has 8048 bp.

6. Do not exceed 40 mL per 50 mL centrifuge tube.
7. Overnight is acceptable.
8. Use a vortex mixer to aid dissolution.
9. The final volume ≤1.5 mL.
10. Ensure each column's concentration is half that of the preceding column.

Acknowledgments

HP is grateful for support from the National Natural Science Foundation of China (Grant No. 32201100).

References

1. Jiang P, Zhang L, Liu X, Ye C, Zhu P, Tan T, Wang D, Wang Y (2024) Tuning oxidant and antioxidant activities of ceria by anchoring copper single-site for antibacterial application. Nat Commun 15(1):1010. https://doi.org/10.1038/s41467-024-45255-6
2. Piddock LJV, Malpani R, Hennessy A (2024) Challenges and opportunities with antibiotic discovery and exploratory research. ACS Infect Dis 10(8):2445–2447. https://doi.org/10.1021/acsinfecdis.4c00530
3. Yang P, Li J, Song Z, Chen B, Li S (2025) Phage and enzyme therapies in wound infections: from lab to bedside. Chin Med J (Engl) 138(17):2102–2115. https://doi.org/10.1097/CM9.0000000000003626
4. Smith GP (1985) Filamentous fusion phage: novel expression vectors that display cloned antigens on the virion surface. Science 228(4705):1315–1317. https://doi.org/10.1126/science.4001944
5. Smith GP, Petrenko VA (1997) Phage display. Chem Rev 97(2):391–410. https://doi.org/10.1021/cr960065d
6. Zhang H, Fu L, Leiliang X, Qu C, Wu W, Wen R, Huang N, He Q, Cheng Q, Liu G,

Cheng Y (2024) Beyond the gut: the intratumoral microbiome's influence on tumorigenesis and treatment response. Cancer Commun (Lond) 44(10):1130–1167. https://doi.org/10.1002/cac2.12597
7. Fooladi S, Faramarz S, Dabiri S, Kajbafzadeh A, MH, Mehrabani M (2022) An efficient strategy to recellularization of a rat aorta scaffold: an optimized decellularization, detergent removal, and Apelin-13 immobilization. Biomater Res 26(1):46. https://doi.org/10.1186/s40824-022-00295-1
8. Koudelka KJ, Pitek AS, Manchester M, Steinmetz NF (2015) Virus-based nanoparticles as versatile nanomachines. Annu Rev Virol 2(1):379–401. https://doi.org/10.1146/annurev-virology-100114-055141

Check for updates

Chapter 8

Yeast Molecular Display for the Screening and Production of Immunological Proteins Using Nanobody as an Example

Seiji Shibasaki, Wataru Aoki and Mitsuyoshi Ueda

Abstract

Yeast molecular display is a convenient tool for developing and improving recombinant proteins and assessing their functions. Molecular display using *Saccharomyces cerevisiae* has been applied for screening valuable biochemical molecules, including antigens and antibodies. In this chapter, we describe the genetic construction of a yeast molecular display system for a nanobody and its evaluation using fluorescence microscopy and flow cytometry.

Keywords Molecular display, Cell surface, Yeast, Screening, Nanobody

1 Introduction

Microbial technologies using yeast cells have advanced considerably in recent years. For instance, progress in modeling and synthetic biology tools has accelerated the development of yeast cell factories [1]. Proteomic analyses in yeast biotechnology have enabled the identification of proteins with useful pharmaceutical functions [2, 3]. Among genetic manipulation–based technologies, cell surface engineering, or molecular display, which uses the yeast cell surface to immobilize proteins, has been developed for various purposes.

In yeast molecular display, directed evolution combined with high-throughput screening provides a convenient tool that avoids the need for protein concentration and purification [4]. The display of affinity molecules on the cell surface has also been applied to the purification of immunological molecules [5] and as bioadsorbents for toxic environmental compounds [6]. Other valuable molecules, including antigens [7] and HGF [8], have been displayed on the yeast cell surface. Moreover, yeast cells are relatively larger than bacterial cells or phages, making them suitable for producing and selecting desired clones from eukaryotic protein libraries. These yeast molecular display systems are typically based on the same anchoring

Huan Peng and Theam Soon Lim (eds.), *Biomolecular Display Technologies*, Methods in Molecular Biology, vol. 3030,
https://doi.org/10.1007/978-1-0716-5249-7_8,

mechanism, which employs α-agglutinin, an endogenous yeast cell wall protein [9]. In this chapter, we introduce a synthetic anchoring protein, 649-stalk [10], as an alternative to the conventional α-agglutinin for molecular display (Figs. 1 and 2). In addition, we describe another molecular display platform, the SpyTag/SpyCatcher system [11], adapted for yeast cell surfaces (Fig. 3). This system is derived from the CnaB2 domain of the *Streptococcus pyogenes* fibronectin-binding protein FbaB, which contains an internal isopeptide bond [12].

As a protein for display on the yeast cell surface, we focus here on nanobodies. Nanobodies are derived from immunoglobulins and correspond to the VHH domain of camelid heavy-chain antibodies [13]. Their small size (10–15 kDa) offers advantages, such as

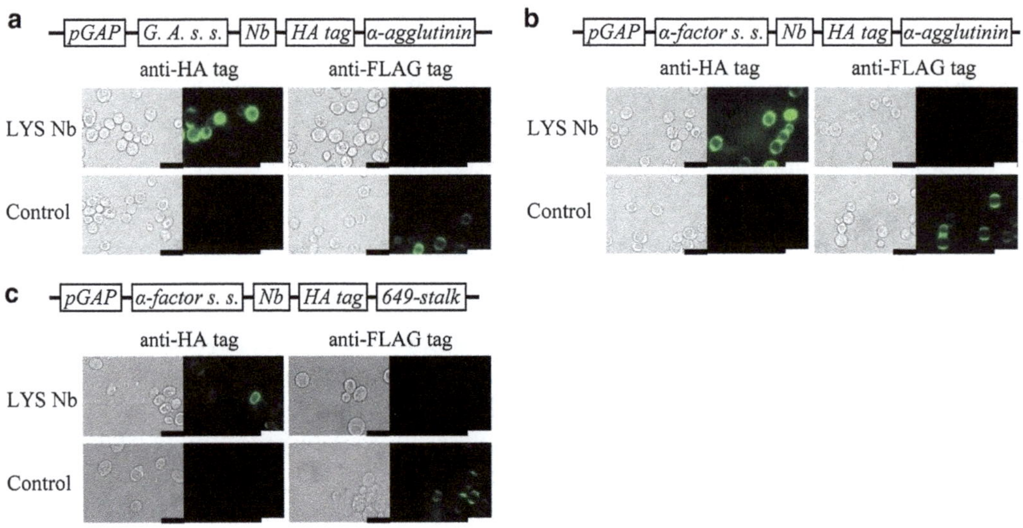

Fig. 1 Immunofluorescence labeling of yeast cells displaying lysozyme nanobody. Yeast cells were stained with either anti-HA tag mouse monoclonal antibody or anti-FLAG tag mouse monoclonal antibody as the primary antibody, followed by Alexa Fluor 488 (AF488)–conjugated anti-mouse monoclonal antibody as the secondary antibody. Gene cassettes for each *LYS Nb* display system are indicated above the micrographs (**a–c**) (*see* **Note 6**). *LYS Nb:* yeast cells with an LYS Nb–encoding plasmid. *Control:* yeast cells containing a plasmid without the nanobody sequence and with a FLAG tag instead of an HA tag. *pGAP*, glyceraldehyde-3-phosphate dehydrogenase promoter; *G.A.s.s.*, secretion signal of glucoamylase from *Rhizopus oryzae*; *α-factor s.s.*, secretion signal of mating factor α preprotein from *S. cerevisiae*; *Nb*, anti-hen egg-white lysozyme nanobody; *α-agglutinin*, 320 C-terminal amino acids of the α-agglutinin gene; *649-stalk*, synthetic anchor protein consisting of 649 amino acids. Scale bars, 10 μm. (Modified and reproduced from [16], with permission from Springer Nature) This figure shows immunofluorescence micrographs of yeast cells displaying a lysozyme nanobody (LYS Nb) using different genetic systems. Micrographs A through C visualize the presence of the nanobody via green fluorescence from Alexa Fluor 488, which targets either an HA or FLAG tag on the cell surface. The labels above each image indicate the specific gene cassettes used, featuring different promoters (pGAP), secretion signals (glucoamylase or α-factor), and anchor proteins (α-agglutinin or a synthetic 649-stalk). Control cells, which lack the nanobody sequence, show a lack of specific labeling, confirming the accuracy of the display systems.

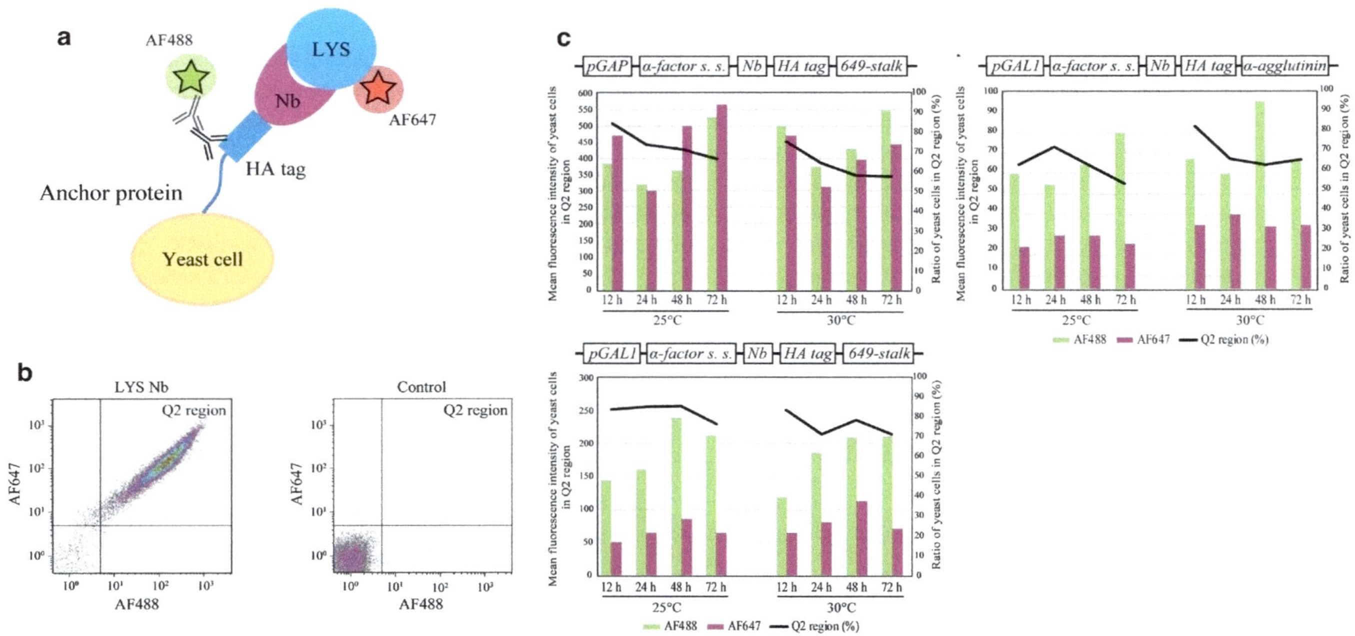

Fig. 2 Evaluation of culture conditions on display efficiency. (**a**) Schematic of lysozyme nanobody and immunofluorescent staining. Yeast cells were cultured at 25°C or 30°C for 72 h, then stained with anti-HA tag mouse monoclonal antibody and AF488-conjugated anti-mouse monoclonal antibody to quantify displayed nanobody levels. Alexa Fluor 647 (AF647)–labeled lysozyme was used to quantify functional nanobodies. *NB*, anti-hen egg-white lysozyme nanobody; *LYS*, hen egg-white lysozyme. (**b**) Representative flow cytometry analysis of yeast cells with display system 1. The Q2 region (%) shows the proportion of yeast cells with strong AF488 and AF647 signals. Bar graphs display mean fluorescence intensity in the Q2 region, and black lines indicate the ratio of yeast cells in Q2. (Modified and reproduced from [16], with permission from Springer Nature) This figure evaluates how different culture temperatures affect the display and function of a lysozyme nanobody on yeast. Panel A provides a schematic of the experimental setup, where the total amount of nanobody is measured using AF488-labeled antibodies (targeting the HA tag), while the amount of functional, binding-capable nanobody is measured using AF647-labeled lysozyme. Panel B presents flow cytometry data for display system 1 at 25°C and 30°C. The Q2 region of the scatter plots identifies the percentage of cells that successfully display functional nanobodies, while the accompanying bar graphs compare the mean fluorescence intensity and the ratio of cells in this high-performing population across the two temperatures.

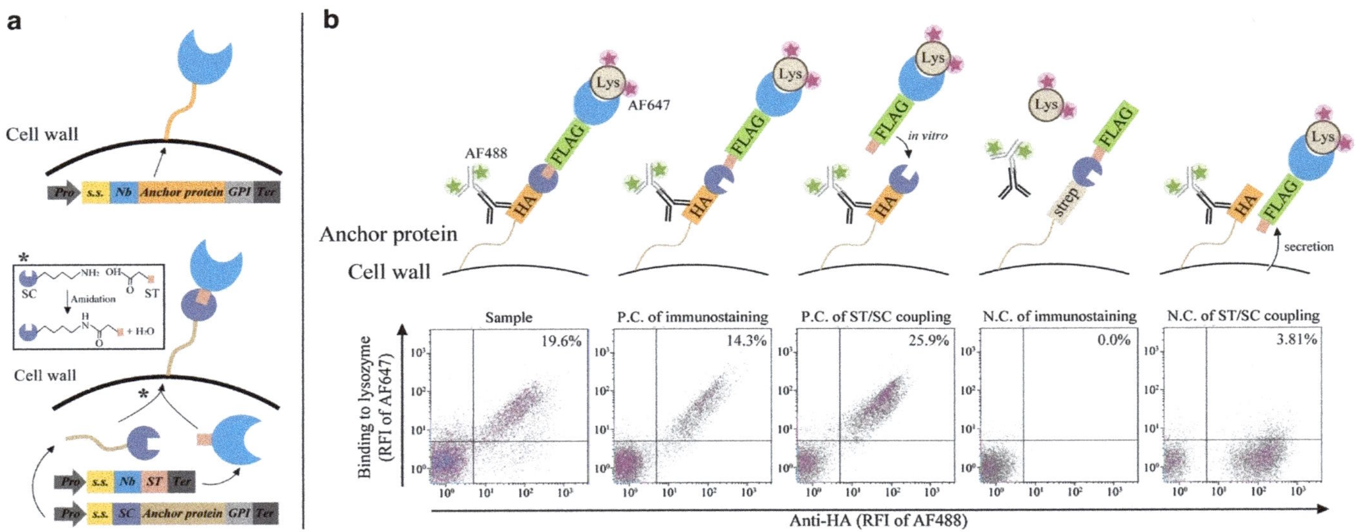

Fig. 3 Yeast surface display of nanobodies generated by SpyTag/SpyCatcher-based protein ligation. (**a**) Schematic of conventional (upper) and SpyTag/SpyCatcher-based (lower) yeast surface display. The inset shows intracellular isopeptide bond formation between SpyCatcher (Lys31) and SpyTag (Asp117). (**b**) Confirmation of anti-lysozyme nanobody surface display via SpyTag/SpyCatcher ligation in vivo and in vitro. Samples were stained with mouse anti-HA tag antibody, AF488-conjugated anti-mouse antibody, and AF647-labeled lysozyme. Ratios of yeast cells are indicated in the upper right (UR) of each graph. Data represent two independent experiments. *Pro*, promoter; *s.s.*, secretion signal; *Nb*, nanobody; *GPI*, glycosylphosphatidylinositol attachment signal; *Ter*, terminator; *ST*, SpyTag; *SC*, SpyCatcher; *N.C.*, negative control; *Lys*, hen egg-white lysozyme; *RFI*, relative fluorescence intensity. (Modified and reproduced from [17], with permission from Springer Nature) This figure illustrates a method for displaying nanobodies on yeast using SpyTag/SpyCatcher ligation. Panel A compares the conventional display method with the SpyTag/SpyCatcher system, where an intracellular isopeptide bond forms between the two components to link the nanobody to the cell surface. Panel B confirms the success of this ligation both in vivo and in vitro using flow cytometry. The graphs plot total nanobody display (AF488) against functional lysozyme binding (AF647), with the upper-right (UR) quadrant indicating the percentage of cells successfully displaying functional nanobodies.

improved penetration into tumors and inflamed tissues compared to the penetrability of larger antibodies, such as human IgG1 (160 kDa) [13–15]. In this chapter, we also describe methods to evaluate nanobody display and antigen binding using fluorescence microscopy and flow cytometry [16, 17].

2 Materials

2.1 Strain

1. *Escherichia coli* DH5α [F⁻ *Φ80lacZ*Δ*M*15 Δ(*lacZYA-argF*) *U169 endA1 recA1 hsdR17*(r_K^-, m_K^+) *deoR supE44 thi-1* λ⁻ gyr*A96 relA1*]
2. *Saccharomyces cerevisiae* BY4741 (*MATa, his3*Δ*1, leu2*Δ*0, met15*Δ*0, ura3*Δ*0*)
3. *Pichia pastoris* strain GS115 (*his4*Δ *Mut*⁺)

2.2 Vectors

1. *S. cerevisiae* surface display vector pULD1 [7, 16, 17]
2. pPIC9K *Pichia* Vector (Thermo Fisher Scientific, MA, USA)

2.3 Media and Buffers

1. Luria–Bertani (LB) media: 1% (w/v) tryptone, 0.5% (w/v) yeast extract, and 1% (w/v) sodium chloride.
2. Yeast extract–peptone–dextrose (YPD) medium: 1% (w/v) yeast extract, 2% (w/v) glucose, and 2% (w/v) peptone.
3. Synthetic dextrose medium (SDC glucose + HML): 0.67% (w/v) yeast nitrogen base without amino acids, 2% (w/v) glucose, 0.5% (w/v) casamino acids, 0.002% (w/v) L-histidine, 0.003% (w/v) L-leucine, 0.003% (w/v) L-methionine, adjusted to pH 6.0 with 1 N NaOH.
4. Minimal dextrose solid medium: 1.34% (w/v) yeast nitrogen base without amino acids, 2% (w/v) glucose, and 2% (w/v) agar.
5. Buffered glycerol-complex (BMGY) medium: 1% (w/v) yeast extract, 2% (w/v) peptone, 1% (w/v) glycerol, 0.1 M potassium phosphate buffer pH 6.0, 2.68% (w/v) yeast nitrogen base without amino acids and 400 μg/mL biotin.
6. Buffered methanol-complex Medium (BMMY) medium: 1% (w/v) yeast extract, 2% (w/v) peptone 0.1 M potassium phosphate buffer pH 6.0, 2.68% (w/v) yeast nitrogen base without amino acids, 400 μg/mL biotin and 0.5% (v/v) methanol.

2.4 Reagents and Tubes

1. In-Fusion Cloning Kit (Takara Bio USA Inc., Shiga, Japan).
2. FastGene Gel/PCR Extraction Kit (NIPPON Genetics).
3. EZ Yeast Transformation II Kit (Zymo Research, Irvine, CA, USA).

4. Restriction enzyme, SacI (Toyobo, Osaka, Japan).
5. Amicon Ultra-15 Centrifugal Filters Ultracel-3K (Merck Millipore, Burlington, MA, USA).
6. Alexa Fluor 647 Microscale Protein Labelling Kit (Invitrogen Corporation, Carlsbad, CA, USA).
7. Mouse monoclonal anti-HA-tag (Nacalai Tesque, Kyoto, Japan) and mouse monoclonal anti-FLAG M2 antibodies (Sigma-Aldrich) were used.
8. Alexa Fluor 488 (AF488)-conjugated goat anti-mouse IgG secondary antibodies were purchased from Invitrogen, CA, USA).
9. MinElute PCR Purification Kit (QIAGEN, Hilden, Germany).

2.5 Equipment

1. Rotary shaker (WKN-2210, Wakenyaku, Kyoto, Japan).
2. Inverted microscope (IX71, Olympus, Tokyo, Japan). Green fluorescence from AF488 can be detected using a U-MNIBA2 mirror unit with a BP470–490 excitation filter, a DM505 dichroic mirror, and a BA 510-–550 emission filter (Olympus). Alternatively, a confocal laser scanning fluorescence microscope equipped with 488 and 561 nm lasers can be used.
3. Flow cytometer (equipped with 488 and 561 nm lasers).

3 Methods

3.1 Simple Molecular Display of a Nanobody on the Yeast Cell Surface

1. Synthesize DNA fragments of the improved α-factor secretion signal [18], anti-hen egg-white lysozyme nanobody cAbLys3 [19], and 649-stalk (649 amino acids) [10] using a commercial gene synthesis service, e.g., gBlocks Gene Fragment (Integrated DNA Technologies, Coralville, IA, USA).
2. Ligate the above gene fragments using an In-Fusion Cloning Kit (*see* **Note 1**).
3. Introduce the ligated gene into competent *E. coli* DH5α cells.
4. Cultivate transformed *E. coli* in LB medium containing 100 μg/mL ampicillin.
5. After confirming the appropriate DNA sequence in the cloned plasmid, purify the constructed plasmid using a spin column (FastGene Gel/PCR Extraction Kit).
6. To introduce the constructed plasmid into *S. cerevisiae* BY4741 (host strain for cell surface display of nanobodies), prepare competent cells using the Frozen-EZ Yeast Transformation II Kit (*see* **Note 2**).

7. Select transformants on synthetic dextrose complete (SDC) glucose + HML solid medium containing 2% (w/v) agar.
8. Preculture selected colonies in liquid SDC glucose + HML medium at 30°C and 250 rpm for 24 h.
9. Measure the optical density of the preculture at 600 nm (OD600) and initiate main cultures at OD600 = 0.1.

3.2 Molecular Display of a Nanobody on the Yeast Cell Surface Using the SpyTag/Spy Catcher System

1. Synthesize DNA fragments of the secretion signal, anti-hen egg-white lysozyme nanobody cAbLys3, and 649-stalk as described in Sect. 3.1.
2. Construct a plasmid for the secretory production of lysozyme nanobody fused with SpyTag. Separately, insert the Spy Catcher sequence between the secretion signal and the anchor protein in the plasmid pULD1. Introduce this pULD1-based plasmid into *S. cerevisiae* as described in Sect. 3.1.
3. Digest the constructed pPIC9K-based plasmid with SacI.
4. Purify the digested plasmid using a MinElute PCR Purification Kit.
5. Introduce the purified plasmid into *Pichia pastoris* using the Frozen-EZ Yeast Transformation II Kit.
6. Screen transformants on minimal dextrose solid medium.
7. Cultivate selected colonies in BMGY medium at 30°C and 250 rpm for 24 h.
8. Transfer the cells to BMMY medium and culture at 30°C and 250 rpm for another 24 h.
9. Centrifuge the cultured BMMY medium to collect the supernatant (*see* **Note 3**).
10. Filter the supernatant for in vitro isopeptide formation using 0.5 μm filters, and concentrate it with Amicon Ultra-15 Centrifugal Filters (Ultracel-3K) at 8000 × *g* for 60 min.
11. Add 10 mL of phosphate-buffered saline (PBS) to the Amicon Ultracel-3K unit and centrifuge at 8000 × *g* for 60 min. Repeat the buffer replacement procedure twice.

3.3 Fluorescence Labeling

3.3.1 Immunofluorescence Staining of Yeast Cell

1. Measure OD600 at each sampling point; approximately 4.5×10^6 cells correspond to an OD600 of 0.3 (OD600 of $1 \approx 1.5 \times 10^7$ yeast cells/mL).
2. Centrifuge cells at 1000 × *g* for 5 min, then wash once with phosphate-buffered saline (PBS, pH 7.2).

3. Resuspend cells in PBS containing 1% bovine serum albumin (BSA; Sigma-Aldrich, MO, USA) and incubate for 30 min at room temperature.
4. Add mouse monoclonal anti-HA tag antibody or mouse monoclonal anti-FLAG M2 antibody at a 1:500 dilution.
5. Incubate the cells at room temperature with gentle shaking on a rotary shaker for 1 h.
6. Wash cells with PBS, then incubate with Alexa Fluor 488 (AF488)-conjugated goat anti-mouse IgG secondary antibody (Invitrogen, CA, USA) diluted 1:1000. Incubate at room temperature with gentle shaking for 1.5 h.
7. Wash cells with PBS and use for microscopic analysis (*see* **Note 4**).

3.3.2 Labeling of Lysozyme

1. Label lysozyme using an Alexa Fluor 647 Microscale Protein Labeling Kit to generate Alexa Fluor 647 (AF647)-labeled lysozyme.
2. Prepare 1 M sodium bicarbonate solution by dissolving in 1 mL deionized water.
3. Transfer 50 μL of a 1 mg/mL lysozyme solution to a reaction tube. Add 5 μL of 1 M sodium bicarbonate and mix by pipetting.
4. Dissolve one vial of Alexa Fluor 647 dye in 10 μL deionized water by pipetting.
5. Add 3 μL of the reactive dye solution to the lysozyme mixture and mix by pipetting.
6. Incubate the reaction for 15 min at room temperature.
7. To separate labeled protein from unreacted dye, load 50 μL of the conjugation reaction mixture onto the center of the resin bed in a spin column.
8. Centrifuge the column with collection tube at 16,000 × *g* for 1 min.
9. Recover purified AF647-labeled protein in PBS from the collection tube.
10. During immunofluorescence staining, add AF647-labeled lysozyme to yeast cells together with the secondary antibody (see Sect. 3.3.1) at a 1:500 dilution (*see* **Note 5**).
11. Wash cells with PBS and resuspend in PBS before flow cytometric analysis.

4 Notes

1. Place DNA sequences for the secretion signal, nanobody, and anchor protein in this order under the promoter.
2. For yeast cell preparation, preculture to mid-log phase in YPD liquid medium at 30°C. Follow the manufacturer's instructions for yeast transformation. The kit suggested here is one option; any commercially available kit may be used.
3. SDS-PAGE is a useful method to confirm secretory production of the anti-hen egg-white lysozyme nanobody by *P. pastoris*. Use culture medium from both nanobody-producing and control cells.
4. Store samples at 4°C before microscopic observation. This staining process can also confirm display of the anchor protein in the SpyTag/SpyCatcher system (Fig. 3).
5. Samples may also be observed under a fluorescence microscope; however, store them in a cool (4°C), dark place protected from light.
6. These experiments examine the function of secretion signal sequences and anchor proteins in displaying lysozyme nanobody on the yeast cell surface.

References

1. Borodina I, Nielsen J (2014) Advances in metabolic engineering of yeast *Saccharomyces cerevisiae* for production of chemicals. Biotechnol J 9(5):609–620
2. Aoki W, Ueda T, Tatsukami Y, Kitahara N, Morisaka H et al (2013) Time-course proteomic profile of *Candida albicans* during adaptation to a fetal serum. Pathog Dis 67(1):67–75
3. Shibasaki S, Aoki W, Nomura T, Karasaki M, Sewaki T, Ueda M (2014) Evaluation of Mdh1 protein as an antigenic candidate for a vaccine against candidiasis. Biocontrol Sci 19(1):51–55
4. Ueda M (2016) Establishment of cell surface engineering and its development. Biosci Biotechnol Biochem 80(7):1243–1253
5. Shibasaki S, Kawabata A, Ishii J, Yagi S, Kadonosono T et al (2007) Construction of a novel synergistic system for production and recovery of secreted recombinant proteins by the cell surface engineering. Appl Microbiol Biotechnol 75(4):821–828
6. Shibasaki S, Ueda M (2014) Bioadsorption strategies with yeast molecular display technology. Biocontrol Sci 19(4):157–164
7. Shibasaki S, Aoki W, Nomura T, Miyoshi A, Tafuku S et al (2013) An oral vaccine against candidiasis generated by a yeast molecular display system. Pathog Dis 69(3):262–268
8. Shibasaki S, Nakatani Y, Taketani K, Karasaki M, Matsui K et al (2022) Construction of HGF-displaying yeast by cell surface engineering. Microorganisms 10(7):1373
9. Shibasaki S, Ueda M (2023) Progress of molecular display technology using *Saccharomyces cerevisiae* to achieve sustainable development goals. Microorganisms 11(1):125
10. McMahon C, Baier AS, Pascolutti R, Wegrecki M, Zheng S et al (2018) Yeast surface display platform for rapid discovery of conformationally selective nanobodies. Nat Struct Mol Biol 25(3):289–296
11. Gallus S, Peschke T, Paulsen M, Burgahn T, Niemeyer CM, Rabe KS (2020) Surface display of complex enzymes by in situ SpyCatcher-SpyTag interaction. ChemBioChem 21(15):2126–2131
12. Zakeri B, Fierer JO, Celik E, Chittock EC, Schwarz-Linek U et al (2012) Peptide tag forming a rapid covalent bond to a protein

through engineering a bacterial adhesin. Proc Natl Acad Sci U S A 109(12):E690–E697
13. Koch-Nolte F (2024) Nanobody-based heavy chain antibodies and chimeric antibodies. Immunol Rev 328(1):466–472
14. Saelens X, Schepens B (2021) Single-domain antibodies make a difference. Science 371(6530):681–682
15. Salvador JP, Vilaplana L, Marco MP (2019) Nanobody: outstanding features for diagnostic and therapeutic applications. Anal Bioanal Chem 411(9):1703–1713
16. Kajiwara K, Aoki W, Ueda M (2020) Evaluation of the yeast surface display system for screening of functional nanobodies. AMB Express 10(1):51
17. Kajiwara K, Aoki W, Koike N, Ueda M (2021) Development of a yeast cell surface display method using the SpyTag/SpyCatcher system. Sci Rep 11(1):11059
18. Rakestraw JA, Sazinsky SL, Piatesi A, Antipov E, Wittrup KD (2009) Directed evolution of a secretory leader for the improved expression of heterologous proteins and full-length antibodies in *Saccharomyces cerevisiae*. Biotechnol Bioeng 103(6):1192–1201
19. Lauwereys M, Arbabi Ghahroudi M, Desmyter A, Kinne J, Hölzer W et al (1998) Potent enzyme inhibitors derived from dromedary heavy-chain antibodies. EMBO J 17(13):3512–3520

Part III

Ligand Discovery and Application

Check for updates

Chapter 9

Application of Phage-Displayed Peptide Library for Epitope Mapping

Belle Li Ling, Angela Chiew Wen Ch'ng, Yee Siew Choong and Theam Soon Lim

Abstract

Antibodies, central components of the adaptive immune system, possess the remarkable ability to specifically recognize and bind to foreign substances known as antigens. This recognition occurs through the interaction of the antibody's antigen-binding site, or paratope, with a specific region on the antigen called the epitope. Understanding the precise nature of these interactions, particularly the identification and characterization of epitopes, is of paramount importance for a wide array of biomedical applications. The mapping of antibody epitopes, the process of experimentally identifying the binding site of an antibody on its target antigen, provides critical insights into antibody function and its diverse applications. Peptide phage display provides a convenient and rapid method to identify epitopes of specific monoclonal antibodies. This protocol highlights the use of a peptide phage display library for epitope identification of a recombinant monoclonal antibody.

Keywords Epitope mapping, Biopanning, Peptide library, Monoclonal antibodies, Phage display

1 Introduction

Understanding how antibodies recognize their targets is essential in immunology, diagnostics, and therapeutic development. Central to this understanding is the identification of epitopes—the specific molecular regions on an antigen that are bound by antibodies. Epitope mapping provides a detailed view of these interaction sites, offering insights into immune recognition and antigenic variability.

Epitopes can be linear or conformational [1]. Linear epitopes consist of a continuous sequence of amino acids in the primary structure of the antigen, often accessible in denatured or unfolded forms. Mapping of linear epitopes can often be accomplished by aligning selected peptide sequences directly to the antigen's primary amino acid sequence, revealing exact or homologous binding sites. On the other hand, conformational epitopes are composed of amino

Huan Peng and Theam Soon Lim (eds.), *Biomolecular Display Technologies*, Methods in Molecular Biology, vol. 3030,
https://doi.org/10.1007/978-1-0716-5249-7_9,

acid residues that are distant in the primary sequence but brought together by the antigen's three-dimensional structure. These are more challenging to identify as the corresponding mimotopes may not share sequence similarity with the actual binding site but instead replicate key structural or chemical features [2, 3].

Methods to map epitopes include X-ray crystallography of antigen–antibody complexes, mutagenesis studies and peptide scanning arrays, but these methods can be time-consuming, low-throughput, or require prior structural knowledge [1]. In contrast, phage display technology offers a rapid, high-throughput and versatile platform for epitope mapping, particularly well-suited for identifying both linear and conformational epitopes via the selection of peptide mimotopes.

In phage display, a highly diverse library of peptides, encoded by a phagemid vector, is expressed on the surface of filamentous bacteriophage particles. This library is screened against the target antibody, specifically binding phage is amplified in bacterial cells and used for subsequent rounds of screening. This is termed biopanning and allows for the enrichment of phage carrying specific peptide binders to the epitope [4]. The selected peptide sequences can then be easily determined by sequencing the phagemid, analyzed for conserved motifs and interpreted to infer the probable binding region on the antigen. When multiple peptides across independently selected clones converge upon a similar motif, this motif is considered a strong candidate for mimicking the natural epitope [1].

Phage-displayed peptide libraries have been successfully used to map epitopes for a wide range of targets including viral protein, bacterial toxin, and tumor antigen [5–7]. This technique not only aids in characterizing antibody–antigen interactions but also facilitates the design of epitope-based vaccines, antibody therapeutics, and diagnostic assays.

This chapter describes the methodology for screening an in-house phage-displayed 20-mer peptide library through biopanning to identify antibody-binding peptide sequences for epitope mapping applications. Figure 1 highlights the process involved in epitope mapping of a monoclonal antibody using peptide phage display.

2 Materials

2.1 Phage-Displayed Peptide Library Packaging

1. 40% (w/v) Glucose: 40 g D-(+)-glucose in 100 mL of dH_2O, autoclave and store at 4°C.
2. 50 mg/mL Ampicillin stock solution: 2.5 g ampicillin sodium salt in 50 mL of 50% (v/v) ethanol, filter sterilize and store at −20°C.
3. M13KO7 helper phage.
4. 80% (v/v) Glycerol: 40 mL glycerol in 10 mL dH_2O, autoclave and store at room temperature.

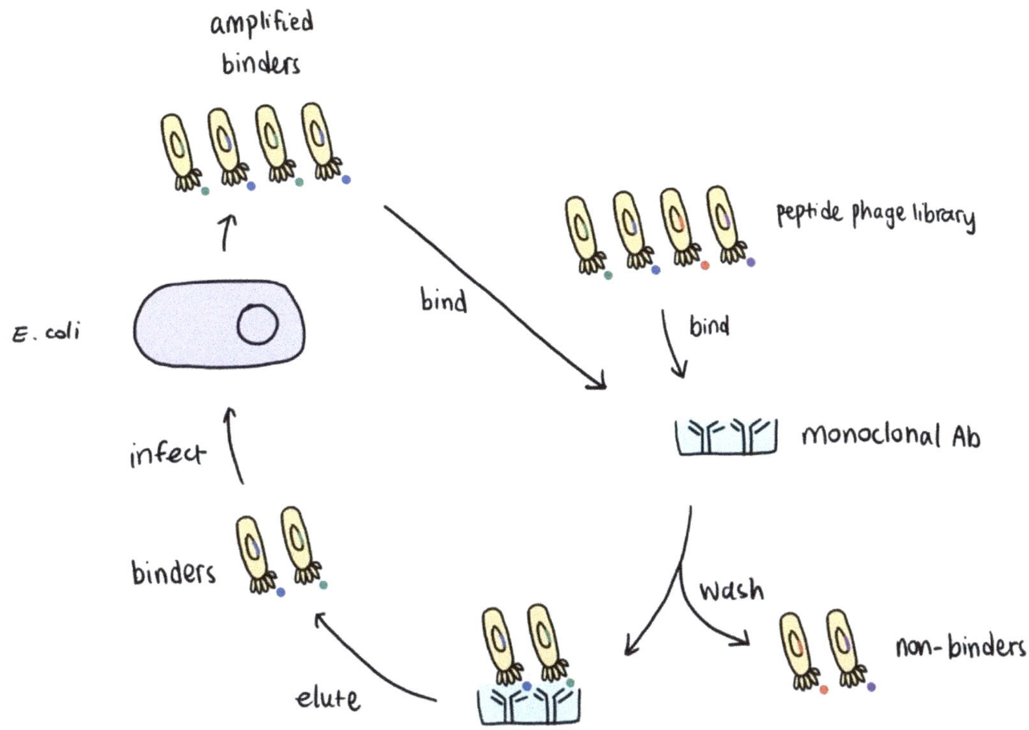

Fig. 1 Biopanning process for epitope mapping

5. 30 mg/mL Kanamycin stock solution: 1.5 g kanamycin sulphate in 50 mL dH_2O, filter sterilize and store at −20°C.
6. PEG/NaCl: 200 g polyethylene glycol 6000 (PEG 6000) and 146 g NaCl in 1 L dH_2O, autoclave and store at room temperature.
7. 10× Phosphate-buffered saline (PBS), pH 7.4: 8 g NaCl, 0.2 g KCl, 1.44 g $Na_2HPO_4{\cdot}2H_2O$, 0.24 g KH_2PO_4 in 1 L dH_2O, autoclave and store at room temperature.

2.2 Target Antibody Expression

1. 40% (w/v) Glucose: 40 g D-(+)-glucose in 100 mL of dH_2O, autoclave and store at 4°C.
2. 50 mg/mL Ampicillin stock solution: 2.5 g ampicillin sodium salt in 50 mL of 50% (v/v) ethanol, filter sterilize and store at −20°C.
3. 100 mM Isopropyl β-D-1-thiogalactopyranoside (IPTG) solution: 0.238 g IPTG in 10 mL dH_2O, filter sterilize and store at −20°C.
4. 1× TES buffer: 42.8 g sucrose, 0.047 g EDTA disodium salt, 6.05 g Tris base in 250 mL dH_2O, adjust pH to 8.0, autoclave and store at 4°C.
5. Lysis buffer: 6.9 g NaH_2PO_4, 17.54 g NaCl, 0.68 g imidazole in 1 L dH_2O, adjust pH to 7.4, autoclave and store at room temperature.

6. Binding buffer: 2.76 g NaH_2PO_4, 29.22 g NaCl, 1.362 g imidazole in 1 L dH_2O, adjust pH to 7.4, autoclave and store at room temperature.
7. Elution buffer: 2.76 g NaH_2PO_4, 29.22 g NaCl, 34 g imidazole in 1 L dH_2O, adjust pH to 7.4, autoclave and store at room temperature.
8. Ni-NTA agarose resin (Qiagen, Germany).
9. Protein assay CBB solution (Nacalai Tesque, Japan).

2.3 Polyclonal Peptide Selection

2.3.1 Biopanning of Peptide Library

1. High-binding 96-well Stripwell polystyrene microplates (Corning, USA).
2. 10× Phosphate-buffered saline (PBS), pH 7.4: 8 g NaCl, 0.2 g KCl, 1.44 g $Na_2HPO_4{\cdot}2H_2O$, 0.24 g KH_2PO_4 in 1 L dH_2O, autoclave and store at room temperature.
3. Maxibinding 5 mL Immunotubes (SPL, South Korea).
4. 0.1% PBST: 1 mL Tween 20 in 1 L 1× PBS.
5. 2% PTM: 2 g skim milk in 100 mL 0.1% PBST.
6. 2 M Glycine, pH 2.2: 1.5 g glycine in 100 mL dH_2O, adjust pH to 2.2 with HCl.
7. 1 M Tris-HCl, pH 9.1: 12.11 g Tris in 100 mL dH_2O, adjust pH to 9.1 with HCl.
8. TG1 electrocompetent cells.
9. 40% (w/v) Glucose: 40 g D-(+)-glucose in 100 mL of dH_2O, autoclave and store at 4°C.
10. 50 mg/mL Ampicillin stock solution: 2.5 g ampicillin sodium salt in 50 mL of 50% (v/v) ethanol, filter sterilize and store at −20°C.
11. M13KO7 helper phage.
12. 30 mg/mL Kanamycin stock solution: 1.5 g kanamycin sulphate in 50 mL dH_2O, filter sterilize and store at −20°C.
13. PEG/NaCl: 200 g polyethylene glycol 6000 (PEG 6000) and 146 g NaCl in 1 L dH_2O, autoclave and store at room temperature.

2.3.2 Phage Titration

1. 10× Phosphate-buffered saline (PBS), pH 7.4: 8 g NaCl, 0.2 g KCl, 1.44 g $Na_2HPO_4{\cdot}2H_2O$, 0.24 g KH_2PO_4 in 1 L dH_2O, autoclave and store at room temperature.
2. TG1 electrocompetent cells.
3. 2×YT/glu/amp agar plate: 15.5 g of 2×YT and 7.5 g of agar in 100 mL dH_2O, autoclave, add 2% (v/v) glucose and 100 μg/mL ampicillin.

4. 2×YT/kan agar plate: 15.5 g of 2×YT and 7.5 g of agar in 100 mL dH_2O, autoclave, add 60 µg/mL kanamycin.

2.3.3 Polyclonal Peptide Phage ELISA

1. High-binding 96-well Stripwell polystyrene microplates (Corning, USA).
2. 10× Phosphate-buffered saline (PBS), pH 7.4: 8 g NaCl, 0.2 g KCl, 1.44 g $Na_2HPO_4 \cdot 2H_2O$, 0.24 g KH_2PO_4 in 1 L dH_2O, autoclave and store at room temperature.
3. 1 mg/mL Bovine serum albumin (BSA) solution: 1 mg lyophilized BSA in 1 mL 1× PBS, store at 4°C for short-term use or −20°C for long-term use.
4. 0.1% PBST: 1 mL Tween 20 in 1 L PBS.
5. 2% PTM: 2 g skim milk in 100 mL PBST.
6. Anti-M13 horseradish peroxidase (HRP): prepare 1:1000 dilution in 2% PTM before use.
7. 2,2'-Azino-bis(3-ethylbenzothiazoline-6-sulponic acid) (ABTS) solution (Roche, USA): prepare buffer by dissolving 0.836 g ABTS buffer powder in 50 mL sterilized dH_2O, then dissolve one ABTS tablet in the buffer completely and store at 4°C in the dark.

2.4 Monoclonal Peptide Selection

2.4.1 Isolation of Monoclonal Peptide Clones

1. 10× Phosphate-buffered saline (PBS), pH 7.4: 8 g NaCl, 0.2 g KCl, 1.44 g $Na_2HPO_4 \cdot 2H_2O$, 0.24 g KH_2PO_4 in 1 L dH_2O, autoclave and store at room temperature.
2. TG1 electrocompetent cell.
3. 2×YT/glu/amp plate: 15.5 g 2×YT and 7.5 g agar in 500 mL dH_2O, autoclave and add 2% glucose and 100 µg/mL ampicillin.
4. 40% (w/v) Glucose: 40 g D-(+)-glucose in 100 mL of dH_2O, autoclave and store at 4 °C.
5. 50 mg/mL Ampicillin stock solution: 2.5 g ampicillin sodium salt in 50 mL of 50% (v/v) ethanol, filter sterilize and store at −20°C.
6. M13KO7 helper phage.
7. 30 mg/mL Kanamycin stock solution: 1.5 g kanamycin sulphate in 50 mL dH_2O, filter sterilize and store at −20°C.

2.4.2 Monoclonal Peptide Phage ELISA

1. High-binding 96-well Microlon ELISA plates (Greiner Bio-One, Austria).
2. 0.1% PBST: 1 mL Tween 20 in 1 L PBS.
3. 2% PTM: 2 g skim milk in 100 mL PBST.
4. Anti-M13 horseradish peroxidase (HRP): prepare 1:1000 dilution in 2% PTM before use.

Table 1
Primer sequence for the amplification of peptide sequence in colony PCR

Primer name	Primer Sequence
LMB3 Fw	5′-CAGGAAACAGCTATGAC-3′
p3 Rv	5′-GTTAGCGTAACGATCTAA-3′

5. 2,2'-Azino-bis(3-ethylbenzothiazoline-6-sulponic acid) (ABTS) solution (Roche, USA): prepare buffer by dissolving 0.836 g ABTS buffer powder in 50 mL sterilized dH_2O, then dissolve one ABTS tablet in the buffer completely and store at 4°C in the dark.

2.4.3 Colony PCR

1. DreamTaq DNA polymerase (Thermo Scientific, USA).
2. 10× DreamTaq buffer (Thermo Scientific, USA).
3. Forward and reverse primers for the amplification of peptide sequence (*see* Table 1).
4. 10 mM dNTP mixture.
5. Agarose.
6. 10× TBE buffer, pH 8.0: 108 g Tris, 55 g boric acid, and 7.4 g EDTA in 1 L dH_2O, autoclave and store at room temperature.

3 Methods

3.1 Phage-Displayed Peptide Library Packaging

The peptide library used for this protocol is based on a 20-mer peptide phagemid library developed previously. The library design utilizes a 20-mer random peptide sequence introduced between the pelB leader peptide and the pIII protein in a phagemid setup. The peptide insert for the peptide library consists of 20 repeats of NNK [8]. However, this library is a phagemid-based system instead of the conventional phage vector system utilized by the Ph.D.-12™ (New England Biolabs) library. Nevertheless, this protocol can be adopted for phage-based peptide libraries with changes to the packaging and rescue protocols following the protocol provided by the supplier.

1. Thaw a 1 mL library stock and culture it in 200 mL of prewarmed 2×YT broth with 2% glucose and 100 μg/mL ampicillin. Shake the culture at 200 rpm, 37°C until OD_{600} reaches 0.5 (*see* **Note 1**).
2. Take 100 mL of the culture and add 2×10^{11} CFU of M13KO7 helper phage (*see* **Note 2**). Incubate the infected culture at 37°C for 30 min. To make glycerol stock of the remaining culture, incubate it at 37°C, 200 rpm for 2 h, centrifuge at 7000× *g* for 10 min, and resuspend the cell pellet in 10 mL fresh 2×YT

(*see* **Note 3**). Add 2% glucose, 100 µg/mL ampicillin and 15% glycerol to the culture and aliquot it into cryotubes with 1 mL each. Keep the glycerol stock at −80°C.

3. Centrifuge the infected culture at 3000×*g* for 10 min and resuspend the cell pellet in 100 mL of 2×YT medium with 0.1% glucose, 100 µg/mL ampicillin, and 60 µg/mL kanamycin. Incubate overnight at 30°C with shaking at 180 rpm for phage packaging.
4. Centrifuge the overnight culture at 7000×*g* for 10 min and transfer the phage-containing supernatant into clean new tubes.
5. Add 0.25 vol of PEG/NaCl to the supernatant and incubate on ice for 1 h.
6. Centrifuge the supernatant at 10,000×*g* for 30 min at 4°C to pellet the phage (*see* **Note 4**). Resuspend the phage pellet in 4 mL PBS.
7. Aliquot the phage into 1.5 mL microcentrifuge tubes and centrifuge at 13,000 rpm for 10 min to pellet any bacterial debris and insoluble contaminants. Transfer the supernatant into new tubes and keep at 4°C.

3.2 Target Antibody Expression

This protocol is based on the use of recombinant monoclonal antibodies as the target for biopanning. The recombinant monoclonal antibody will first be expressed and purified. A suitable expression system should be chosen to ensure proper folding and functionality of the antibody. The antibody is also typically fused with a purification tag to allow for easy purification via affinity chromatography. The purified antibody is then quantified and coated on a surface for phage biopanning. In this protocol, a single-chain variable fragment (ScFv) monoclonal antibody fused with a His-tag is used as the target antibody for epitope mapping (*see* **Note 5**).

1. Culture the glycerol stock of the transformed cell with the expression plasmid harboring the antibody gene in 5 mL 2× YT with 2% glucose and 100 µg/mL ampicillin. Shake the culture at 200 rpm, 37°C overnight.
2. Subculture the overnight culture in 500 mL of 2×YT with 2% glucose and 100 µg/mL ampicillin. Shake at 200 rpm, 37°C until OD_{600} reaches 0.6–0.8.
3. Add 1 mM of IPTG to induce expression. Incubate the culture at 30°C overnight with shaking at 160 rpm.
4. Centrifuge the cell culture at 7000×*g* for 10 min and resuspend the pellet in 2 mL of ice-cold 1× TES buffer. Add another 3 mL ice-cold 0.2× TES buffer and incubate on ice for 1 h (*see* **Note 6**).
5. Centrifuge at 7000×*g* for 10 min and collect the periplasmic fraction in a new tube.

6. Wash the Ni-NTA column with five CV dH_2O and equilibrate with five CV binding buffer (*see* **Note 7**).
7. Incubate the periplasmic fraction in the column with rotation for 1 h (*see* **Note 8**).
8. Wash the column with five CV of binding buffer to remove nonspecifically or weakly bound proteins.
9. Elute the column with 1 mL of elution buffer. Repeat five times and collect each elution in a separate 1.5 mL microcentrifuge tube (*see* **Note 9**).
10. Run SDS-PAGE with the eluted fractions to confirm the presence of the target antibody.
11. Determine the concentration of the eluted antibody via Bradford assay (*see* **Note 10**).

3.3 Peptide Selection

The peptide phage library will have a diverse set of peptide-displaying phages. The selection process will enrich peptide motifs based on their ability to bind to the target antibody.

3.3.1 Biopanning of Peptide Library

Binders of a target can be screened from a library through biopanning. Multiple rounds of biopanning with increasing selection stringency are done to enrich a population of phage displaying peptide binders. Generally, three to five rounds are sufficient to achieve reasonable enrichment, but additional rounds can be carried out if a clear enrichment pattern is not visible. The amount and specificity of eluted phage from each round is validated via phage titration and polyclonal ELISA, respectively.

1. Coat a microtiter well with 10 μg of target antibody in PBS at a final volume of 100 μL. Shake the well for 10 min and incubate at 4°C overnight.
2. Block an immunotube with 2% PTM and incubate at 4°C overnight.
3. Wash the microtiter well and immunotube with 0.1% PBST three times (*see* **Note 11**).
4. Block the microtiter well with 300 μL of 2% PTM with shaking (~600 rpm) for 1 h.
5. Add 10^{11} CFU of phage library to the immunotube and adjust the volume to 100 μL with PBS. Then, add 100 μL of 2% PTM and incubate with rotation for 1 h.
6. Wash the microtiter well with 0.1% PBST three times.
7. Transfer the preincubated library from the immunotube to the microtiter well. Incubate with shaking for 2 h.
8. Wash the microtiter well with 0.1% PBST three times to remove unbound or weakly bound phage. Increase the washing steps by three times for every subsequent round of panning.

9. Elute bound phage with 100 μL 0.2 M glycine, pH 2.2 with shaking for 10 min, then immediately neutralize with 10 μL 1 M Tris-HCl, pH 9.1 to achieve pH 7.
10. Take 10 μL of eluted phage to perform phage titration. Infect 2 mL of TG1 culture at OD_{600} ~0.5 with the remaining phage in a 50 mL Falcon tube at 37°C for 30 min.
11. Incubate the phage-infected TG1 culture at 37°C for 30 min, then supply the culture with 2% glucose and 100 μg/mL ampicillin. Continue incubating the culture at 37°C with 200 rpm shaking for 2 h.
12. Dilute the TG1 culture with 2 mL 2×YT medium, mix well and take out 2 mL of diluted culture to be prepared as stock (*see* **Note 12**).
13. Infect the remaining 2 mL of culture with 10^{10} CFU of M13KO7 helper phage. Incubate at 37°C for 30 min.
14. Centrifuge the culture at 9000×*g* for 10 min and resuspend the cell pellet in 2 mL fresh 2×YT medium. Add 0.1% glucose, 100 μ g/mL ampicillin and 60 μg/mL kanamycin. Culture the cells at 30°C with shaking at 200 rpm overnight for phage packaging.
15. Centrifuge the overnight culture at 9000×*g* for 10 min and transfer phage-containing supernatant to a new tube.
16. Add 0.25 vol of PEG/NaCl to the supernatant and incubate on ice for 1 h. Centrifuge at 10,000×*g* for 30 min at 4°C to obtain phage pellet. Resuspend the pellet in 1 mL of PBS. Take 10 μL of phage to determine the amplified phage titer and keep the remaining phage at 4°C to be used in subsequent rounds of panning.

3.3.2 Phage Titration

1. Perform ten-fold serial dilutions by transferring 10 μL eluted phage to 90 μL PBS in 1.5 mL microcentrifuge tubes. Vortex to mix thoroughly. Repeat this process sequentially to obtain dilutions from 10^{-1} to 10^{-10}.
2. Add 100 μL of TG1 cells at OD_{600} ~0.5 to each tube of diluted phage. Incubate at 37°C for 30 min for infection to occur.
3. Spot 10 μL of the infected cells on a 2×YT/glu/amp agar plate and a 2×YT/kan agar plate (*see* **Note 13**). Incubate at 37°C overnight. Colonies on the 2×YT-amp agar plate represent library phage particles that carry the ampicillin-resistant phagemid. Colonies on the 2×YT-kan agar plate indicate background contamination.
4. Calculate the phage titer using the formula:

$$\text{phage titer}\left(\text{CFU/mL}\right) = \frac{\text{number of colonies} \times \text{dilution factor}}{\text{volume spotted}}$$

3.3.3 Polyclonal Peptide Phage ELISA

1. Coat a microtiter well for each round of eluted phage with 10 μ g of target antibody in PBS at a final volume of 100 μL. Also coat corresponding numbers of wells with the same amount of BSA to detect nonspecific background binders. Shake the wells for 10 min and incubate at 4°C overnight.
2. Wash the microtiter wells three times with 0.1% PBST.
3. Block each microtiter well with 300 μL of 2% PTM with shaking for 1 h, then wash the wells three times with 0.1% PBST.
4. To each well, add 50 μL of phage and 50 μL of 2% PTM. Shake the wells at 600 rpm for 2 h for phage to bind to the coated antibody.
5. Wash the microtiter wells three times with 0.1% PBST to remove unbound or weakly bound phage.
6. Add 100 μL of anti-M13-HRP to each microtiter well. Incubate for 1 h with shaking at 600 rpm, then wash the wells with 0.1% PBST for three times.
7. Add 100 μL of ABTS solution to each well and cover with aluminium foil. Shake the wells at 600 rpm and measure absorbance at 405 nm with a spectrophotometer after 1 h.

3.4 Monoclonal Peptide Phage Selection

After obtaining a suitably enriched phage pool displaying polyclonal peptide binders through successive rounds of biopanning, the next step is to isolate monoclonal peptide binders to identify unique peptide sequences with specific binding properties.

3.4.1 Isolation of Monoclonal Peptide Clones

1. Make ten-fold serial dilutions of the appropriately enriched phage from 10^{-1} to 10^{-8} using PBS as the diluent.
2. Infect 100 μL of TG1 cells at OD_{600} ~0.5 with each serial diluted phage. Incubate at 37°C for 30 min for infection to occur.
3. Centrifuge the infected cells at 3500×*g* for 10 min and resuspend the cell pellet in 100 μL of 2×YT medium to concentrate the cells.
4. Spread the cells on 2×YT/glu/amp plates evenly (*see* **Note 14**). Incubate the plates at 37°C overnight to obtain cell colonies.
5. Randomly pick 92 single colonies with sterilized toothpicks and inoculate them into 200 μL of 2×YT medium with 2% glucose and 100 μg/mL ampicillin on a 96-well microtiter cell culture plate (*see* **Note 15**). Leave two wells as positive controls and two as negative controls. Inoculate cells expressing anti-ubiquitin in the positive control wells (*see* **Note 16**). Incubate the microtiter plate at 37°C with shaking at 800 rpm overnight.
6. Subculture 10 μL of the overnight culture into 90 μL of 2×YT medium with 2% glucose and 100 μg/mL ampicillin on a new 96-well microtiter cell culture plate (*see* **Note 17**). Incubate the plate at 37°C with shaking at 800 rpm for 1 h.

7. Infect each well with 10^9 CFU of M13KO7 helper phage and incubate the plate at 37°C for 30 min.
8. Centrifuge the microtiter plate at 3500 rpm for 15 min. Carefully aspirate and discard the supernatant with a multichannel pipette. Resuspend the pellets in 200 μL of 2×YT medium with 100 μg/mL ampicillin and 60 μg/mL kanamycin. Incubate the plate at 30°C overnight with shaking at 800 rpm.
9. Centrifuge the overnight culture at 3500 rpm for 15 min to obtain phage-containing supernatant.

3.4.2 Monoclonal Phage Peptide ELISA

1. Coat a 96-well ELISA plate with 10 μg of target antibody except the positive control wells, which will be coated with 10 μg of ubiquitin. Coat another 96-well ELISA plate with 10 μg of BSA to detect background signals. Shake the wells for 10 min and incubate at 4°C overnight.
2. Carry out ELISA with the steps described in Sect. 3.3.3.
3. Identify positive clones with good signal to background ratio for sequencing.

3.4.3 Colony PCR and Gel Electrophoresis

Colony PCR and gel electrophoresis are performed on positive clones to confirm the insert of peptide-encoding sequence in the phagemid before sequencing.

1. Pick some glycerol stock of the selected positive clones from Sect. 3.4.1 with a sterilized toothpick and dissolve in 10 μL of dH_2O in a 1.5 mL microcentrifuge tube. This would be used as the DNA template.
2. Setup each PCR reaction with 1× DreamTaq buffer, 0.2 mM dNTPs, 0.5 μM forward primer, 0.5 μM reverse primer, 2 μL DNA template, 1 U DreamTaq DNA polymerase, and dH_2O in a total volume of 20 μL (*see* **Note 18**).
3. Run PCR: initial denaturation at 95°C (5 min), 30 cycles of amplification with denaturation at 95°C (30 s), annealing at 55°C (30 s), and elongation at 72°C (1.5 min), followed by a final elongation step at 72°C (5 min).
4. Separate the amplified PCR products by gel electrophoresis (1.2% agarose gel in 0.5× TBE buffer). View the gel under UV illumination to confirm insertion of peptide sequence. Send the colonies with the correct band size for sequencing. The expected band size for successful insertion of the 20-mer peptide sequence is 340 bp and for positive control, 419 bp.

3.5 Sequence Analysis

To ensure the reliability of biopanning results, peptide sequences may be analyzed first using the SAROTUP suite (https://i.uestc.edu.cn/sarotup3/index.html), which helps identify and exclude target-unrelated peptides [9]. These peptides appear in the screening results due to nonspecific binding or growth bias rather than genuine affinity for the intended target. Target-related peptide sequences can then be aligned with multiple sequence alignment tools such as Clustal Omega (https://www.ebi.ac.uk/jdispatcher/msa/clustalo) to identify common motifs, conserved residues, or sequence patterns indicative of epitope recognition [10]. For linear epitopes, motif sequences obtained from the peptides can often be directly aligned to the primary sequence of the antigen of interest. Meanwhile to identify conformational epitopes, the identified motifs can be mapped onto the antigen surface using structural modeling software such as PyMOL, Chimera, and PEP-SiteFinder [11–13]. Surface-exposed regions enriched with chemical or spatial similarities to the motif may suggest possible locations of conformational epitopes.

4 Notes

1. This should give a starting OD_{600} of 0.1. This ensures that cells have enough time to grow into the exponential phase for downstream applications. Normally, 2–4 h are needed for the culture to reach OD_{600} of 0.5. To be safe, check the reading with a spectrophotometer every 1 h to predict growth trend. Note that growth is exponential, and therefore, should be monitored closely after OD_{600} reaches ~0.3 to avoid overshooting.
2. A multiplicity of infection (MOI) of 20 is used to ensure that there are enough phage particles to infect each bacterial cell, maximizing the chances of efficient phage uptake and library amplification. The volume of helper phage that needs to be added can be calculated as follows, where 10^8 CFU/mL is the concentration of cells at OD_{600} 0.5.

$$\text{volume of phage (mL)} = \frac{\text{MOI} \times 10^8\ \text{CFU/mL} \times \text{volume of cell (mL)}}{\text{phage titre (CFU/mL)}}$$

3. Standardizing the initiating OD_{600} of cell culture growth is important to ensure experimental consistency and optimal phage amplification. In this protocol, cultures are initiated at an OD_{600} of approximately 0.1. To make sure, dilute 5 μL of the stock culture in 995 μL of 2×YT (1:200 dilution) and measure the OD_{600}. If the OD_{600} is approximately 0.1, this means that a 1:200 dilution would be used to culture the cell stock in future use.

4. Centrifugation at 3500×*g* is sufficient to pellet phage particles but higher speeds are found to improve recovery. Centrifugation is done at 4°C because PEG precipitates more efficiently at low temperatures and phage particles are more stable at 4°C.
5. This protocol can also be used with hybridoma-derived monoclonal antibodies purified using protein A columns. Recombinant antibodies expressed using other systems such as yeast and mammalian cells can also be applied in a similar fashion.
6. Adding 0.2× TES buffer introduces osmotic shock that releases the content of the periplasm of the cells. Using 0.2× TES buffer instead of dH_2O or $MgCl_2$ solution results in a gentler osmotic shock, which can give a cleaner periplasmic extract by reducing cell lysis and cytoplasmic contamination.
7. The column is typically equilibrated with the same buffer used for the wash step to maintain consistent conditions during protein binding and removal of nonspecifically bound contaminants.
8. In this protocol, the target antibody is purified from the periplasmic fraction due to the presence of the pelB leader sequence, which directs the expressed antibody to the periplasm. If the antibody is found to be insoluble or forms inclusion bodies, extraction from the total cell pellet using a denaturing agent like urea is required, followed by stepwise dialysis or dilution for refolding under controlled conditions. If the solubility of the antibody is uncertain, an SDS-PAGE analysis of the periplasmic and insoluble fractions should be run to determine where the majority of the target antibody is located.
9. Specifically bound antibodies are eluted from the column with increasing concentration of imidazole in the buffers. Imidazole competes with the His-tag for binding to Ni^{2+} ions on the resin. Alternatively, antibodies can also be eluted from the column using pH gradient where decreasing pH reduces the affinity of His-tag for Ni^{2+} ions.
10. Alternative assays like the BCA protein assay or UV absorbance at 280 nm may be used to determine eluted antibody concentration. Bradford assay is employed here due to its speed and sensitivity.
11. Use a plate washer to wash the microtiter well. For the immunotube, wash manually using a squirt bottle filled with 0.1% PBST. Gently tap them on dry paper towel to remove residue. Care must be taken to ensure the bubbles during washing are not carried over to the next step.

12. Culture the cells overnight together with the helper phage-infected culture. The next day, aliquot appropriate amount into 1.5 mL microcentrifuge tubes, add 20% glycerol to each tube and keep at −80°C as stock. As needed, the cells can be revived and infected with M13KO7 helper phage to produce the phage population enriched after a panning round.
13. Also spot 10 μL of TG1 cells and 10 μL of PBS used as the diluent to check for contamination. No colony growth should be observed. If colonies are present in the controls, the infection should be repeated as this indicates contamination.
14. Place some beads on the agar plate, pipette the cell culture and swirl the plate back and forth until the cell culture is spread evenly over the plate and is dry. Alternatively, use bent glass rod or other similar applicators to spread the cell culture.
15. If the number of positive hits is low, additional clones may need to be picked.
16. In this protocol, anti-ubiquitin is used as a positive control by coating wells with purified ubiquitin. This setup serves to confirm that the ELISA is functioning properly. Alternative positive control systems such as anti-His antibody against tagged proteins or previously validated monoclonal antibodies against known targets can be used.
17. Gently resuspend the overnight cultures before transferring to avoid sedimentation of cells at the bottom of the wells. Each overnight culture should be transferred into the same corresponding well on the new microtiter plate as monoclones will be identified by their well position. Multichannel pipette may be used but care must be taken to avoid cross-contamination between wells. Add 20% glycerol to the remaining overnight culture and store the microtiter plate at −80°C as stock.
18. Include a positive control and a negative control to confirm the colony PCR is working normally. For positive control, use ~20 ng of the empty plasmid without the insert. Briefly centrifuge the PCR tubes to ensure that all components are collected at the bottom and properly mixed before running PCR.

Acknowledgments

The authors would like to acknowledge the support of Malaysian Ministry for Higher Education through the Fundamental Research Grant Scheme (FRGS/1/2024/STG01/USM/02/10).

References

1. Nilvebrant J, Rockberg J (2018) An introduction to epitope mapping. Methods Mol Biol Clifton NJ 1785:1–10
2. Meloen RH, Puijk WC, Slootstra JW (2000) Mimotopes: realization of an unlikely concept. J Mol Recognit 13:352–359
3. Zhang C, Li Y, Tang W et al (2016) The relationship between B-cell epitope and mimotope sequences. Protein Pept Lett 23:132–141
4. Ehrlich GK, Berthold W, Bailon P (2000) Phage display technology. Affinity selection by biopanning. Methods Mol Biol Clifton NJ 147:195–208
5. Förster-Waldl E, Riemer AB, Dehof AK et al (2005) Isolation and structural analysis of peptide mimotopes for the disialoganglioside GD2, a neuroblastoma tumor antigen. Mol Immunol 42:319–325
6. Palma M (2023) Epitopes and mimotopes identification using phage display for vaccine development against infectious pathogens. Vaccines 11:1176
7. Yu RK, Usuki S, Itokazu Y et al (2016) Novel GM1 ganglioside-like peptide mimics prevent the association of cholera toxin to human intestinal epithelial cells in vitro. Glycobiology 26:63–73
8. Chin CF, Lai JY, Choong YS et al (2017) Delineation of B-cell epitopes of Salmonella enterica serovar Typhi Hemolysin E: potential antibody therapeutic target. Sci Rep 7:2176
9. Huang J, Ru B, Li S et al (2010) SAROTUP: scanner and reporter of target-unrelated peptides. J Biomed Biotechnol 2010:101932
10. Sievers F, Wilm A, Dineen D et al (2011) Fast, scalable generation of high-quality protein multiple sequence alignments using Clustal Omega. Mol Syst Biol 7:539
11. Seeliger D, de Groot BL (2010) Ligand docking and binding site analysis with PyMOL and Autodock/Vina. J Comput Aided Mol Des 24(5):417–22
12. Pettersen EF, Goddard TD, Huang CC et al (2004) UCSF Chimera—a visualization system for exploratory research and analysis. J Comput Chem 25:1605–1612
13. Saladin A, Rey J, Thévenet P et al (2014) PEP-SiteFinder: a tool for the blind identification of peptide binding sites on protein surfaces. Nucleic Acids Res 42:W221–226

Chapter 10

Phage Display Biopanning Strategy for Discovery of Nanoparticle-Binding Peptides

Piotr Golec and Grzegorz Węgrzyn

Abstract

The phage display technology allows to select peptides, exposed on the surface of bacteriophage virions, which can specifically bind to virtually any materials, including proteins, lipids, carbohydrates, and other organic macromolecules, as well as metals or metal oxides. In this chapter, we describe and discuss procedures for effective selection of peptides characterized with affinity to metallic or metal oxide nanoparticles. The use of a peptide library displayed on virions of the M13 bacteriophage, the most commonly used phage display system, is presented. Specific notes indicate what are crucial steps in the procedure, what should be avoided and why, and what should be done if common problems appear. The scheme of the biopanning process, the crucial step in selecting specific peptides, which bind to nanoparticles composed of metals or metal oxides, is presented and discussed.

Keywords Phage display, Biopanning, Peptide library, Nanoparticles, M13 bacteriophage, Binding efficiency, Targeted binding

1 Introduction

Phage display (PD) is a powerful molecular biology technique in which peptides, proteins, or antibody fragments are presented on the surface of bacteriophages—viruses that infect bacteria [1]. The method was first described in 1985 by George P. Smith, who demonstrated that short peptides could be displayed on the surface of the filamentous phage M13 by inserting the corresponding coding sequence into the viral genome [2]. In 2018, Smith was awarded the Nobel Prize in Chemistry, shared with Frances Arnold and Sir Gregory Winter, "*for the phage display of peptides and antibodies.*"

Phage display allows for the creation of highly diverse phage libraries, containing billions of unique peptides, or antibody fragments exposed on virion particles [3]. Each individual phage in such a library displays a different peptide, creating a vast reservoir of potential ligands capable of binding to a specific biological or

Huan Peng and Theam Soon Lim (eds.), *Biomolecular Display Technologies*, Methods in Molecular Biology, vol. 3030,
https://doi.org/10.1007/978-1-0716-5249-7_10,

nonbiological target, such as a protein, receptor, cell, small molecule, metal surface, or nanoparticle [4–8].

The selection of desirable binders from a phage library is performed through a process known as biopanning, which involves: (i) incubation of phages form the peptide library with a target material, (ii) removal of nonbinding phages via washing steps, (iii) recovery of phages that display peptides capable specific binding of target material, and (iv) amplification of the recovered phages and using them through subsequent rounds of biopanning, or (v) isolation of phage DNA followed by sequencing of the inserted peptide-encoding region. As a result, one obtains phage clones displaying peptides or antibody fragments with high affinity and specificity toward the selected target material.

Phage display has been used in a wide spectrum of applications, including fields such as biotechnology, diagnostics, and medicine. In recent years, it has also become an increasingly important tool in nanotechnology, particularly for identifying peptides that bind to or modify nanomaterials [8–11]. In this chapter, we demonstrate how to identify peptides with affinity towards metallic or metal oxide nanoparticles using a peptide library displayed on the M13 bacteriophage.

2 Materials

2.1 Bacterial Strain and Phage Display Library with Sequencing Primer

Prepare all buffers using ultrapure water (resistivity of 18 MΩ cm at 25°C, obtained by further purifying deionized water) and molecular biology grade reagents. Prepare and sterilize all buffers by autoclaving, then store at room temperature. Follow all applicable waste disposal regulations when discarding materials.

1. *Escherichia coli* K12 ER2738: F′*proA*$^{+}$*B*$^{+}$ *lacI*^{q} *Δ(lacZ)M15 zzf::Tn*10(Tet^{R})/ *fhuA2 glnV Δ(lac-proAB) thi-1 Δ(hsdS-mcrB)5*, New England Biolabs, #E4104.
2. Phage Display Peptide Library: the Ph.D^{TM}-12 Phage Display Peptide Library Kit v2 (New England Biolabs, #E8111L) (*see* **Note 1**).
3. The 96 gIII sequencing primer: 5′-CCCTCATAGTTAG CGTAACG-3′, supplied with Ph.D^{TM}-12 Phage Display Peptide Library Kit v2 (New England Biolabs).

2.2 Culture Media

1. LB; 1% bacto-tryptone, 0.5% yeast extract, 0.05% NaCl.
2. LB-agar; 1% bacto-tryptone, 0.5% yeast extract, 0.5% NaCl, 1.5% agar.
3. Top agar (soft-agar); 1% bacto-tryptone, 0.5% yeast extract, 0.5% NaCl, 0.7% agar.

2.3 Buffers and Solutions

1. Gly-HCl buffer; 0.2 M glycine solution, pH 2.2, adjusted with HCl.
2. PEG/NaCl; 20% polyethylene glycol (PEG 8000), 2.5 M NaCl.
3. TBS buffer; 50 mM Tris-HCl (pH 7.5), 150 mM NaCl.
4. TBST buffer; 50 mM Tris-HCl (pH 7.5), 150 mM NaCl, 0.1% Tween-20.
5. Tris-HCl buffer (pH 9.1); 1 M Tris solution, pH 9.0, adjusted with HCl.

3 Methods

All steps of the biopanning procedure should be performed at room temperature unless otherwise specified. A schematic overview of the key stages of the biopanning workflow is presented in Fig. 1.

3.1 Preparing Nanoparticle-Based Target Material for Biopanning

1. Prepare 10 mg of the nanoparticles in the form of a nanopowder in sterile, 1.5 mL centrifuge tube (*see* **Note 2**).
2. Suspend the nanoparticles in 1 mL of the TBST buffer and vortex for 1 min (*see* **Note 3**).
3. Incubate for 30 min at room temperature (RT) with gentle mixing (*see* **Note 4**).
4. Wash the nanoparticles 6 × 1 mL of TBST by performing alternating steps of centrifugation and resuspension in TBST (*see* **Note 5**).
5. After the final wash, resuspend the nanoparticles in 1 mL of TBST and use in biopanning (Sect. 3.2) or evaluation of binding efficiency (Sect. 3.4) procedures (*see* **Note 6**).

3.2 Performing Biopanning to Select Target-Binding Peptides from a Phage Display Library

1. Add 10 μL of Phage Display Peptide Library to nanoparticles, washed and suspended in TBST (*see* **Note 7**).
2. Incubate the mixture at RT with gentle mixing for 30 min (*see* **Note 4**).
3. Wash the mixture with 10 × 1 mL of TBST (*see* **Note 5**).
4. After last cycle of washing, resuspend the nanoparticle pellet in 1 mL of Gly-HCl buffer (*see* **Note 8**).
5. Incubate the mixture for 5–10 min at RT with gentle rocking (*see* **Note 9**).
6. Centrifuge at 4000×*g* for 1–5 min at RT (*see* **Note 10**).
7. Collect and transfer the supernatant containing eluted phages to a new tube (*see* **Note 11**).

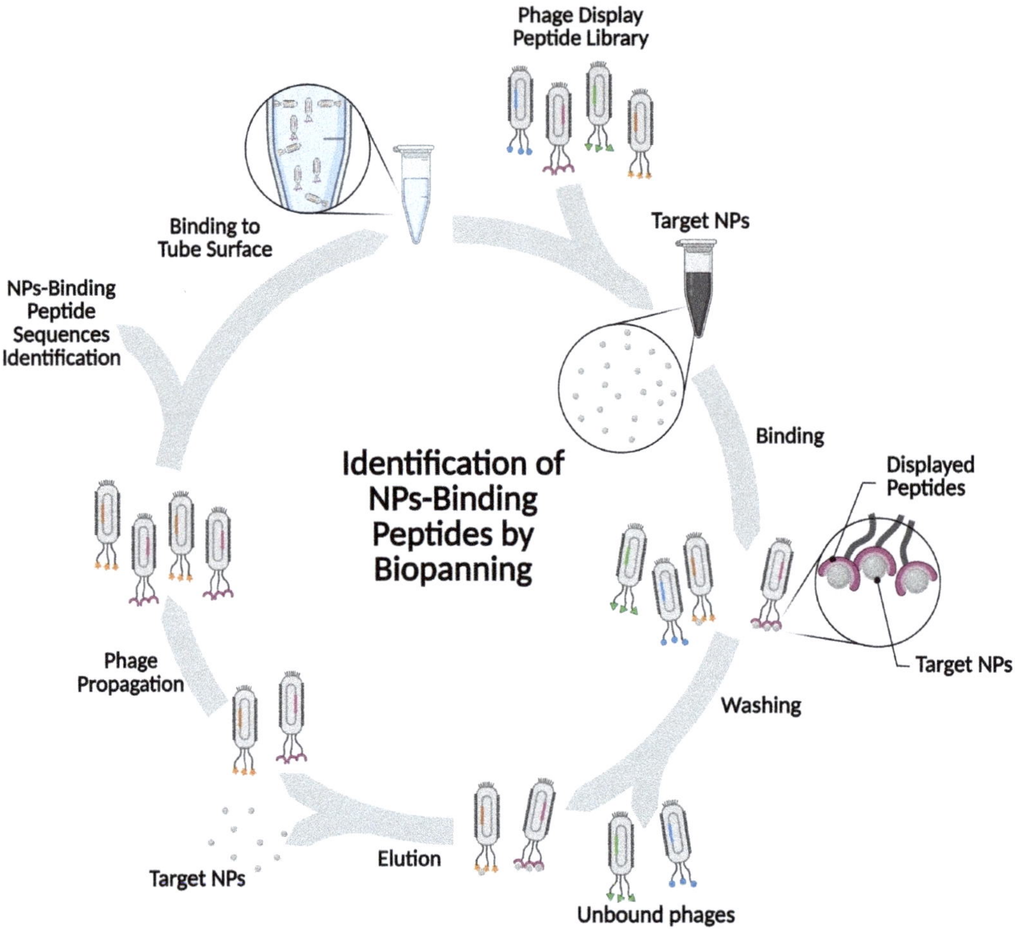

Fig. 1 Schematic representation of the biopanning procedure for identifying peptides binding to nanoparticles (NPs). The process begins with the addition of phages to the target NPs. These can include either the original phage display peptide library or phages amplified after previous rounds of biopanning, following removal of clones binding nonspecifically to the surface of the centrifuge tube. Phages displaying peptides bind to the target NPs, after which unbound phages are removed by washing. In the elution step, the interaction between peptide-displaying phages and the NPs is disrupted, allowing recovery of bound phages. The eluted phages are then amplified in *Escherichia coli*. After three rounds of selection, individual phage clones are isolated, single-stranded DNA is extracted, and the peptide-coding sequences are identified by Sanger sequencing. The figure was prepared with BioRender.com

8. Immediately neutralize the eluate with the Tris-HCl buffer (pH 9.1) at a ratio of 150 μL Tris-HCl per 1000 μL of Gly-HCl (*see* **Note 12**).
9. Use the neutralized eluate for phage propagation in *Escherichia coli* K12 ER2738 liquid culture (*see* **Note 13**).
10. Concentrate and clean-up of propagated phages for next biopanning round by PEG precipitation. Add one-fifth volume of the PEG/NaCl buffer. Incubate at 4°C for 1 h and then

centrifuge at 12,000×*g* for 15 min at 4°C. Discard supernatant and resuspend the pellet containing phages in 1 mL of the TBS buffer. Use the phages for next biopanning rounds (at least three rounds) (*see* **Note 14**).

11. Start the second and third round of biopanning with binding of phages to a clean tube. Add 10 μL of propagated, concentrated and purified phages to a clean centrifuge tube containing 1 mL of TBST only. Incubate for 30–60 min. Collect all supernatant and use it for resuspension of target nanoparticles. Then, follow the second or third round of biopanning procedure starting from point two (*see* **Note 15**).

3.3 Amplifying Phage Clones and Sequencing the Peptide-Encoding Region

1. Following the final round of biopanning, perform serial decimal dilutions of eluted and neutralized phages in TBS (*see* **Note 16**).
2. Perform full-plate titration of phages on double layer LB-agar plates, with X-Gal/IPTG incorporated into the bottom layer (*see* **Note 17**).
3. Incubate the plates overnight at 37°C (*see* **Note 18**).
4. Select individual blue plaques, each representing a single phage clone displaying a potentially unique peptide for propagation in a liquid bacterial culture (*see* **Note 19**).
5. Pick individual plaques with a sterile pipette tip and transfer each into 13 mL tube containing 2 mL of exponentially growing *E. coli* K12 ER2738 culture in LB medium (*see* **Note 20**).
6. Incubate at 37°C with vigorous shaking for 5 h (*see* **Note 21**).
7. Centrifuge cultures at 12,000×*g* for 10 min to remove bacterial cells.
8. Transfer the supernatant to a fresh tube and precipitate phage particles by PEG precipitation. Add one-fifth volume of the PEG/NaCl buffer. Incubate at 4°C and then centrifuge at 12,000×*g* for 15 min at 4°C. Discard supernatant and resuspend a pellet containing phages in the TBS buffer. Use the phages for single-stranded DNA (ssDNA) isolation or to evaluating binding efficiency (Sect. 3.4) (*see* **Note 14**).
9. Isolate ssDNA from phage particles following the protocol described previously [12].
10. Assess ssDNA quality and concentration spectrophotometrically (*see* **Note 22**).
11. Perform Sanger sequencing using the 96 gIII sequencing primer.
12. Analyze the resulting sequences to identify peptide-encoding regions (*see* **Note 23**).

3.4 Evaluating Binding Efficiency and Selecting High-Affinity Peptide Candidates

1. Prepare a phage suspension at a concentration of approximately 1×10^8 plaque-forming units (pfu)/mL in TBS buffer using phage clones presenting candidate peptides with nanomaterial-binding properties (*see* **Note 24**).
2. Add 10 μL of the phage suspension, presenting individual peptide (designated as *Input phages*, I) to the nanoparticle suspension, prepared in TBST (*see* **Note 25**).
3. Incubate for 30 min at RT with gentle mixing (*see* **Note 26**).
4. Wash the mixture 10×1 mL of TBST (*see* **Note 5**).
5. After the last cycle of washing, resuspend the nanoparticle pellet in 1 mL of Gly-HCl buffer to elute attached phages (designated as *Output phages*, O) (*see* **Note 8**).
6. Incubate the mixture for 5–10 min at RT with gentle rocking (*see* **Note 9**).
7. Centrifuge at $4000 \times g$ for 1–5 min at RT (*see* **Note 10**).
8. Collect and transfer the supernatant containing eluted phages to a new tube (*see* **Note 11**).
9. Neutralize immediately with Tris-HCl (pH 9.1) buffer (*see* **Note 12**).
10. Titrate the neutralized *Output* phages on double layer LB/X-Gal/IPTG agar plates to determine phage concentration.
11. Calculate binding efficiency as the ratio of *Output* to *Input* phage titers (O/I).

4 Notes

1. The Ph.D.™ system from New England Biolabs includes the 12-residue linear peptide library (NEB #E8111L), as well as two additional formats: a 7-residue linear library (NEB #E8211S) and a 7-residue disulfide-constrained library (NEB #E8212S). Each library exhibits slightly different binding and structural properties; therefore, selection of the appropriate library should be based on a thorough review of the technical specifications. On December 15, 2022, NEB replaced the previous version of the 12-mer library with an updated kit (Ph.D.™-12 Phage Display Peptide Library Kit v2).
2. Nanoparticles are often presuspended in water or a stabilizing buffer. In such cases, a volume of the nanoparticle suspension equivalent to 10 mg of nanoparticle powder should be used.
3. Nanoparticles suspended in TBST should not undergo excessive aggregation; they should form a stable suspension rather than settling as a precipitate. If aggregation is observed, an

alternative approach should be considered, such as replacing the nanoparticle powder with a solid support made of the target material (e.g., a foil or plate). In this case, a clean target material plate (approximately 1 × 1 cm in size) should be immersed in TBST. Another case involves the stable adsorption of nanoparticles onto the inner surface of a centrifuge tube. In such a case, nanoparticles adhered to the tube wall can also be exploited during the biopanning process as the target material.

4. Placing the sample on an orbital shaker is preferable over using a rocking shaker. Orbital motion ensures more uniform and efficient mixing that promotes better contact between phages and the nanomaterial, thereby enhancing binding efficiency.
5. The centrifugation speed during washing steps should be optimized individually for each type of nanomaterial. After each centrifugation, the nanoparticles should form a loose pellet that can be easily resuspended into a uniform suspension. If the centrifugation speed is too low, significant loss of nanomaterial may occur. Conversely, if the speed is too high, the nanomaterial may form a compact pellet that is difficult to resuspend. Typically, brief centrifugation for 1 min at 1000–2000 rpm is sufficient. Avoid excessive removal of the supernatant, as this may result in the accidental uptake of nanoparticles with bound phages into the pipette tip, leading to the loss of both target material and peptide-displaying phages. It is preferable to leave a small volume of TBST buffer above the pellet rather than to risk aspirating the nanoparticle suspension.
6. Nanoparticle suspensions should be freshly prepared on the day the biopanning procedure is planned to be conducted. Avoid long-term storage to minimize aggregation.
7. A standard M13 phage display peptide library has a typical concentration of approximately 1×10^{13} pfu/mL, with each unique peptide variant represented by about 100 copies. Therefore, using 10 μL of the library in the first round of biopanning should, in theory, provide at least one copy of each peptide. However, to increase the likelihood that all peptide variants are present in the initial screening, the volume of the library can be safely increased (e.g., to 50–100 μL).
8. Resuspend the phages in the Gly-HCl buffer by gently pipetting with an automatic pipette. Avoid vigorous mixing by using vortex.
9. An incubation time of approximately 5 min is generally sufficient for effective phage elution under acidic conditions. Extending the incubation period may improve the recovery of bound phages; however, prolonged exposure of M13 phages

to low pH can adversely affect their structural integrity and infectivity. Incubation times exceeding 15 min are not recommended, as significant inactivation of phage particles has been observed under such conditions. Additionally, acidic environment may compromise the stability of certain nanoparticle targets, potentially leading to aggregation or partial dissolution. If low pH elution proves ineffective or introduces unwanted effects on either the phage or the target material, alternative elution strategies using milder or more selective buffers should be considered. Examples of alternative elution buffers include TBS supplemented with 1 M NaCl, TBS with 0.1%–0.5% Tween-20 or 0.1% SDS, 10 mM EDTA, 100 mM imidazole, 0.1 M citrate buffer at pH 2.5, and 0.1 M Na_2CO_3 at pH 10.5.

10. Centrifugation at this stage should be optimized based on the specific properties of the nanoparticle material and the overall biopanning procedure. In contrast to the washing steps used for nanoparticle-bound phages, this centrifugation should typically be performed at higher speeds. The main objective of this step is to effectively separate the phages from the nanoparticle matrix.
11. Withdraw as much of the supernatant as possible without disturbing the nanoparticle pellet. Avoid aspirating the pellet, as residual nanoparticles may rebind phages during subsequent steps and interfere with accurate analysis.
12. For convenience, prealiquot Tris-HCl buffer (pH 9.1) into microcentrifuge tubes and add the collected eluate directly to the buffer to achieve immediate neutralization.
13. It is recommended to assess elution efficiency prior to phage amplification using a standard plaque assay. Phage amplification should be performed by infecting 20 mL of the *E. coli* culture growing at the early exponential phase, followed by incubation with vigorous shaking to ensure proper aeration for at least 5 h. Prior to infection, briefly pause shaking to allow regeneration of F pili, which are essential for efficient M13 phage infection.
14. Overnight incubation on ice is recommended, as it significantly enhances the efficiency of the process. Prior to centrifugation, mark the side of the microcentrifuge tube where the phage pellet is expected to form. After centrifugation, the phage pellet may be invisible or barely detectable. Resuspend the phages in the TBS buffer by gentle pipetting. Do not vortex at this stage, as phages are sensitive to mechanical damage.
15. Use microcentrifuge tubes identical to those employed during the nanoparticle-phage binding step. This is important because, at this stage, phages that bind nonspecifically to the tube material are being removed. When removing the

supernatant, avoid touching the inner walls of the tube with the pipette tip to prevent aspirating phages that may have adhered to the tube surface.

16. Prepare serial dilutions immediately after the neutralization step. A five-step ten-fold dilution series in TBS is usually sufficient for downstream titration. Retain the remaining eluate and store it at 4°C for further use.
17. For each dilution, prepare a double-layer agar plate. Combine 4 mL of top agar (LB soft agar), 200 μL of an overnight *E. coli* K12 ER2738 culture, and 10 μL of the diluted eluate. Pour the mixture evenly over the surface of a prepoured LB-agar plate containing X-Gal/IPTG, added at a ratio of 1000 μL X-Gal/IPTG per 1000 mL of LB agar. Ensure that the bottom agar layer is not overly dry, as this may impair plaque formation. To avoid over-drying, use plates that have been poured and allowed to dry at room temperature overnight.
18. Incubate the plates inverted (agar side down) to prevent condensation of water (arising due to the evaporation and precipitation processes) on the agar surface, which could interfere with plaque visualization and accurate counting.
19. Select at least 20 individual blue plaques that differ in diameter, ensuring diversity in phage clone representation.
20. Use 1000 μL pipette tips with the narrow end cut to a diameter of approximately 3 mm, then sterilized prior to use. Excise selected plaques using the modified tips and transfer each into 2–3 mL of *E. coli* K12 ER2738 culture for amplification.
21. Incubation may be extended overnight if necessary, without negatively affecting phage amplification.
22. The concentration of ssDNA is typically low, ranging from a few to several dozens of ng/μL; however, this is sufficient for Sanger sequencing.
23. During sequence analysis, utilize a characteristic feature of the peptide library—three glycine residues located literally at the beginning of the peptide sequence displayed on the phage surface.
24. Use phages amplified from individual plaques, following the procedure described earlier. It is recommended to perform binding efficiency analysis after sequencing of the peptide-encoding regions. Some peptide sequences may be repeated among multiple amplified phage clones, while others may lack an identifiable peptide insert. This sequencing step allows for a reduction in the number of phage clones subjected to binding analysis, focusing only on unique and sequence-confirmed variants.
25. For each phage variant displaying a unique peptide, perform a control titration by adding 10 μL of phage suspension to

1 mL of TBST. This dilution will serve as the defined *input phages* (pfu/mL) for subsequent binding efficiency analysis.

26. Use the same incubation parameters as applied during the biopanning procedure.

Acknowledgments

This work was supported by the National Science Center (Poland) within the project grant no. 2016/23/B/NZ6/02537 (to P.G.).

References

1. Pierzynowska K, Morcinek-Orłowska J, Gaffke L, Jaroszewicz W, Skowron PM, Węgrzyn G (2024) Applications of the phage display technology in molecular biology, biotechnology and medicine. Crit Rev Microbiol 50:450–490. https://doi.org/10.1080/1040841X.2023.2219741
2. Smith GP (1985) Filamentous fusion phage: novel expression vectors that display cloned antigens on the virion surface. Science 228:1315–1317. https://doi.org/10.1126/science.4001944
3. Carle V, Kong XD, Comberlato A, Edwards C, Díaz-Perlas C, Heinis C (2021) Generation of a 100-billion cyclic peptide phage display library having a high skeletal diversity. Protein Eng Des Sel 34:gzab018. https://doi.org/10.1093/protein/gzab018
4. Wood AC, Johnson EC, Prasad RRR, Sullivan MV, Turner NW, Armes SP, Staniland SS, Foster JA (2024) Phage display against 2D metal–organic nanosheets as a new route to highly selective biomolecular recognition surfaces. Small 13:e2406339. https://doi.org/10.1002/smll.202406339
5. Jin H, Gao X, Xiao L, He H, Cheng S, Zhang C, Hou Y, Song F, Su X, Gao Q, Lu Z, Yang R, Song X, Yang J, Duan W, Hou Y (2021) Screening and identification of a specific peptide binding to breast cancer cells from a phage-displayed peptide library. Biotechnol Lett 43:153–164. https://doi.org/10.1007/s10529-020-03044-3
6. Yang F, Liu L, Neuenschwander PF, Idell S, Vankayalapati R, Jain KG, Du K, Ji H, Yi G (2022) Phage display-derived peptide for the specific binding of SARS-CoV-2. ACS Omega 7:3203–3211. https://doi.org/10.1021/acsomega.1c04873
7. Cheng Y, Qi J, Liu K, Zhou C, Wang W, Zuo Y, Zhang P, Liang S, Wang Y, Chen P, Tang C, Liu Z (2022) Characterization of a novel affinity binding ligand for tyrosine nitrated peptides from a phage-displayed peptide library. Talanta 241:123225. https://doi.org/10.1016/j.talanta.2022.123225
8. Karczewska-Golec J, Sadowska K, Golec P, Karczewski J, Węgrzyn G (2024) Engineered M13-derived bacteriophages capable of gold nanoparticle synthesis and nanogold manipulations. Int J Mol Sci 25:11222. https://doi.org/10.3390/ijms252011222
9. Golec P, Żelechowska K, Karczewska-Golec J, Karczewski J, Leśniewski A, Łoś M, Węgrzyn G, Kłonkowski AM (2017) Bacteriophages as factories for Eu2O3 nanoparticle synthesis. Bioconjug Chem 28:1834–1841. https://doi.org/10.1021/acs.bioconjchem.7b00119
10. Golec P, Karczewska-Golec J, Węgrzyn G (2016) Phage display-selected peptides for binding and synthesis of nanoparticles: ZnO as an example. Biotechnologia 97:145–151. https://doi.org/10.5114/bta.2016.60784
11. Żelechowska K, Karczewska-Golec J, Karczewski J, Łoś M, Kłonkowski AM, Węgrzyn G, Golec P (2016) Phage-directed synthesis of photoluminescent zinc oxide nanoparticles under benign conditions. Bioconjug Chem 27:1999–2006. https://doi.org/10.1021/acs.bioconjchem.6b00196
12. Wilson RK (1993) High-throughput purification of M13 templates for DNA sequencing. Biotechniques 15:414–422

Check for updates

Chapter 11

De Novo Discovery of Prenylated Macrocyclic Peptide Ligands

Sota Uchida, Hiroaki Suga and Yuki Goto

Abstract

Prenylated peptides, endowed with hydrophobic prenyl groups, are widely found as secondary metabolites in nature. To develop de novo artificial prenylated peptide ligands with selective affinity for a target protein of choice, a random prenylated peptide library can be constructed through the combination of a custom-made in vitro translation system and a peptide prenyltransferase, which is subsequently applied to mRNA display screening. In this chapter, we describe protocols for constructing a prenylated thioether-closed macrocyclic peptide library and conducting mRNA display screening to identify selective ligands.

Keywords Macrocyclic peptide, Prenylation, Pseudo natural product peptides, RiPPs, RaPID system, mRNA display, In vitro selection, FIT system, Translation

1 Introduction

Prenylated peptides represent a promising scaffold for developing biologically active ligands. Prenyl groups endow these peptides with unique chemical properties inaccessible through the canonical set of proteinogenic amino acids [1–5], resulting in enhanced binding affinity, target selectivity, proteolytic stability, and membrane permeability [6]. Prenylated peptides are widespread as natural products across diverse taxa, and are most notably exemplified by cyanobactins, a family of ribosomally synthesized and posttranslationally modified peptides (RiPPs) produced by cyanobacteria [7–18].

The prenylation of cyanobactins is catalyzed by a family of cyanobactin prenyltransferases. These enzymes generally exhibit broad substrate tolerance toward diverse peptide sequences, highlighting their potential as versatile biocatalysts for the synthesis of nonnatural designer prenylated peptides [13–27]. As an example, we combined the Trp-modifying cyanobactin prenyltransferase KgpF [14, 21] with a custom-made cell-free translation system, referred to as the

Huan Peng and Theam Soon Lim (eds.), *Biomolecular Display Technologies*, Methods in Molecular Biology, vol. 3030, https://doi.org/10.1007/978-1-0716-5249-7_11,

Flexible In vitro Translation (FIT) system [28], thereby establishing a synthetic platform termed FIT-KgpF [6]. KgpF is involved in the biosynthesis of kawaguchipeptin A and stereoselectively dimethylallylates the C3 position of tryptophan and bridges the C2 carbon to the main-chain nitrogen, forming a tricyclic prenylated pyrroloindoline (PrPI) residue [14, 21]. KgpF accepts not only its native substrate but also a wide range of artificial thioether-closed macrocyclic peptides (teMPs) translated by the FIT system, demonstrating the broad synthetic capability of this platform. Thus, by designing mRNAs with appropriate codon randomization and subjecting them to FIT-KgpF in combination with mRNA display [29–31], highly diverse libraries of prenylated teMPs can be constructed and explored. This discovery platform, referred to as the KgpF-RaPID system, has enabled the development of pseudonatural prenylated peptides targeting proteins of interest.

A representative design of the mRNA libraries used in the KgpF-RaPID selection is shown in Fig. 1. The mRNA design incorporates three key features: (i) the AUG start codon is reprogrammed with ^{ClAc}DY for macrocyclization, (ii) the UGG (Trp) codon can be positioned at different sites within the randomized region, and (iii) the codon upstream of the UGG is restricted to RYU codons, where R = G or A and Y = C or U, which encode the KgpF-preferred residues Val, Ala, Thr, or Ile. Prior to translation, mRNAs are conjugated at the 3′ end with a puromycin linker, enabling the fusion of the translated cyclic peptides with their encoding mRNAs. Following reverse transcription, the cyclic peptides are modified by KgpF, yielding an mRNA/cDNA-tagged prenylated teMP (^{PrPI}teMP) library. The desired binders are then collected by affinity-based selection using magnetic beads immobilized with the target protein. The cDNA tagged onto the recovered peptide binders is amplified by PCR and transcribed to regenerate the next-round mRNA library. Iterative selection enriches cDNAs encoding high-affinity ligands, and next generation sequencing of these cDNAs allows identification of the pseudonatural prenylated peptides that bind the target proteins.

Each selection round can be conducted in 2 days, and the entire screening campaign is typically completed within 2–3 weeks after five to seven rounds. The utility of the KgpF-RaPID workflow is illustrated by the case of the cofactor-independent phosphoglycerate mutase from *Caenorhabditis elegans* (CeiPGM) [6]. This application yielded several ligands that bound the target in a prenyl-dependent manner. It has been demonstrated that one of them inhibited CeiPGM with an IC_{50} of 30 nM and was efficiently internalized into cells. The KgpF-RaPID system offers a versatile platform enabling the de novo discovery of pseudonatural prenylated peptides with potential therapeutic relevance.

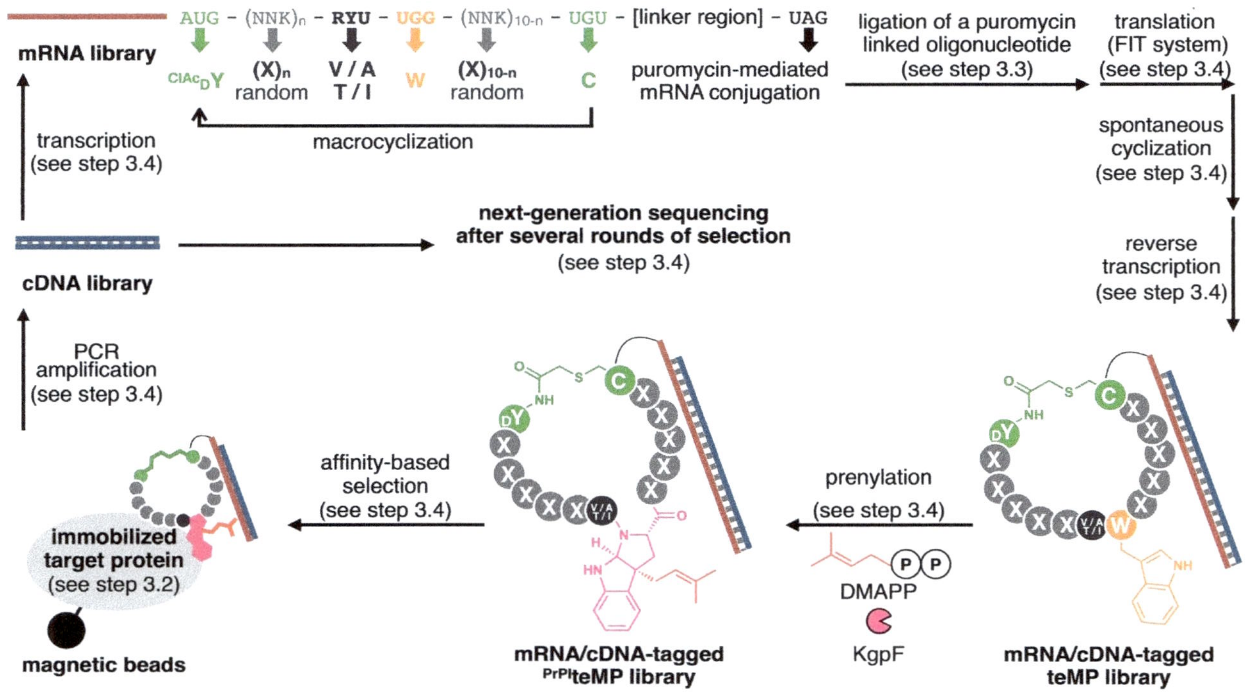

Fig. 1 Schematic representation of the KgpF-RaPID system. The scheme illustrates a typical selection cycle. See Sect. 3 for the details

2 Materials

All procedures should be performed under RNase-free conditions, using RNase-free tubes, pipettes, pipette tips, and water. Gloves should always be worn.

2.1 Synthesis of N-ClAc-D-Tyrosyl-tRNA^{fMet}$_{CAU}$

1. 1.7 mL microcentrifuge tubes.
2. 500 mM HEPES–KOH buffer (pH 7.5).
3. Flexizyme: Prepare an artificial tRNA-acylating ribozyme, eFx, by in vitro transcription according to the previously described method (*see* **Note 1**) [28, 32].
4. tRNA^{fMet}$_{CAU}$: Prepare an engineered initiator tRNA by in vitro transcription according to the previously described method [33].
5. A heat block.
6. 3 M $MgCl_2$.
7. 25 mM *N*-ClAc-D-tyrosine in dimethyl sulfoxide (DMSO): Chemically synthesize this D-tyrosine derivative, whose amino group is chloroacetylated and carboxyl group is derivatized as cyanomethyl ester. Dissolve it in DMSO to make a 25 mM solution (*see* **Note 1**) [32].
8. 0.3 M acidic sodium acetate (NaOAc): Dilute 1 mL of 3 M NaOAc–acetic acid (AcOH) buffer (pH 5.2) with 9 mL of water.
9. Ethanol (pure reagent grade).
10. A centrifuge.
11. 70% ethanol containing 0.1 M acidic NaOAc: Combine 333 μL of 3 M NaOAc (pH 5.2) and 2.67 mL of water with 7 mL of ethanol.
12. 70% ethanol: Combine 3 mL of water with 7 mL of ethanol.

2.2 Immobilization of the Target Protein onto Magnetic Beads

1. 0.6 mL microcentrifuge tubes.
2. His-tagged target protein of interest: Express and purify the protein using an appropriate protocol (*see* **Note 2**), or obtain it from a commercial source. The required amount will depend on the specific protein.
3. Magnetic nickel-nitrilotriacetic acid (Ni-NTA) beads (*see* **Note 2**).
4. 1× TBS–T: 50 mM Tris–HCl (pH 7.5), 150 mM NaCl, 0.05% (v/v) Tween 20.
5. A tube rotator.
6. A neodymium magnet.

2.3 Construction of a Puromycin-Conjugated mRNA Library

1. 0.6 mL microcentrifuge tubes.
2. mRNA library: Construct an mRNA library of choice (*see* **Notes 3–5**).
3. Puromycin-tagged oligonucleotide linker: Design and synthesize an oligonucleotide with a 3′-terminal puromycin modification (*see* **Note 6**).
4. T4 RNA ligase: Express and purify T4 RNA ligase heterologously in *E. coli* as described previously [34].
5. T4 RNA ligase buffer: 50 mM Tris–HCl (pH 7.5), 10 mM $MgCl_2$, 10 mM dithiothreitol (DTT), 1 mM adenosine triphosphate (ATP), and 20% DMSO.
6. Ligation stop buffer: 0.6 M NaCl, 10 mM ethylenediaminetetraacetic acid (EDTA) (pH 8.0).
7. Phenol/chloroform/isoamyl alcohol: Combine 50 mL of phenol saturated with TE buffer [10 mM Tris–HCl (pH 8.0), 1 mM EDTA], 48 mL of chloroform, and 2 mL of isoamyl alcohol.
8. A centrifuge.
9. Chloroform/isoamyl alcohol: Combine 96 mL of chloroform with 4 mL of isoamyl alcohol.
10. Tissues.

2.4 Preparation of Prenylated Macrocyclic Peptide–mRNA Fusion Library and Selection of Active Species

1. 0.6 mL microcentrifuge tubes.
2. Methionine-free FIT reaction mixture: 50 mM HEPES–KOH (pH 7.6), 100 mM potassium acetate, 12.3 mM magnesium acetate, 2 mM ATP, 2 mM guanosine triphosphate (GTP), 1 mM cytosine triphosphate (CTP), 1 mM uridine triphosphate (UTP), 20 mM creatine phosphate, 2 mM spermidine, 1 mM DTT, 1.5 mg/mL *E. coli* total tRNA, 1.2 μM *E. coli* ribosome, 0.6 μM methionyl-tRNA formyltransferase, 2.7 μM IF1, 0.4 μM IF2, 1.5 μM IF3, 0.26 μM EF-G, 10 μM EF-Tu, 0.66 μM EF-Ts, 0.25 μM RF2, 0.17 μM RF3, 0.5 μM RRF, 4 μg/mL creatine kinase, 3 μg/mL myokinase, 0.1 μM inorganic pyrophosphatase, 0.1 μM nucleotide diphosphate kinase, and 0.1 μM T7 RNA polymerase, 0.73 μM AlaRS, 0.03 μM ArgRS, 0.38 μM AsnRS, 0.13 μM AspRS, 0.02 μM CysRS, 0.06 μM GlnRS, 0.23 μM GluRS, 0.09 μM GlyRS, 0.02 μM HisRS, 0.4 μM IleRS, 0.04 μM LeuRS, 0.11 μM LysRS, 0.03 μM MetRS, 0.68 μM PheRS, 0.16 μM ProRS, 0.04 μM SerRS, 0.09 μM ThrRS, 0.03 μM TrpRS, 0.02 μM TyrRS, and 0.02 μM ValRS, 0.5 mM alanine, 0.5 mM cysteine, 0.5 mM aspartic acid, 0.5 mM glutamic acid, 0.5 mM phenylalanine, 0.5 mM glycine, 0.5 mM histidine, 0.5 mM isoleucine, 0.5 mM lysine, 0.5 mM leucine, 0.5 mM asparagine, 0.5 mM

proline, 0.5 mM glutamine, 0.5 mM arginine, 0.5 mM serine, 0.5 mM threonine, 0.5 mM valine, 0.5 mM tryptophan, and 0.5 mM tyrosine.

3. An air incubator.
4. 100 mM EDTA: Combine 2 mL of 0.5 M EDTA (pH 8.0) with 8 mL of water.
5. Reverse primer: Design and synthesize the reverse primer as appropriate (*see* **Note 4** and Fig. 1).
6. Reverse transcriptase (RTase): M-MLV reverse transcriptase, RNase H minus, point mutant (Promega).
7. Reverse transcription mix (RT mix): 75 mM Tris–HCl (pH 8.3), 0.75 mM deoxynucleoside triphosphates (dNTPs), 45 mM $Mg(OAc)_2$, 30 mM KOH, and 15 U/μL RTase.
8. KgpF prenyltransferase: Express and purify KgpF prenyltransferase heterologously in *E. coli* as described previously [6]. According to the protocol in Sect. 3.2, immobilize it on magnetic Ni-NTA beads instead of the target protein (*see* **Note 7**).
9. 50 mM Dimethylallyl diphosphate (DMAPP): Dissolve 15 mg of DMAPP in 1 mL of water.
10. A tube rotator.
11. 50 mM Tryptophan: Dissolve 10 mg of tryptophan in 1 mL of water.
12. A neodymium magnet
13. A 1.2 mL column.
14. Sephadex G-25: Equilibrate Sephadex G-25 fine with 1× TBS–T and thoroughly wash it with 1× TBS–T.
15. Forward primer: Design and synthesize the forward primer as appropriate (*see* **Note 4** and Fig. 1).
16. Polymerase-free PCR mixture: 50 mM KCl, 10 mM Tris–HCl (pH 9.0), 0.1% (v/v) Triton X-100, 2.5 mM $MgCl_2$, 0.5 mM dNTP, 0.25 μM forward primer, and 0.25 μM reverse primer.
17. A heat block.
18. *Taq* DNA polymerase: Express and purify *Taq* DNA polymerase heterologously in *E. coli* as described previously [35]. It may also be obtained from a commercial source.
19. A thermal cycler.
20. 3% agarose gel: Combine 3% agarose containing 1× TAE buffer (40 mM Tris, 20 mM acetate, and 1 mM EDTA) and 0.25 μg/mL ethidium bromide. Heat to dissolve the agarose, cast it in the electrophoresis apparatus, and allow it to solidify upon cooling.
21. 1× TAE buffer: 40 mM Tris, 20 mM acetate, and 1 mM EDTA.

22. DNA ladder.
23. DNA loading dye.
24. Electrophoresis equipment for agarose gels.
25. A UV light source or a gel imager.
26. 3 M NaCl
27. A centrifuge.
28. Ethanol.
29. Tissues.
30. RNase inhibitor: RNasin Plus (Promega).
31. 1.25× transcription mixture: 50 mM Tris–HCl (pH 8.0), 1.25 mM spermidine, 0.013% (v/v) Triton X-100, 12.5 mM DTT, 4.3 mM NTPs (pH 8.0), 0.5 U/μL RNase inhibitor, 0.3 μM T7 RNA polymerase. Freshly prepare this solution before each transcription reaction.
32. Transcription stop buffer: 0.6 M NaCl, 50 mM EDTA (pH 8.0).
33. 300 mM NaCl: Dilute 1 mL of 3 M NaCl with 9 mL of water.
34. Isopropanol.
35. A UV spectrometer.
36. A next-generation sequencer: MiSeq system (Illumina), or sequencing may be outsourced to a commercial service.

3 Methods

3.1 Synthesis of N-ClAc-D-Tyrosyl-tRNA$^{fMet}_{CAU}$

1. In a 1.7 mL microcentrifuge tube, combine 30 μL of 500 mM HEPES–KOH buffer (pH 7.5), 30 μL of 250 μM flexizyme, 30 μL of 250 μM tRNA$^{fMet}_{CAU}$, and 90 μL of water.
2. Place the tube in a preheated heat block at 95°C for 2 min. After heating, allow the solution to gradually cool at room temperature for 5 min.
3. Add 60 μL of 3 M $MgCl_2$ to the reaction mixture, incubate at room temperature for 5 min, and then transfer to ice for an additional 3 min.
4. Add 60 μL of 25 mM *N*-ClAc-D-tyrosine in DMSO to the tube. Mix gently but thoroughly.
5. Incubate the reaction mixture on ice for 2 h.
6. To quench the reaction, add 1.2 mL of 0.3 M acidic NaOAc and 3 mL of ethanol (*see* **Note 8**).
7. Centrifuge the mixture at 15,000 × *g* for 15 min at 25°C. Carefully discard the supernatant.

8. Add 750 µL of 70% ethanol containing 0.1 M acidic NaOAc. Vortex vigorously to resuspend the pellet.
9. Centrifuge the mixture at 15,000 × *g* for 5 min at 25°C. Carefully discard the supernatant.
10. Repeat Steps 8 and 9 (*see* **Note 9**).
11. Add 750 µL of 70% ethanol to wash the pellet.
12. Centrifuge the mixture at 15,000 × *g* for 3 min at 25°C, then carefully discard the supernatant.
13. Leave the tube open, loosely covered with a tissue, to allow the RNA pellet to air dry at room temperature for approximately 5 min.

3.2 Immobilization of the Target Protein onto Magnetic Beads

1. In a 0.6 mL microcentrifuge tube, combine 750 pmol of His-tagged target protein of interest with 600 µg of magnetic Ni-NTA beads in 150 µL of 1× TBS–T (*see* **Note 10**).
2. Incubate the suspension on a tube rotator at 4°C for 30 min.
3. Separate the beads using a neodymium magnet, and carefully discard the supernatant.
4. Resuspend the beads in 300 µL of 1× TBS–T, separate the beads, and discard the supernatant.
5. Wash the beads twice as described in Step 4.

3.3 Construction of a Puromycin-Conjugated mRNA Library

1. In a 0.6 mL microcentrifuge tube, combine 200 pmol of the mRNA library, 300 pmol of puromycin-tagged oligonucleotide linker, and 60 pmol of T4 RNA ligase in 200 µL of T4 RNA ligase buffer.
2. Incubate the reaction mixture at 25°C for 30 min.
3. Terminate the reaction by adding 200 µL of ligation stop buffer.
4. Add 400 µL of phenol/chloroform/isoamyl alcohol, and mix vigorously.
5. Centrifuge the mixture at 15,000 × *g* for 5 min at 25°C.
6. Collect the upper phase, add 400 µL of chloroform/isoamyl alcohol, and mix vigorously.
7. Centrifuge the mixture at 15,000 × *g* for 5 min at 25°C.
8. Collect the upper phase and add 800 µL of ethanol to the sample.
9. Centrifuge the mixture at 15,000 × *g* for 15 min at 25°C.
10. Discard the supernatant and wash the pellet with 70% ethanol.
11. Leave the tube open and loosely covered with a tissue to allow the RNA pellet to air dry at room temperature for approximately 5 min.
12. Resuspend the RNA pellet in 30 µL of water.

3.4 Preparation of Prenylated Macrocyclic Peptide–mRNA Fusion Library and Selection of Active Species

1. In a 0.6 mL microcentrifuge tube, combine 180 pmol of puromycin-tagged mRNA library and 7500 pmol of *N*-ClAc-D-tyrosyl-$tRNA^{fMet}{}_{CAU}$ in 150 μL of methionine-free FIT reaction mixture.
2. Incubate the reaction mixture in an air incubator, first at 37°C for 30 min and then at 25°C for 12 min.
3. Add 30 μL of 100 mM EDTA to the sample and incubate the mixture at 37°C for 30 min.
4. Add 500 pmol of the reverse primer into 100 μL of RT mix and incubate the mixture at 42°C in an air incubator for 1 h.
5. Add 21 nmol of KgpF prenyltransferase immobilized onto magnetic Ni-NTA beads and 12 μL of 50 mM DMAPP to the resulting mRNA/cDNA-tagged teMP library.
6. Incubate the reaction mixture on a tube rotator at 4°C for 14 h.
7. Add tryptophan (final concentration: 1 mM) and incubate the mixture at 4°C for 1 h.
8. Separate the beads using a neodymium magnet and collect the supernatant containing the mRNA/cDNA-tagged ^{PrPI}teMP library (*see* **Note 7**).
9. Desalt the reaction mixture using a 1.2 mL column packed with 1 mL of Sephadex G-25 equilibrated in 1× TBS–T.
10. Add 3.2 mg of magnetic Ni-NTA beads to the desalted sample and gently rotate the mixture at 4°C for 30 min.
11. Separate the beads using a neodymium magnet, and carefully discard the supernatant (*see* **Note 11**).
12. Add 600 μg of magnetic Ni-NTA beads preloaded with the target protein (prepared in Sect. 3.2) to the supernatant and incubate the mixture on a tube rotator at 4°C for 30 min.
13. Separate the beads using a neodymium magnet, and carefully discard the supernatant.
14. Wash the beads three times with 100 μL of 1× TBS–T.
15. Resuspend the washed beads in 400 μL of polymerase-free PCR mixture.
16. Incubate the tube in a heat block at 95°C for 5 min, then collect the resulting supernatant.
17. Add 6 μL of *Taq* polymerase solution to the collected supernatant and perform PCR amplification using a thermal cycler under conditions tailored to the specific primers and library used.
18. Verify successful amplification using 3% agarose gel electrophoresis (135 V, ~10 min).
19. Add 40 μL of 3 M NaCl and 440 μL of phenol/chloroform/isoamyl alcohol to the sample, and mix vigorously.

20. Centrifuge the mixture at 15,000 × *g* for 5 min at 25°C, and carefully collect the aqueous phase.
21. Add 440 μL of chloroform/isoamyl alcohol to the sample and mix vigorously.
22. Centrifuge the mixture at 15,000 × *g* for 5 min at 25°C, and collect the aqueous phase.
23. Add 880 μL of ethanol to the sample and centrifuge the mixture at 15,000 × *g* for 15 min at 25°C.
24. Discard the supernatant and wash the pellet once with 70% ethanol.
25. Air-dry the RNA pellet at room temperature for 5 min with the tube lid open, loosely covered with a tissue.
26. Resuspend the RNA pellet in 40 μL of water.
27. Combine 2 μL of the resulting RNA solution with 8 μL of 1.25× transcription mixture.
28. Incubate the mixture at 37°C for 16 h.
29. Add 10 μL of transcription stop buffer and 20 μL of phenol/chloroform/isoamyl alcohol and mix vigorously.
30. Centrifuge the mixture at 15,000 × *g* for 5 min at 25°C, and collect the aqueous phase.
31. Add 20 μL of chloroform/isoamyl alcohol to the sample and mix vigorously.
32. Centrifuge the mixture at 15,000 × *g* for 5 min at 25°C, and collect the aqueous phase.
33. Add 16 μL of isopropanol to the sample, and centrifuge the mixture at 15,000 × *g* for 5 min at 25°C.
34. Discard the supernatant and wash the pellet once with 70% ethanol.
35. Air-dry the RNA pellet at room temperature for 5 min with the tube open, loosely covered with a tissue.
36. Resuspend the RNA pellet in 20 μL of 300 mM NaCl.
37. Add 16 μL of isopropanol to the RNA solution, then centrifuge the mixture at 15,000 × *g* for 5 min at 25°C.
38. Repeat Steps 34 and 35.
39. Resuspend the RNA pellet in 5 μL of water.
40. Measure absorbance at 260 nm using a UV spectrophotometer to determine the RNA concentration.
41. Dilute the RNA solution to a final concentration of 10 μM with water.
42. Generate a puromycin-tagged mRNA library from the RNA prepared in Step 41 according to the procedure described in Sect. 3.3.

43. Repeat Steps 1–14 at a reduced scale (e.g., 3 pmol mRNA library in a 2.5 μL FIT reaction).
44. Add 100 μL of polymerase-free PCR mixture to the washed beads.
45. Repeat Steps 16–26 using one-quarter of the original reaction volume.
46. Repeat Steps 27–42.
47. Repeat Steps 43–46 for four to six additional cycles.
48. Sequence the resulting DNA using a next-generation sequencer according to the manufacturer's instructions.

4 Notes

1. Amino acids other than *N*-ClAc-D-tyrosine may also be used. In such cases, the appropriate variant of Flexizyme, such as eFx, dFx, or aFx, should be selected.
2. Alternative immobilization tags, such as a biotin tag or a Fc tag, may be introduced into the target protein in place of a His tag. In such cases, the corresponding magnetic beads, rather than Ni-NTA beads, should be used.
3. To enable macrocyclization of the peptide library, the open reading frame must include a cysteine codon (UGU or UGC) positioned at the C-terminus of the randomized sequence. The cysteine thiol spontaneously reacts with the N-terminal chloroacetyl moiety, yielding a thioether-closed macrocyclic scaffold. A representative mRNA design is shown in Fig. 1.
4. The 5′ and 3′ UTRs of the mRNA library can be freely designed, provided that peptide translation efficiency is maintained. The Shine–Dalgarno sequence must be incorporated in the 5′ UTR to ensure efficient ribosome binding. An example design is illustrated in Fig. 1. Primer sequences for reverse transcription and PCR should be appropriately designed according to the 5′ and 3′ UTR sequences.
5. To introduce the PrPI scaffold, the open reading frame must include a tryptophan codon (UGG) within the randomized region, serving as the precursor for PrPI formation. In addition, to maintain efficient prenylation, the residue immediately upstream of the tryptophan is preferably fixed to residues such as Val, Ala, Thr, Ile, or Pro [6]. A representative design is shown in Fig. 1.
6. The puromycin linker should be designed to be complementary to the 3′ UTR of the mRNA library to improve the ligation efficiency.

7. KgpF is immobilized on beads and removed prior to affinity-based selection to prevent interference with downstream selection procedures. If the target protein carries an immobilization tag other than a His tag, this immobilization step may be omitted.
8. Ethanol precipitation and subsequent washing steps (Steps 6–9 in Sect. 3.1) should be performed at room temperature. Performing these procedures at lower temperatures may cause undesirable salt precipitation.
9. The washing steps (Steps 8 and 9 in Sect. 3.1) are essential for efficient translation in subsequent steps. Residual magnesium or sodium ions due to insufficient washing can significantly impair translation efficiency.
10. The ratio of target protein to magnetic beads should be empirically optimized so that the bead surface is sufficiently saturated with the target protein. While TBS–T is commonly used, other suitable buffer systems may also be employed and can be supplemented with cofactors or detergents to maintain protein stability and activity.
11. Steps 10 and 11 of Sect. 3.4 are intended to eliminate bead-binding peptides from the library, as well as His-tagged proteins present in the translation mixture. These steps may be repeated, if necessary.

Acknowledgments

We thank S. Inoue for her contributions to the development of the methods presented in this chapter. This work was partially supported by KAKENHI grants (JP23H04546, JP24K01634, JP24H01754, and JP24K21760 to Y.G.; JP20H05618 to H.S.) from the Japan Society for the Promotion of Science, and by Adopting Sustainable Partnerships for Innovative Research Ecosystem program (JPMJAP2418) of the Japan Science and Technology Agency to Y.G.

References

1. Elshahawi SI, Cao H, Shaaban KA, Ponomareva LV, Subramanian T, Farman ML, Spielmann HP, Phillips Jr GN, Thorson JS, Singh S (2017) Structure and specificity of a permissive bacterial C-prenyltransferase. Nat Chem Biol 13(4):366–368
2. Offerman SC, Kadirvel M, Abusara OH, Bryant JL, Telfer BA, Brown G, Freeman S, White A, Williams KJ, Aojula HS (2017) N-tert-prenylation of the indole ring improves the cytotoxicity of a short antagonist G analogue against small cell lung cancer. MedChemComm 8(3):551–558
3. Gelb MH, Brunsveld L, Hrycyna CA, Michaelis S, Tamanoi F, Van Voorhis WC, Waldmann H (2006) Therapeutic intervention based on protein prenylation and associated modifications. Nat Chem Biol 2(10):518–528
4. Palsuledesai CC, Distefano MD (2015) Protein prenylation: enzymes, therapeutics, and

biotechnology applications. ACS Chem Biol 10(1):51–62
5. Wang M, Casey PJ (2016) Protein prenylation: unique fats make their mark on biology. Nat Rev Mol Cell Biol 17(2):110–122
6. Inoue S, Thanh Nguyen D, Hamada K, Okuma R, Okada C, Okada M, Abe I, Sengoku T, Goto Y, Suga H (2024) De novo discovery of pseudo-natural prenylated macrocyclic peptide ligands. Angew Chem Int Ed 63(36):e202409973
7. Phan C-S, Matsuda K, Balloo N, Fujita K, Wakimoto T, Okino T (2021) Argicyclamides A–C unveil enzymatic basis for guanidine bis-prenylation. J Am Chem Soc 143(27):10083–10087
8. Montalbán-López M, Scott TA, Ramesh S, Rahman IR, Van Heel AJ, Viel JH, Bandarian V, Dittmann E, Genilloud O, Goto Y (2021) New developments in RiPP discovery, enzymology and engineering. Nat Prod Rep 38(1):130–239
9. Arnison PG, Bibb MJ, Bierbaum G, Bowers AA, Bugni TS, Bulaj G, Camarero JA, Campopiano DJ, Challis GL, Clardy J (2013) Ribosomally synthesized and post-translationally modified peptide natural products: overview and recommendations for a universal nomenclature. Nat Prod Rep 30(1):108–160
10. Donia MS, Schmidt EW (2011) Linking chemistry and genetics in the growing cyanobactin natural products family. Chem Biol 18(4):508–519
11. Mattila A, Andsten R-M, Jumppanen M, Assante M, Jokela J, Wahlsten M, Mikula KM, Sigindere C, Kwak DH, Gugger M (2019) Biosynthesis of the bis-prenylated alkaloids muscoride A and B. ACS Chem Biol 14(12):2683–2690
12. Donia MS, Ravel J, Schmidt EW (2008) A global assembly line for cyanobactins. Nat Chem Biol 4(6):341–343
13. Clemente C, Johnson N, Ouyang X, Popin RV, Dall'Angelo S, Wahlsten M, Jokela J, Colombano A, Nardone B, Fewer DP (2022) Biochemical characterization of a cyanobactin arginine-N-prenylase from the autumnalamide biosynthetic pathway. Chem Commun 58(86):12054–12057
14. Parajuli A, Kwak DH, Dalponte L, Leikoski N, Galica T, Umeobika U, Trembleau L, Bent A, Sivonen K, Wahlsten M (2016) A unique tryptophan C-prenyltransferase from the Kawaguchipeptin biosynthetic pathway. Angew Chem Int Ed 55(11):3596–3599
15. Purushothaman M, Sarkar S, Morita M, Gugger M, Schmidt EW, Morinaka BI (2021) Genome-mining-based discovery of the cyclic peptide tolypamide and TolF, a Ser/Thr forward O-prenyltransferase. Angew Chem Int Ed 60(15):8460–8465
16. Dalponte L, Parajuli A, Younger E, Mattila A, Jokela J, Wahlsten M, Leikoski N, Sivonen K, Jarmusch SA, Houssen WE (2018) N-prenylation of tryptophan by an aromatic prenyltransferase from the cyanobactin biosynthetic pathway. Biochemistry 57(50):6860–6867
17. Morita M, Hao Y, Jokela JK, Sardar D, Lin Z, Sivonen K, Nair SK, Schmidt EW (2018) Post-translational tyrosine geranylation in cyanobactin biosynthesis. J Am Chem Soc 140(19):6044–6048
18. McIntosh JA, Donia MS, Nair SK, Schmidt EW (2011) Enzymatic basis of ribosomal peptide prenylation in cyanobacteria. J Am Chem Soc 133(34):13698–13705
19. Cong Y, Scesa PD, Schmidt EW (2022) AgeMTPT, a catalyst for peptide N-terminal modification. ACS Synth Biol 11(11):3699–3705
20. Hao Y, Pierce E, Roe D, Morita M, McIntosh JA, Agarwal V, Cheatham IIITE, Schmidt EW, Nair SK (2016) Molecular basis for the broad substrate selectivity of a peptide prenyltransferase. Natl Acad Sci 113(49):14037–14042
21. Okada M, Sugita T, Akita K, Nakashima Y, Tian T, Li C, Mori T, Abe I (2016) Stereospecific prenylation of tryptophan by a cyanobacterial post-translational modification enzyme. Org Biomol Chem 14(40):9639–9644
22. Ruffner DE, Schmidt EW, Heemstra JR (2015) Assessing the combinatorial potential of the RiPP cyanobactin tru pathway. ACS Synth Biol 4(4):482–492
23. Tianero MDB, Donia MS, Young TS, Schultz PG, Schmidt EW (2012) Ribosomal route to small-molecule diversity. J Am Chem Soc 134(1):418–425
24. Zhang Y, Hamada K, Nguyen DT, Inoue S, Satake M, Kobayashi S, Okada C, Ogata K, Okada M, Sengoku T (2022) LimF is a versatile prenyltransferase for histidine-C-geranylation on diverse non-natural substrates. Nat Catal 5(8):682–693
25. Sardar D, Lin Z, Schmidt EW (2015) Modularity of RiPP enzymes enables designed synthesis of decorated peptides. Chem Biol 22(7):907–916
26. Zhang Y, Goto Y, Suga H (2023) Discovery, biochemical characterization, and bioengineering of cyanobactin prenyltransferases. Trends Biochem Sci 48(4):360–374
27. Zheng Y, Cong Y, Schmidt EW, Nair SK (2022) Catalysts for the enzymatic lipidation of peptides. Acc Chem Res 55(9):1313–1323
28. Goto Y, Katoh T, Suga H (2011) Flexizymes for genetic code reprogramming. Nat Protoc 6(6):779–790
29. Nemoto N, Miyamoto-Sato E, Husimi Y, Yanagawa H (1997) In vitro virus: bonding of mRNA bearing puromycin at the 3′-terminal end to the C-terminal end of its encoded protein on the ribosome in vitro. FEBS Lett 414(2):405–408

30. Roberts RW, Szostak JW (1997) RNA-peptide fusions for the in vitro selection of peptides and proteins. Natl Acad Sci 94(23):12297–12302
31. Goto Y, Suga H (2021) The RaPID platform for the discovery of pseudo-natural macrocyclic peptides. Acc Chem Res 54(18):3604–3617
32. Murakami H, Ohta A, Ashigai H, Suga H (2006) A highly flexible tRNA acylation method for non-natural polypeptide synthesis. Nat Methods 3(5):357–359
33. Goto Y, Ohta A, Sako Y, Yamagishi Y, Murakami H, Suga H (2008) Reprogramming the translation initiation for the synthesis of physiologically stable cyclic peptides. ACS Chem Biol 3(2):120–129
34. Wang QS, Unrau PJ (2002) Purification of histidine-tagged T4 RNA ligase from *E. coli*. Biotechniques 33(6):1256–1260
35. Pluthero FG (1993) Rapid purification of high-activity Taq DNA polymerase. Nucleic Acids Res 21(20):4850

Chapter 12

Methods for the In Vitro Selection of Protein and Peptide Libraries Using mRNA Display

Colin M. Leaf, Pearl Qi, Richard W. Roberts and Terry T. Takahashi

Abstract

mRNA display is a powerful in vitro selection technique that enables the discovery of peptide and protein ligands from libraries exceeding 10 trillion unique sequences. The technique allows for exquisite control over binding stringency and specificity, and it is highly amenable to high-throughput ligand profiling and integration with machine learning approaches. Here, we describe general methods for performing mRNA display selections.

Keywords mRNA display, In vitro selection, Directed evolution, RNA-protein fusion, Combinatorial chemistry, Ligand discovery, Protein engineering

1 Introduction

Techniques that enable the rapid identification and engineering of peptides or proteins have broad applications, including the development of therapeutic leads, diagnostic reagents, and molecular tools. mRNA display enables the selection of peptide or protein binders by linking an in vitro translated polypeptide to its encoding mRNA through a puromycin-based covalent linkage (Fig. 1) [1]. This physical genotype–phenotype fusion enables iterative cycles of selection, amplification, and diversification—collectively enabling the directed evolution of ligands from libraries that can exceed 10^{14} unique sequences. mRNA display has been applied to a wide range of target classes, including proteins, nucleic acids, small molecules, and catalytic motifs, and supports a variety of selection formats depending on the biochemical context [2, 3].

Several variants of mRNA display have been developed, all of which rely on puromycin to link genotype to phenotype, but differ in chemical structure and method of attaching the puromycin linker

The authors "Colin M. Leaf" and "Pearl Qi" contributed equally to this manuscript.

Huan Peng and Theam Soon Lim (eds.), *Biomolecular Display Technologies*, Methods in Molecular Biology, vol. 3030,
https://doi.org/10.1007/978-1-0716-5249-7_12,

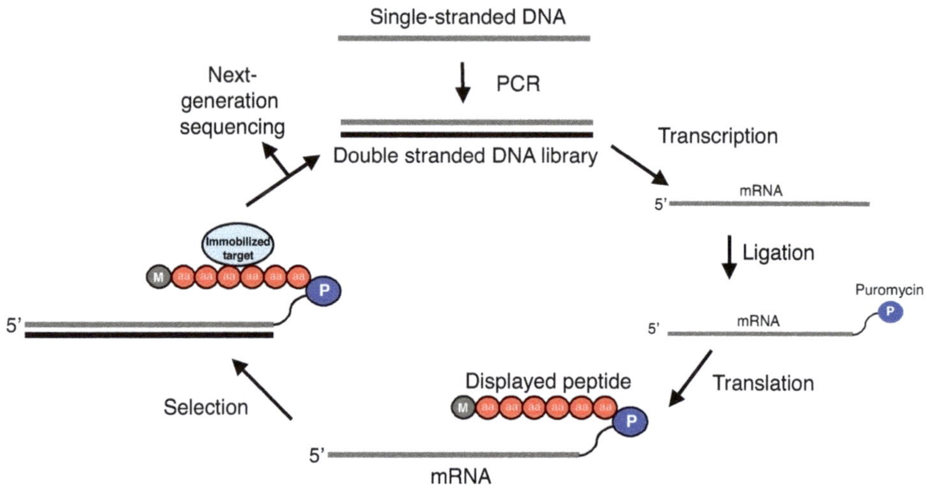

Fig. 1 An mRNA display selection cycle. ssDNA is PCR amplified (Sect. 3.2) into dsDNA. The dsDNA library is transcribed into mRNA by T7 RNA polymerase (Sect. 3.3), and a pF30P linker is ligated to the 3' end of the mRNA (Sect. 3.4). The ligated template is translated in vitro (Sect. 3.5), purified, reverse transcribed, and sieved against an immobilized target (Sect. 3.6). PCR regenerates a dsDNA library and the cycle is repeated (Sect. 3.7)

to the mRNA. These include mRNA display [2], cDNA display [4], and TRAP display [5]. Platform choice may depend on the stability, efficiency, and workflow compatibility needed for a given application. The scope of mRNA display has also been expanded through the use of sense suppression [6], nonsense suppression [7, 8], and flexizymes, which enable the incorporation of unnatural amino acids into mRNA display [9, 10].

Coupling mRNA display with next-generation sequencing (NGS) allows population-level tracking of millions of variants, enabling analysis of binding motifs and rare sequences. This approach underlies high-throughput sequencing kinetics (HTSK), which supports quantitative ranking of association and dissociation rates of thousands of ligands without the need for individual binding assays to be performed [11].

The quantitative and large-scale nature of HTSK data also facilitates machine learning-driven optimization. Denoising diffusion implicit models (DDIMs) trained on HTSK datasets can generate novel peptide ligands that demonstrate high-affinity binding despite being absent from the original library [12]. Furthermore, the output of the DDIM model can be coupled with predictive models to estimate binding affinity prior to synthesis (unpublished observations), enabling a prioritization step that refines candidate selection before experimental validation. The closed-loop integration of generation and prediction provides a scalable framework for de novo ligand discovery.

mRNA display can also be adapted to probe characteristics other than affinity, such as protease resistance [13]. By introducing proteolytic digestion prior to reverse transcription, it is possible to engineer more protease resistant sequences [14]. Sequences can also be analyzed for susceptibility to protease digestion, as one can selectively recover sequences that remain full-length after digestion, enabling quantitative analysis of sequence-dependent stability [15]. When combined with kinetic data and machine learning (ML) models, these approaches allow multiparameter optimization of ligand candidates with respect to affinity, stability, and ultimately therapeutic potential.

The following section details a basic protocol for the discovery of ligands using mRNA display (Fig. 1). While the fundamental workflow remains experimentally intensive, the method is scalable and highly adaptable. The initial selection typically requires 1–4 weeks to complete, with convergence achieved in as few as one to two rounds for low-diversity libraries, and up to ten or more rounds for complex naive libraries. The largest technical challenge in mRNA display, as with all in vitro selection techniques, is the serial nature of the experiments: early-stage errors will propagate through to later steps, and it is difficult to detect these errors until several rounds have been performed. New users are advised to first perform small-scale pilot selections with internal controls and limited diversity to ensure that all steps are working optimally. Diagnostic selections using libraries randomizing one or two positions of a known binder can also be useful for troubleshooting and benchmarking experimental fidelity [16].

2 Materials

2.1 Urea PAGE Purification of Nucleic Acids

1. 2× Formamide loading buffer: 80% (v/v) ddH_2O, 20% formamide, add bromophenol blue until dark purple. Store at 4°C (*see* **Note 1**).
2. Twenty five percent acrylamide/bis solution (19:1) containing 7.5 M urea in ddH_2O, 7.5 M urea in ddH_2O, and 10× gel buffer (7.5 M urea, 890 mM Tris base, 890 mM boric acid, and 20 mM EDTA pH 8.0) (Sequagel® system, National Diagnostics, Atlanta, GA, cat# EC-833): The solutions can be stored at room temperature for >12 months. Unpolymerized acrylamide is a neurotoxin; wear gloves and avoid exposure.
3. Ammonium persulfate (APS): prepare a 10% solution (w/v) in ddH_2O and store at 4°C for up to a month.
4. *N,N,N',N'*-Tetramethylethylenediamine (TEMED) (various suppliers). Store at 4°C.
5. Vertical gel electrophoresis apparatus capable of running gels >15 cm long (ThermoFisher Scientific, cat# P10DS-2 or similar) including 1.5 mm spacers, comb, and glass plates.
6. 5× TBE Buffer: 445 mM Tris base, 445 mM boric acid, and 10 mM EDTA pH 8.0. Filter through a 0.45 μm filter to prevent precipitation. Store at room temperature.

7. Pur-A-Lyzer Maxi 6000 Dialysis Kit (Millipore-Sigma cat# PURX60100).
8. Pur-A-Lyzer Supporting Trays for Electro elution (Millipore-Sigma, cat# PURXT).
9. Electrophoresis chamber capable of holding the Pur-A-Lyzer Maxi.
10. Saran wrap.
11. 20×20 cm glass-backed TLC plate with fluorescent dye excitable at 254 nm.
12. Amicon Ultra Centrifugal Filters, 3, 10, and 30 kDa.

2.2 Phenol Extraction/Ethanol Precipitation

1. Phenol/Chloroform/Isoamyl Alcohol (25:24:1 v/v; *see* **Note 2**).
2. Sodium Acetate: 3 M NaOAc, pH adjusted to 5.2. Store at room temperature.
3. 100% ethanol. Store at −20°C.
4. 95% (v/v) ethanol, 5% (v/v) ddH_2O. Store at 4°C.
5. 1× TE buffer: 10 mM Tris-HCl, pH 8.0, and 0.5 mM EDTA pH 8.0. Store at 4°C.

2.3 PCR

1. Taq DNA polymerase (various suppliers) or other thermostable polymerase (*see* **Note 3**). Store at −20°C.
2. 10× PCR Buffer: 100 mM Tris-HCl, pH 9.0 at room temperature, 500 mM KCl, 20 mM $MgCl_2$, 1% (v/v) Triton X-100. Aliquot and store at −20°C.
3. 10× dNTP solution (various suppliers): 2 mM of each dNTP pH adjusted to 7–8. Aliquot and store at −20°C.
4. Appropriate 5' and 3' library primers (various suppliers) at 100 μM. Store at −20°C.
5. 20× SB: 200 mM NaOH, pH adjusted to 8.0 with boric acid [17].
6. 5× TBE Buffer: See above. Store at room temperature.
7. Low melt agarose for small DNA fragments (various suppliers).
8. 5× SB Loading Buffer: Add 2.5 mL of 20× SB, 2.5 mL of ddH_2O, 6.3 g of glycerol, and add bromophenol blue until dark purple (*see* **Note 1**).
9. 100 bp DNA ladder (New England Biolabs, cat# N3231L).
10. 10 mg/mL Ethidium bromide solution (various suppliers). Store in a dark bottle. Ethidium bromide is a mutagen. Wear gloves and avoid exposure. Dispose of ethidium bromide waste accordingly.
11. Gel box for agarose gels (Bio-rad Sub-cell GT, cat# 1704466, or similar), including gel tray, 0.75 mm thick 15-well comb (*see* **Note 4**), preparative gel comb, and casting apparatus.

12. Agarose Gel Extraction Kit (Qiagen, or other vendor).

2.4 Transcription

1. T7 RNA Polymerase (various suppliers; *see* **Note 3**). Store at −20°C.
2. 5× Transcription Buffer: 400 mM HEPES-KOH, pH 7.5, 10 mM spermidine, 200 mM DTT, and 125 mM $MgCl_2$. Aliquot and store at −20°C
3. 5× NTP Solution: 20 mM each NTP, pH adjusted to 7–8 with NaOH (check pH with pH paper). It is easiest to make solutions of 5 mL or larger. Aliquot and store at −20°C.
4. 0.5 M EDTA: Adjust pH to 8.0 with NaOH (roughly, 2 g of NaOH per 100 mL) and sterile filter. Store at room temperature.
5. Sephadex G-25 DNA grade (Cytiva, cat# 17057202).
6. Pierce centrifuge columns: 5 mL (ThermoFisher Scientific, cat# 89897).

2.5 Ligation

1. T4 DNA Ligase (New England Biolabs or other supplier). Store at −20°C. (*see* **Note 3**).
2. 10× T4 DNA Ligase buffer: 50 mM Tris-HCl pH 7.5, 10 mM $MgCl_2$, 1 mM ATP, and 10 mM DTT. Store at −20°C.

2.6 Translation

1. Rabbit reticulocyte lysate (Promega, cat# L4960). The kit contains nuclease treated reticulocyte lysate and amino acid mixtures. Alternatively, reticulocyte-rich rabbit blood can be purchased from Green Hectares (https://greenhectares.com) and nuclease treated. Store at −80°C.
2. ^{35}S-methionine, in vitro translation grade, >800 Ci/mmol (Revvity, Waltham, MA, or other supplier). Store at 4°C.
3. 2.5 M KOAc. Sterile filter. Store at −20°C.
4. 25 mM $Mg(OAc)_2$. Sterile filter. Store at −20°C.
5. 12.5× Translation buffer *with* methionine: 250 mM Hepes-KOH pH 7.6, 100 mM creatine phosphate, 25 mM DTT, 312.5 μM of each amino acid. Store at −80°C.
6. 12.5× Translation buffer *without* methionine: 250 mM Hepes-KOH pH 7.6, 100 mM creatine phosphate, 25 mM DTT, 312.5 μM of each amino acid except for methionine. This buffer is for use with ^{35}S-methionine for radiolabeling experiments. Store at −80°C.
7. 1 M $MgCl_2$. Sterile filter. Store at room temperature.
8. 2.5 M KCl. Sterile filter. Store at room temperature.

2.7 Selection

1. POROS Oligo $(dT)_{25}$ Affinity Resin (ThermoFisher Scientific, cat# A48605). Store at 4°C. Do not freeze.
2. 1× Isolation Buffer: 100 mM Tris-HCl, pH 8.0, 1 M NaCl, 0.2% (v/v) Triton X-100. Sterile filter and store at 4°C.

3. RNase A, DNase, and protease-free (ThermoFisher Scientific, cat#EN0531).
4. Spin-X Filters, cellulose acetate, 0.45 μm (Corning).
5. Superscript IV reverse transcriptase (ThermoFisher Scientific, cat# 18091050): Supplied as a kit containing buffers, dNTPs, and RT enzymes. Other reverse transcriptases may be used, but should be RNase H^- to avoid degradation of the mRNA during reverse transcription.
6. 100 μM 3' library primer.
7. Sephadex G-50 DNA grade (Cytiva, cat# **17057301**).
8. Pierce Centrifuge Columns, 2 mL (ThermoFisher Scientific, cat# 89896).
9. Neutravidin agarose (ThermoFisher Scientific, cat# 29200) supplied as a 50/50 (v/v) slurry. Store at 4°C. (*see* **Note 5**).
10. Selection target (*see* **Note 6**).
11. Selection buffer (*see* **Note** 7).
12. 2 mM Biotin solution: 2 mM D-biotin dissolved in 1× PBS (137 mM NaCl, 2.7 mM KCl, 4.3 mM Na_2HPO_4, and 1.47 mM KH_2PO_4). Sterile filter and store at 4°C.
13. Blocking buffer: 1 mL of selection buffer + 25 μL of 2 mM biotin solution (50 μM biotin, final concentration).

3 Methods

Before beginning an mRNA display selection, a target and library must first be identified. The quality of the target is arguably the most critical determinant of success in an in vitro selection. Target purity and homogeneity is important to avoid enrichment of ligands that bind contaminants or undesired conformations. Proteins should be validated minimally by SDS-PAGE and activity assays post-immobilization. Size-exclusion chromatography is recommended to determine the oligomeric state of the target, detect any undesired aggregation, and isolate the correct oligomeric species. Posttranslational modifications (PTMs) should also be considered, as previous selections have produced PTM-specific ligands [18]. Typically, 1 mg of protein is sufficient for an entire selection, though it is possible to use lower amounts of target as actual usage depends on the target and the library complexity.

Library design involves balancing sequence length, codon usage, and diversity. Random peptide libraries using NNS codons (where S=G or C) are standard and have yielded picomolar ligands [11] (*see* **Note 8**). Longer constructs have been used successfully, but pose challenges due to lower fusion efficiency and higher stop codon frequency [19–21].

Libraries can be generated by chemical synthesis, via mutagenic PCR [22], by DNA shuffling [23], or can be from natural sources [24]. For chemical synthesis of libraries, phosphoramidites should be premixed in a defined ratio (A:C:G:T = 3:3:2:2) [25] and used in a separate bottle to avoid bias from different reactivities of the phosphoramidites. Machine mixed nucleotides generally produce uneven randomization and should be avoided. Libraries <37 residues can be synthesized as single oligos; for longer libraries, multiple oligos must be synthesized and ligated together [20, 26] (*see* **Note 9**).

All mRNA display libraries require a 5' constant region, a start codon, and a 3' constant region (Fig. 2a). The most common 5' constant region for selections using the rabbit reticulocyte translation system use the sequence (5'-TAATACGACTCACTATAGGGACAATTACTATTTACAATTACA-3'). This sequence contains the T7 RNA Polymerase promoter sequence (5'-TAATACGACTCACTATA-3') necessary for in vitro transcription, a GGG transcription start sequence preferred by T7 RNA Polymerase, and a translation enhancer sequence derived from Tobacco Mosaic Virus (ΔTMV). Other RNA polymerases can be used, but the T7 RNA Polymerase is robust and affordable. The start codon ATG follows the 5' constant region and is necessary for translation initiation. For *E. coli*-based translation systems, e.g., the PURE system [27], a Shine-Dalgarno sequence (5'-AGGAGGT-3') [28] should be substituted for the Δ TMV sequence above and placed an appropriate distance from the start codon. The epsilon sequence [29] has been reported to increase translation yield in reconstituted translation systems [30]. The 3' constant region is more flexible; sequences unlikely to contribute

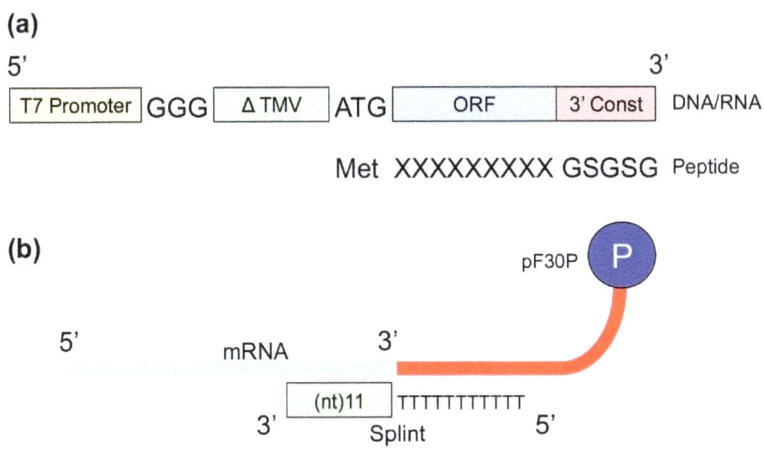

Fig. 2 (**a**) Typical design of an mRNA display library. The 5' constant region contains a T7 promoter for transcription initiation, a GGG transcription start sequence, and a ΔTMV translation enhancer sequence. The translation begins at the initiator Met codon followed by an open reading frame (ORF) and the 3' constant region. The 5' primer anneals to the 5' constant region, and the 3' primer anneals to the region labeled 3' Const. (**b**) Splint-mediated ligation of mRNA and pF30P. The splint contains the sequence 5'-$(T)_{11}(nt)_{11}$ where $(nt)_{11}$ base pairs to the 3' end of the mRNA

to binding such as $(Gly)_n$ or $(Gly\text{-}Ser)_n$ are commonly used, as are sequences which allow peptide-based purification (e.g., FLAG (DYKDDDDK) or His_6), which aid selection by enriching in frame translation products and improving convergence [26].

Lastly, the complexity of the library should be considered. While higher complexity increases the chances of discovering high-affinity binders, the larger volumes required to achieve such complexities introduce additional challenges during library synthesis, handling of material, and selection. To mitigate some of these technical issues, the first round can be performed multiple times in smaller reactions, then combined after selection. In later rounds, smaller translation volumes are often used due to the ease of handling smaller amounts of material and the reduced diversity after the first round of selection.

3.1 Purification of Nucleic Acids by Urea-PAGE

This protocol describes the preparation of a library from chemically synthesized DNA. As with preparation of the target, the quality of the library preparation is a critical factor for success. Care should be taken to ensure library complexity is preserved during experimental steps, and the library corresponds to how it was designed. Spurious reaction products (incorrect size products, smeary products, etc.) should be avoided, and reaction steps should be optimized to avoid these undesired products.

1. Obtain an appropriate DNA library. Calculate the volume of ddH_2O required to resuspend the DNA based on 50–100 μL of ddH_2O per 100 nmol of DNA. Add an equal volume of 2× Formamide loading buffer.
2. Based on the size of the DNA fragment, prepare an appropriate percentage 1.5 mm-thick urea-polyacrylamide gel according to the manufacturer's recommendations (*see* **Note 10**). Prepare enough gel mixture to have >5 mL excess, then add 1% of the volume of 10% APS and 0.1% of the volume of TEMED. Mix quickly (*see* **Note 11**) and pour the gel. Insert the comb diagonally to avoid trapping air bubbles and allow the gel to polymerize.
3. Prepare 1 L of 1× TBE by dilution of the 5× TBE stock.
4. Assemble the gel in the gel system. Remove the comb and wash the wells with 1× TBE buffer to remove any unpolymerized acrylamide. Prerun the gel at 25 W per gel for 15–30 min (*see* **Note 12**). Prerunning the gel helps to increase gel temperature and helps to keep the nucleic acid denatured.
5. Ensure the gel is disconnected from the power supply, then wash the wells with 1× TBE buffer again to remove any urea that has diffused into the wells. Load 100 μL of sample per lane (*see* **Note 13**). Run the gel at 25 W until the bromophenol blue dye reaches the bottom of the gel. Typically, this will take 60–90 min, depending on the percentage gel. For longer RNAs, run until the xylene cyanol reaches the bottom of the gel, which can take >2 h.

6. Ensure that the gel is disconnected from the power supply. Disassemble the gel apparatus and remove one glass plate. Place a piece of Saran wrap on the gel, invert, then remove the second glass plate, leaving the gel on the Saran wrap. Place on a fluorescent TLC plate and use a handheld UV light to UV shadow the nucleic acid, taking care to minimize the UV exposure to prevent DNA damage. The bands will be dark purple/black against the green plate background (*see* **Note 14**). Excise the bands with a clean razor or glass cover slide (*see* **Note 15**). The gel slices can be stored in a 15 or 50 mL conical tube overnight at −20°C if desired.
7. Insert gel slices into a Pur-A-Lyzer Maxi dialysis tube taking care not to overfill the tube.
8. Prepare 2 L of 0.5× TBE. Fill the dialysis tubes containing gel slices with 0.5× TBE and seal the tube, avoiding any bubbles. The dialysis tubes can then be put in the tube holder for electroelution. Fill the inner chamber of an appropriately sized electrophoresis tank with 0.5× TBE buffer then place tubes in the filled tank such that membranes are totally covered by buffer. Orient the tubes so that the tubes are perpendicular to the current, so that the current can pass through the membranes on the dialyzer tube.
9. Elute the DNA for 2 h at 200 V. Switch the polarity of the leads and run backwards for 10–15 s. Collect the eluent using a P1000 pipette, taking care not to poke a hole in the membranes or collect any gel pieces in the tip. Most of the DNA will be eluted in the first hour, which is usually sufficient; however, a second elution can be performed if desired.
10. Concentrate the eluent with an appropriately sized Amicon Centrifugal Concentrator. Desalt the sample by washing five times with 500 μL ddH_2O. Elute the sample by flipping the concentrator upside down into a new collection tube and spinning at 750×*g* for 2 min (*see* **Note 16**).
11. Determine the DNA concentration by UV absorbance.

3.2 PCR Amplification of DNA

We recommend performing a small-scale PCR reaction before performing a large-scale reaction to ensure that the PCR reaction is robust, as poor amplification can result in unwanted bias in the library. This is especially important to avoid "monster" sequences that solely amplify well [31]. If the PCR reaction is not amplifying well, optimization of the reaction can improve the product yield. However, if the PCR reaction remains poor even after optimization, consider resynthesizing the library, possibly with a different 3' primer. Primer design is critical in PCR and any primers that form primer dimers should especially be avoided.

3.2.1 Initial Small-Scale PCR

1. Obtain a 5' and 3' primer for amplification of the desired template. Resuspend the primers in ddH_2O such that the final concentration is 100 μM and divide into 100 μL aliquots (*see* **Note 17**).
2. Prepare a 1 μM stock of ssDNA template (from Sect. 3.1).
3. Prepare a PCR reaction in a 0.65 mL tube containing 1 pmol of ssDNA template (1 μL of 1 μM), 100 pmol of each primer (1 μL of each 100 μM primer), 10 μL of 10× dNTP mix, 10 μL of 10× PCR mix, and add ddH_2O to 99 μL (*see* **Note 18**).
4. Place the tube on a PCR block and preheat the reaction to 94°C. Once the reaction reaches 94°C, add 1 μL of Taq to the tube. Perform six cycles of PCR of 94°C for 30 s, 55°C for 30 s, and 72°C for 45 s. (*see* **Note 19**).
5. While the reaction is cycling, prepare a 2% agarose gel with the low melting point (LMP) agarose. This protocol is for the Bio-rad mini-sub cell GT but can be adapted for other systems. Place the gel tray into the casting apparatus (or tape the ends). Weigh 1 g of LMP agarose, place in a 125 mL Erlenmeyer flask, then add 50 mL of 1× SB buffer or 1× TBE buffer. Microwave until the agarose is dissolved, stirring occasionally. Caution is advised since the solution can easily boil over. Cool the flask under running tap water while swirling until it can comfortably be touched (~55°C), then add 2 μL of 10 mg/mL ethidium bromide. Before the gel hardens, pour the solution into the gel tray, place the comb into the gel, and allow it to harden (*see* **Note 20**).
6. After the reaction is completed, remove the tube from the thermocycler.
7. Mix 1 μL of 100 bp DNA ladder with 1 μL of 5× SB Loading buffer and load on the gel. Mix 1 μL of 5× SB Loading buffer with 4 μL of PCR product and load on an adjacent lane (*see* **Note 21**). Run the gel for 4 min at 300 V if using SB buffer (or 7 min at 220 V for 1× TBE gels), then image the gel. Longer run times may be required for longer templates (*see* **Note 22**).
8. Evaluate the PCR reaction by comparing the density of the product band to that of the nearest-sized band of the 100 bp DNA ladder. Examples of an ideal PCR reaction, and commonly observed issues are shown in Fig. 3. The PCR product should be roughly the same intensity as the corresponding band of the 100 bp ladder, and qualitatively the PCR product should be one band of the correct size (Fig. 3a). Double-banding, smearing, incorrectly-sized products, or primer dimer all indicate that the PCR reaction should be optimized (*see* **Note 23**) (Fig. 3b, c).

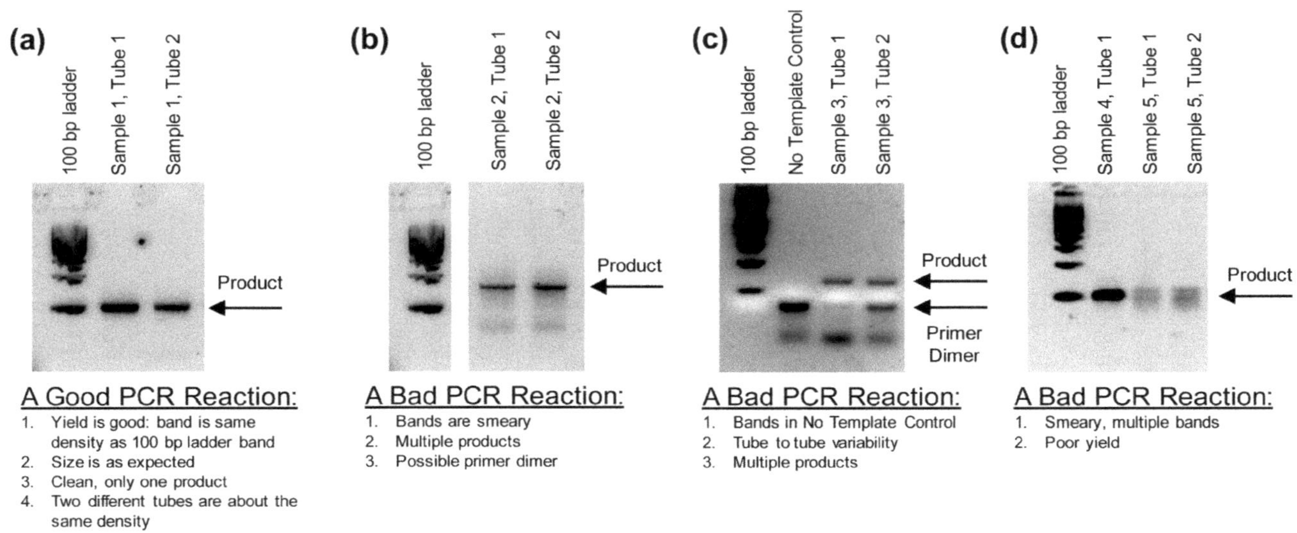

Fig. 3 (**a**) An example of a successful PCR reaction of a library. A single band at the expected size is observed, and multiple tubes from the PCR reaction yield the same amount of product. (**b**) An example of an PCR reaction that may need optimization. Here, the bands are smeary, and there are multiple products including possible primer dimer. The PCR reaction may need optimization (Sect. 3.2.2). (**c**) An example of a PCR reaction where the 3' primer may need to be redesigned. There is a band in the no-template control that shows significant primer dimer. Variability is also seen when comparing one tube to another. (**d**) An example of a PCR reaction that may need optimization or resynthesis of the DNA template. There are multiple bands in the Sample five tubes, and the product bands are smeary. There may be multiple priming sites in the template or the template was not synthesized or purified correctly

3.2.2 Optimization of the PCR Reaction (as Necessary)

If PCR optimization is necessary, several factors can be optimized including template concentration, primer concentration, dNTP concentration, magnesium concentration, Taq concentration, and annealing temperature.

1. Prepare a series of PCR reaction mixes in 0.65 mL tubes containing 1–8 pmol of ssDNA template (1–8 μL of 1 μM), 100–200 pmol of each primer (1 μL of 100–200 μM primer), 10 μL of 10× dNTP mix, 10 μL of 10× PCR mix, and add ddH_2O to 99 μL.
2. If desired, the annealing temperature (45–65°C), dNTP concentration (0.1–0.3 mM final concentration), magnesium concentration (0.5–3 mM), and Taq can be also be varied.
3. Perform the PCR cycling and analysis as described in Sect. 3.2.1.
4. If the PCR product is still not optimal, first recheck the design of the library and primer sequences. If these are correct, sequence and analyze the library as in Sect. 3.2.3 to ensure the synthetic library corresponds to the design. The ssDNA template can also be run on a denaturing gel as in Sect. 3.1 to ensure it is one band—roughly 250 pmol of a 100-nt ssDNA template can be loaded and visualized via UV-shadowing. Consider resynthesizing and/or redesigning the library if all these efforts fail.

3.2.3 Sequencing the Rd 0 Library

The library should be analyzed by DNA sequencing to ensure that the library corresponds to what was designed. This can be performed concurrently with PCR optimization and can be helpful to determine the reason for undesired PCR products. While Sanger sequencing can be used for analysis, we recommend next generation sequencing for ease of use and higher number of sequences for a marginal increase in cost.

1. Pour a preparative agarose gel using a preparative gel comb. Gel purify an entire 100 μL PCR reaction (*see* **Note 24**). Visualize the band using a handheld UV lamp and excise with a clean razor. Minimize UV exposure and wear proper PPE (gloves, face shield, etc.).
2. Extract the DNA from the gel slice using a gel extraction kit according to the manufacturer's specifications.
3. Submit the gel-purified DNA sample for DNA sequencing. We recommend sending the DNA to Plasmidsaurus (https://plasmidsaurus.com/) or similar sequencing facility. Most sequencing facility minimums for nanopore sequencing are in excess of a thousand reads for a purified PCR product, which is more than sufficient to determine if the library was designed and synthesized correctly.

4. Analyze the sequencing data. The majority of the sequences should be in frame and verified that random positions are reasonably close to the designed A, T, C, G percentages. If sequencing reveals undesigned bias, consider resynthesizing the library.

3.2.4 Preparation of a Large-Scale Library

Determine the size of the library required for selection; typical libraries range from 10^{12} to 10^{14} molecules. While larger libraries theoretically search a large fraction of sequence space, we typically use libraries of 10^{12} molecules to avoid the additional experimental difficulty and complications of larger libraries. A library of this size is usually sufficient to find initial high affinity ligands, which can be further improved using mRNA display or traditional design techniques.

1. Assuming that each DNA sequence entering the PCR is unique, the pool complexity will be the number of molecules entering the PCR multiplied by the fraction of molecules extendable (*see* **Note 25**), also called a pool equivalent. Calculate the number of 100 μL reactions needed to obtain the desired pool complexity (e.g., a single 100 μL reaction with 1 pmol template that is 20% extendable contains ~1.2×10^{11} molecules; a pool of 1×10^{12} molecules would require ~0.83 mL of PCR).
2. Perform a large-scale PCR reaction. If more than ten tubes are loaded onto the PCR block, change the cycling reaction to 2 min at 94°C, 2 min at 55°C, and 4 min at 72°C to adjust for the increased mass that must be cycled (*see* **Note 26**).
3. Run an agarose gel to check the quality of the PCR product. Several representative tubes should be checked to ensure the amplification across the entire PCR block was even.

3.2.5 Phenol Extraction/Ethanol Precipitation of Nucleic Acids

Phenol extraction followed by ethanol precipitation is used to clean up the sample. PCR purification columns can be used instead and are faster than phenol extraction/ethanol precipitation, however, in some cases poor yields or salty samples have been observed with cleanup columns.

1. Pool the PCR reactions in 1.7 mL tubes. Add a maximum of 0.5 mL to each tube. Add an equal volume of phenol/chloroform/isoamyl alcohol and vortex. **Caution!** Phenol can cause severe chemical burns—wear proper Personal Protection Equipment (PPE) and have a phenol spill kit and phenol-specific first aid kit.
2. Spin for 30–60 s at top speed in a centrifuge to separate the organic and aqueous layers. Remove (save) the top aqueous layer (*see* **Note 27**) and transfer to a new 1.7 mL tube.
3. Add 1/10 volume of 3 M NaOAc, pH 5.2, then add two to three volumes of −20°C 100% ethanol.
4. Allow the DNA to incubate at −20°C for 15–30 min.

5. Spin at top speed (14–15 K RPM) in a 4°C centrifuge (*see* **Note 28**).
6. Remove and discard the supernatant with an aspirator or pipette. Do not disturb the pellet. The pellet should appear white and approximately 1–2 mm in length. Wash the pellet by adding 1 mL of 95% ethanol, inverting the tube, then remove the supernatant without disturbing the pellet.
7. Dry the pellet by placing the tube in a Speedvac or by allowing the tube to air dry upside down on a Kimwipe. Alternatively, leave the open tube on a 65°C heat block covered with a Kimwipe until dry.
8. Resuspend the pellet in 10 mM Tris-HCl, pH 8.0, or other similar buffer. (*see* **Note 29**).

3.2.6 Quantification of the Large-Scale Library

1. Run a dilution series of the dsDNA pool (e.g., 1/4, 1/8, 1/16, etc.) on an agarose gel and compare the dsDNA product to the nearest-sized band of the 100 bp ladder to determine the concentration of dsDNA (in ng/μL; *see* **Note 30**).
2. Determine the number of pool equivalents that have been synthesized (i.e., the number of times the initial pool has been amplified). For a six cycle PCR, theoretically 32 pool equivalents should have been synthesized (the first cycle of PCR does not amplify DNA, but rather makes the ssDNA template double-stranded), however, the actual number can range from ~5 to 20. The dsDNA pool can be stored at −20°C indefinitely.

3.3 In Vitro Transcription

1. In order to preserve the complexity of the library, at least three pool equivalents must be carried through each subsequent step until the affinity selection step. Calculate the volume of the transcription reaction required to retain the pool complexity, assuming a final template DNA concentration in the transcription reaction of 100 nM. For example, a pool of 1×10^{13} molecules would require ~50 pmol to be carried through in a 0.5 mL transcription (*see* **Note 31**).
2. Prepare the transcription reaction; per mL add the dsDNA PCR product from Sect. 3.2.6 to a final concentration of 100 nM, 200 μL of 5× NTP buffer, 200 μL of 5× Transcription buffer, and ddH_2O to 1 mL (*see* **Notes 32 and 33**). Heat the reaction to 65°C for 5 min, then cool on ice. Once cool, add 10 μL of T7 RNA polymerase, gently invert the tube several times to ensure complete mixing, and incubate at 37°C for 2–4 h to overnight. Formation of a white magnesium pyrophosphate precipitate indicates successful transcription. Generally, most of the product is generated within

1–2 h, however, longer incubations will yield more product. Occasionally, nonspecific products have been observed after longer incubations.

3. After setting up the transcription reaction, prepare the G-25 Sephadex resin for desalting. Per 1 mL of transcription (or less), weigh 1 g of Sephadex G-25 and add 8 mL of ddH_2O in a 15 mL conical tube. Swell the resin by rotating for >30 min. Avoid swelling the resin >24 h as it will clog the column in the following steps.
4. After the transcription reaction is complete, add 1/10 volume of 0.5 M EDTA, pH 8.0 and vortex until the white precipitate is dissolved.
5. Phenol extract as in Sect. 3.2.5, but do not ethanol precipitate (*see* **Note 34**).
6. Place an empty 5 mL spin desalting column into a 15 mL conical tube. Add the 8 mL of preswollen resin slurry to the column. Let the column drain until it stops dripping, then discard the filtrate. Spin at 750×*g* for 2 min, then discard the filtrate. Transfer the desalting column to a new 15 mL conical tube. Add the aqueous layer from phenol extraction to the center of the desalting column slowly. Spin at 750×*g* for 2 min, and keep the filtrate (*see* **Note 35**).
7. Gel purify the mRNA on an appropriate percentage denaturing gel (*see* **Note 10**). Up to 2 mL of transcription reaction can be loaded on a 1.5 mm gel, depending on the quality of the mRNA. Electroelute the purified mRNA as in Sect. 3.1, and ethanol precipitate and quantitate the mRNA as in Sect. 3.2.5. The mRNA can be stored at −20°C indefinitely.

3.4 Ligation of the Puromycin Linker

1. Synthesize a DNA splint that contains the sequence 5'-$(T)_{11}(nt)_{11}$-3' where the $(nt)_{11}$ region base pairs to the 3' end of the mRNA (*see* **Notes 36 and 37**). Resuspend the splint in ddH_2O to a final concentration of 500 μM.
2. Synthesize the pF30P linker. The linker may be ordered from a number of commercial sources (e.g., Integrated DNA Technologies or the Keck Biotechnology Resource Laboratory, New Haven, CT). Order a 1 μmol scale synthesis of the sequence $8(A)_{21}777ACC6$, where 8 is chemical phosphorylation reagent, 7 is spacer phosphoramidite 9, and 6 is puromycin CPG (*see* **Note 38**). Purify the pF30P via urea-PAGE using a 12% Urea gel, electroelute, and concentrate using an Amicon 3 kDa MWCO filter (*see* **Note 16**). Dilute the sample to 100–200 μL with ddH_2O and determine the concentration using an $\varepsilon = 294{,}200\ M^{-1}cm^{-1}$. Dilute the pF30P to 500 μM.

3. Determine the volume of translation required to carry three pool equivalents through the translation and purification steps to just before the affinity selection step. Assume an overall yield of 3% through all steps from translation to right before the affinity selection step (*see* **Note 39**). For example, for a pool of 1×10^{12} molecules, ~170 pmol should be translated in order for 3×10^{12} molecules to enter the selective step.
4. Calculate the minimum volume of ligation reaction required, based on the number of pmol required for translation. Assume a conservative yield of 20% of input mRNA (e.g., a yield of 1000 pmol per 500 μL of ligation reaction). For a pool of 1×10^{12}, roughly 0.1 mL of ligation would be required. However, it is typically better to perform at least 0.25–0.5 mL ligation reactions so that there is enough ligated material to perform optimization experiments or the first round of selection several times.
5. Prepare the large-scale ligation reaction; a 0.5 mL ligation contains 10 μM mRNA, 15 μM splint (500 μM stock), 10 μM pF30P (500 μM stock), 50 μL 10× ligase buffer, and ddH_2O to 487.5 μL (*see* **Note 40**). Add 12.5 μL of T4 DNA ligase and incubate at room temperature for 30–60 min.
6. Add an equal volume of 2× Formamide loading buffer and gel purify on an appropriate percentage gel as in Sect. 3.1 (*see* **Notes 41 and 42**). A lower amount of formamide buffer can be used if the sample is heated at 65°C for 5–10 min before loading.
7. Lane 1 in Fig. 4 shows an example of an ideal ligation. The ligation product should appear as a single band above the transcription, and should be slightly less than equal to the transcription band in size and intensity (~40% conversion) (Fig. 4a).
8. Excise the ligated product and electroelute as in Sect. 3.1.
9. Determine the concentration of the mRNA-pF30P ligated template by UV. Adjust the concentration to 10 μM.
10. Commonly observed issues with ligation are shown in lanes 2 and 3 of Fig. 4. If poor yield is observed due to insufficient transcription, transcription yield can often by improved by increasing the amount of DNA used. If poor ligation is observed, incubating the ligation reaction at 37°C has shown to improve the ligation efficiency for some templates. However, if these methods fail to improve ligation, redesigning the 3' end is often necessary.

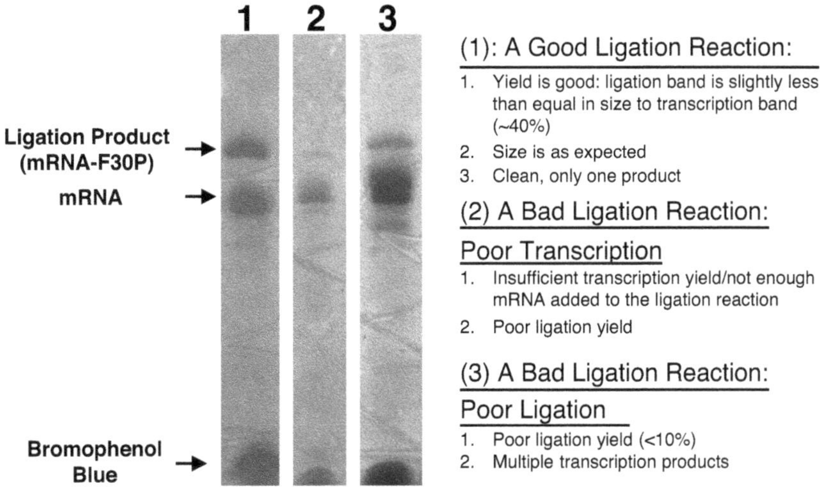

Fig. 4 Comparison between a successful splint-mediated ligation (Lane 1) and commonly observed unsuccessful ligations (Lanes 2 and 3). In the successful ligation in Lane 1, there is a good yield of transcription (lower band) and roughly 40% of the total transcription product is converted to ligated product (upper band). In Lane 2, the ligation yield is worse than Lane 1 but not enough mRNA was synthesized during transcription. There may not be enough DNA template or a smeary PCR product resulting in production of heterogenous mRNA that is also smeary. In Lane 3, the transcription reaction produced a good transcription yield, however, the ligation yield was poor. This is usually due to secondary structure in the 3' region, which prevents the splint from annealing. If this poor yield is observed, performing the ligation at 37°C can improve results, but generally it is best to redesign the 3' region

3.5 *In Vitro Translation*

This section details the preparation of a translation mix using rabbit reticulocyte lysate, though other translation mixes can be used (*see* **Note 43**). The following protocol is for a total cold translation volume of 1 mL, which is a typical translation size for a library of 1×10^{12} members.

1. Prepare the translation reaction. Typically, a larger-scale translation (cold; 1 mL) for selection is performed alongside a smaller-scale translation (50 μL) with ^{35}S-methionine to track binding (hot). The hot reaction is used to monitor the various steps of the selection, as well as test for background and target binding. Adjust the reagent volumes accordingly for larger or smaller translations. Each 1000 μL cold reaction contains 40 μ L of 10 μM ligated template from Sect. 3.4, 40 μL of 2.5 M KOAc, 20 μL 25 mM $Mg(OAc)_2$, 80 μL 12.5× translation mix *with* Methionine, 420 μL of ddH_2O, and 400 μL of treated rabbit reticulocyte lysate.
2. In a separate tube, prepare a 50 μL hot reaction with 2 μL of 10 μM ligated template, 2 μL of 2.5 M KOAc, 1 μL 25 mM $Mg(OAc)_2$, 4 μL 12.5× translation mix *without* Methionine,

2 μL in vitro translation grade ^{35}S-labeled methionine, 19 μL of ddH_2O, and 20 μL of treated rabbit reticulocyte lysate.

3. Incubate both reactions at 30°C for 1 h.
4. After translation, add 2 μL of 1 M $MgCl_2$ and 7 μL of 2.5 M KCl per 25 μL of translation to facilitate fusion formation [32]. Incubate at room temperature for 5–15 min. Alternatively, store at −20°C overnight.

3.6 First Round of Selection

The first round of selection is difficult because there are so few copies of each sequence (average of ~3 copies). If a functional sequence is lost in the first round, it is permanently lost, thus it is important that all the steps of the selection are performing optimally to retain as many sequences as possible. We recommend that a novice user perform a smaller-scale selection (100 μL cold translation) through the PCR amplification step to ensure the selection is working correctly, before proceeding to the large-scale selection.

1. Aliquot 20% of the translation volume (0.2 mL) of the POROS Oligo $(dT)_{25}$ Affinity Resin bead slurry into a 1.7 mL tube. Wash the beads three times with 1 mL isolation buffer (IB), spinning to pellet and discarding the supernatant each time. Add 100 μL of IB to make a 50/50 slurry.
2. Aliquot the slurry into 11 tubes—each with 20 μL of the 50/50 slurry. One tube will be for the hot sample while the remaining tubes will be for the cold sample. Add 980 μL of IB to each tube.
3. To **only** the tube with hot sample add 1 μL of 10 mg/mL RNase A (*see* **Note 44**). This will ensure observed binding is not a result of mRNA aptamer.
4. Add the entire hot sample to one tube. Split the cold sample among the remaining ten tubes and rotate at 4°C for 1 h.
5. While the translation is incubating with dT beads, prepare the target and no target beads (*see* **Note 45**). To prepare the target beads (two binding reactions—one hot and one cold), aliquot 20 μL of a 50/50 slurry of neutravidin agarose in a 1.7 mL tube and wash three times with 1 mL of selection buffer. Add 200 pmol of target and 1 mL of selection buffer and incubate at 4°C for 1 h (*see* **Note 46**). To prepare the no target beads (one binding reaction—only hot), aliquot 10 μL of neutravidin agarose and wash as above (do not add target to this sample). Following the incubation, wash the beads three times with 1 mL of blocking buffer, then add 1 mL of blocking buffer and rotate at 4°C for another hour for both samples. This procedure is enough to prepare target beads for two binding samples—one hot and one cold.
6. Before beginning the dT washing steps, fill two 1.7 mL tubes with ddH_2O and heat at 65°C.

7. Transfer the hot sample to one Spin-X column. Recombine the cold samples into a single Spin-X column (*see* **Note 47**). Spin for 30 s at 1500×*g* and remove the filtrate. For the cold reactions, repeat this process until all the samples are filtered. Wash the beads five times with 500–600 μL IB, spinning and removing the filtrate between washes. After removing the last wash, spin the empty column for 30 s at 1500×*g*.
8. Save the last wash from the hot sample and count it in a scintillation counter. The last wash should be below ~2000 cpm. If not, continue washing until the cpm are below 2000.
9. Transfer the top cup of the Spin-X to a new 1.7 mL tube. Elute the fusions by adding 50 μL of 65°C water, incubating for 1 min, then centrifuging. Repeat for a total of five elutions. The elution volume and number of elutions can be adjusted, but a minimum of three elutions and a minimum volume of 50 μL are necessary for good yields (*see* **Note 48**). Count 1/10 volume of the eluent to determine the total cpm for the entire reaction (*see* **Note 49**).
10. Prepare a binding reaction of 100,000 cpm of hot fusions, 10 μL of 50/50 slurry of target, and add selection buffer to 1 mL. Similarly, prepare a no target control reaction with the no target beads. Incubate both samples at 4°C for 1 h transfer the solutions to a Spin-X filter and wash 3× with 500–600 μ L of selection buffer. Count the supernatant, the washes, and the beads in a scintillation counter. Determine the percent binding by dividing the cpm on the beads by the total number of cpm in the reaction (supernatant + washes + beads) (*see* **Note 50**).
11. While the hot translation is incubating with target, prepare a desalting column (*see* **Note 51**).
12. Swell 0.5 g of Sephadex G-50 in 10 mL of water for >30 min, with rotation.
13. Add the prehydrated G-50 resin to the 2 mL spin column. Allow the sample to drain, then discard the filtrate. Spin at 750×*g* for 2 min, then discard the filtrate.
14. Add the cold reaction to the center of the column and spin at 750×*g* for 2 min., then keep the filtrate.
15. For every 500 μL of cold translation, prepare 490 μL of RT mix (50 μL of 12.5× First strand buffer, 10 μL of 100 μM 3' primer, 50 μL of 10× dNTPs, and 380 μL of elution) (*see* **Note 52**).
16. Heat the RT mix at 65°C for 5–10 min, and place on ice (*see* **Note 53**). Once cooled, remove 1 μL for a negative control RT reaction (–RT). Place the cooled RT mixture at 42°C for 2 min and then add 1 μL of SSIV enzyme per 50 μL of RT

mix, and incubate at 42°C for 60 min. Heat at 65°C to kill the RT enzyme, then cool on ice. Remove 1 μL for a positive control RT reaction (+RT).

17. Combine the RT reaction and target beads (*see* **Notes 54 and 55**). Incubate at 4°C for 1 h.
18. Spin the tube at 1500×*g* for 30 s until the beads settle. Remove the supernatant and wash three times with 1 mL of selection buffer. Add 1 mL of selection buffer, resuspend the beads and transfer to a new tube (*see* **Note 56**). Remove ~ 950 μL supernatant after the last wash.
19. Prepare a 1.4 mL PCR mix with 14 μL of each primer, 140 μL of 10× dNTP mix, 140 μL of 10× PCR mix, and add ddH_2O to 1386 μL. Resuspend the pellet with 990 μL of the mix and aliquot into 10×0.65 mL tubes. Aliquot 99 μL of the mix into a 0.65 mL tube, which will serve as a no template control reaction (*see* **Note 57**). Lastly, add 99 μL of the PCR mix into the –RT and +RT samples.
20. Calculate the initial template concentration in the PCR reaction. For example, for 1 mL of translation, the initial template concentration will be approximately 0.000012 μM assuming a binding efficiency of ~0.1% (*see* **Note 58**). Based on the initial template concentration, calculate the number of cycles needed to amplify the library, assuming a final template concentration of 0.1 μM. Similarly, calculate the initial concentration and cycles required for the +RT reaction.
21. Cycle the PCR reaction according to Sect. 3.2, but stop the reaction three cycles before the number calculated in Step 20. Run 4 μL of the PCR product on a 2% SB or TBE gel to determine if more cycles are necessary (*see* **Note 59**). If there is no product, perform three additional cycles, and check again. If a light band is seen, perform one to four more cycles. Continue until the product band is similar in density to the nearest-sized band of the 100 bp ladder (*see* **Note 60**). The +RT and –RT controls will provide confirmation that the reverse transcription was successful. There should be a > 4 round difference between when the +RT and –RT control reactions show a band.

3.7 Additional Selection Rounds

Once the first round of selection is completed in Sect. 3.6, repeat the following cycle until binding is observed.

1. Phenol extract and ethanol precipitate the enriched pool. Resuspend the DNA pellet in 200 μL of 1× TE buffer or 10 mM Tris-HCl, pH 7.5.
2. Use 100 μL of the resuspended DNA in a 1 mL transcription as in Sect. 3.3 (*see* **Note 61**).

3. Add EDTA, phenol extract and desalt using Sephadex G-25 in a spin column as in Sect. 3.3. After the first round of selection, we typically do not gel purify the RNA before ligation of the puromycin linker.
4. Perform a ligation reaction as in Sect. 3.4, except add no water to the ligation. Instead, add as much volume of desalted mRNA as possible. Gel purify the product as in Sect. 3.1.
5. Perform a 100 μL cold translation and a 50 μL hot translation, dT purify, desalt, and reverse transcribe the sample as in Sect. 3.6.
6. Perform a hot binding assay as described in Sect. 3.6.
7. Incubate with target, wash, elute, then PCR amplify the reaction as in Sect. 3.6. Once binding over background is observed, the library can be sequenced (see Qi et al. Chap. 2). Typically, 10% binding to target with little binding to beads with no target indicates a successful selection. As the selection progresses, the selective pressure can be increased to retain higher affinity sequences and get rid of lower affinity sequences. Selective pressure can be increased in a number of ways, including increasing the temperature, increasing salt, or adding a specific competitor.
8. It is difficult to monitor selection progress as any changes in pool composition or errors are not observed for several rounds. The easiest way to monitor the selection progress is to sequence every round, however, this can be expensive. Plasmidsaurus (https://plasmidsaurus.com/) offers affordable sequencing to gauge changes in pool composition. Alternatively, there are several other crude metrics to gauge selection progress. Generally, the cpm after dT purification should remain the same or increase round over round. The number of PCR cycles should also remain the same or decrease, assuming the same level of selective pressure is applied. However, the number of PCR cycles is not very sensitive to changes in the pool and will often only drop after binding increases significantly in the radioactive binding assay.

4 Notes

1. The amount of bromophenol blue added is not critical as it acts as an electrophoresis marker. Xylene cyanol can also be added if desired. This is particularly useful when gels must be run for hours as in the case of longer mRNAs (e.g., with protein libraries).
2. The phenol/chloroform/isoamyl solution can be purchased premixed or made in house. Pink solutions of phenol indicate oxidation and should be discarded.

3. Plasmids for Taq, T4 DNA Ligase, T7 RNA Polymerase, and MMLV RNaseH- Reverse Transcriptase are available on Addgene (https://www.addgene.org). Significant quantities of these enzymes can be purified making the overall process more affordable.
4. Thin 0.75 mm combs give better resolution but are more difficult to load. Thicker 1.5 mm combs are easier to load, though will give slightly worse resolution.
5. The target may be immobilized by other methods such as neutravidin acrylamide (Ultralink, Pierce), streptavidin agarose, or other biotin-binding matrix. Covalent methods of immobilization include NHS-activated sepharose or agarose, epoxy-activated sepharose, or cyanogen bromide-activated sepharose.
6. Roughly 1–10 μg of a 30 kDa protein will be needed per round of selection (33–330 pmol). However, we recommend at least 1 mg of protein since more protein is required for the first round of selection, as well as for optimization experiments, monitoring selection progress, and analysis of functional sequences.
7. The selection buffer will depend on the specific requirements of the target. We have successfully used buffers such as 25 mM Hepes pH 7.5, 150 mM NaCl, 0.05% (v/v) Tween 20, 0.05% (w/v) Bsa, and 1 μg/mL tRNA. Buffers should have a buffering agent (e.g., Hepes, Tris, or phosphate), a monovalent salt (NaCl or KCl), a non-ionic detergent (Tween−20, NP-40, or Triton X-100), Bsa, and tRNA. Magnesium, reducing agents (DTT or β-mercaptoethanol), or protein specific requirements (such as GDP for G proteins [33]) can also be added, as needed.
8. NNS codons (where N=A/T/G/C and S=G/C) are the best choice for a random codon with relatively even ratios of amino acids and access to all 20 amino acids for a library translated in the rabbit reticulocyte lysate (from *Oryctolagus cuniculus*). NNN codons contain a higher frequency of stop codons. For *E. coli*-based translation systems, NNK (K=G/T) is a better choice for a random codon. Alternatively, trimer codons that offer more flexibility over amino acid ratios and avoid stop codons entirely are available (Glen Research), though are expensive.
9. While it is possible to construct a random library via overlap PCR of two random oligos, ligation is the method of choice to retain pool complexity. Synthetic DNA is often 10%–20% extendable by Taq and PCR of these oligos will result in a significant loss of complexity since only 1%–4% of all sequences will be fully extended (see for example, [26])

10. See Table 1.
11. Do not vortex the gel solution as introducing oxygen will prevent gel polymerization.
12. We find that placing an aluminum plate (~0.17 cm thick) on the glass plates helps to equalize the heat across the gel and reduces smiling.
13. For templates >200 nt, it is sometimes necessary to heat the sample at 95°C for 1–2 min before loading to completely denature the nucleic acid. The sample should be loaded directly from the heat block.
14. For larger or more complex libraries, multiple bands may be seen due to incomplete or extended synthesis products. In such instances, it can be helpful to run either a ssDNA ladder, or ssDNA of a known size to help determine the correct product.
15. Since a DNA synthesis produces much more DNA that is required for downstream steps, it is often better to sacrifice yield by cutting more conservatively to obtain a higher quality product.
16. See Table 2.
17. It is good practice to aliquot and store primers in small volumes since primers can easily be contaminated with template DNA.
18. Filter tips should always be used when setting up PCR reactions to avoid potential contamination, though other precautions such as having dedicated pre-PCR and post-PCR areas and setting PCR reactions up in a laminar flow hood or PCR cabinet are good practice. However, the use of dUTP to prevent PCR contamination should be avoided as it has negative effects on in vitro transcription [34].

Table 1
Acrylamide gel percentages and dye migration in denaturing polyacrylamide gels [40]

Acrylamide percentage	DNA separation (in nucleotides)	Bromophenol blue migration (in nucleotides)	Xylene cyanol migration (in nucleotides)
4	>200	36	155
5	80–200		
6	60–150	26	110
8	40–100	20	75
12	10–50		
20	<20	8	28

Table 2
Centrifugation guidelines for amicon centrifugal concentrators [41]

Membrane nominal molecular weight limit in Daltons (proteins)	Nucleotide cut-off for ssRNA/ssDNA	Nucleotide cut-off for dsRNA/dsDNA
3000	10	10
10,000	30	20
30,000	60	50
50,000	125	100
100,000	300	125

19. It is important to not over-PCR the sample as this will introduce bias in the library and/or introduce incorrect products including primer dimers.
20. Two combs can be added and the 10 cm gel cut in half so that two gels can be made. These can be stored in a sealed plastic bag at 4°C for up to 2 weeks.
21. The gel can be more quickly loaded if 1 μL spots of 5× loading buffer (one spot per sample) are placed on a piece of parafilm. The PCR samples can then be mixed on the parafilm and loaded onto the gel.
22. The gel can be saved as in **Note 20**, and samples loaded on the empty lanes.
23. While it can be tempting to push forward with a suboptimal PCR reaction, it is often worth spending the time to optimize the reaction and/or reorder the library. Over the course of a selection, the library will undergo hundreds of cycles of PCR and any spurious products will make the overall selection more difficult and more likely to fail.
24. We recommend gel purification even if the PCR product looks very clean, however, it can be omitted if the product is clean.
25. Due to errors in synthesis, not all input synthetic DNA will be extendable. Typically, >20% of a 100-mer oligo can be extended by Taq polymerase. The actual fraction can be determined by labeling the complementary primer with ^{32}P, performing one cycle of PCR under excess template conditions, and running the products on a denaturing gel. With modern DNA synthesis being so robust, however, it is no longer needed to determine the fraction of ssDNA template that is extendable.
26. It is possible to load 200 μL into a 0.65 mL tube with a slight loss in product yield. If this is done, the cycling times must be extended and a heated lid on the thermocycler must not be used.

27. Avoid any white precipitate at the organic/aqueous interface. Most of the liquid can be removed by setting a pipette for a smaller volume and backpipetting to remove the last amounts of the aqueous layer.
28. It is good practice to place the tubes in the centrifuge so that the pellet will be known in orientation. For example, place the tubes in the centrifuge so that the tabs of the 1.7 mL tubes face inward.
29. The dsDNA of any random library should always be resuspended in a buffer with a minimal amount (>10 mM) of cationic salt (e.g., 10 mM Tris-HCl or 1× TE) to keep the DNA double stranded. Resuspending in pure ddH_2O can denature the DNA, inhibiting in vitro transcription.
30. Densitometry must be used instead of UV to determine the product yield since some of the primers and dNTPs will also precipitate and will contribute to the UV absorbance of the stock DNA solution.
31. More material can be carried through a step if required. For example, we typically perform at least 1 mL of transcription to make more mRNA than needed. This is often good practice as the reagent cost is minimal and gives enough material for several ligations in case challenges are encountered.
32. Avoid adding the water and dsDNA together first. Water can denature the DNA preventing transcription.
33. Working with RNA requires several basic precautions including wearing gloves and using disposable materials as much as possible. Glassware can be washed with RNase removal solutions [e.g., RNase Zap (ThermoFisher Scientific), and others], however, we tend to exclusively use plasticware. Tips and tubes can be purchased RNase/DNase free and should be used without autoclaving. Water can be DEPC treated, however, many commercially available water purification systems are capable of producing RNase-free water (Millipore-Sigma).
34. The RNA can be DNase treated at this step (see [33]). It is possible to omit this step since any ligated DNA will not be translated and will be removed at the selective step.
35. Desalting the sample before running on a denaturing gel helps to reduce the smearing and improves the gel resolution.
36. Including an N base in the middle of the splint will allow ligation of N and N + 1 products resulting from T7 transcription [32]. It is possible to use different chemistries to ligate the puromycin on the C-terminus [4, 35, 36]. Although the psoralen method [36] may be a quicker ligation procedure that does not require gel purification, we have found

(data not shown) that the psoralen ligation strategy inhibits the reverse transcription reaction by ~50%.

37. Care should be taken such that the region of the 3' primer which anneals to the splint does not have a secondary structure as this will greatly decrease the efficiency of ligation.
38. If ordering from the Keck Oligo Facility at Yale, it is more economical to order multiple 1 µM syntheses of the pF30P. Multiple syntheses more effectively use up the Spacer nine and Chemical phosphorylation reagent. While the upfront cost is greater, the per oligo cost is lower for $7 < 6 < 4 = 5$ syntheses.
39. Ideally, the efficiency of each selection step should be determined experimentally. Conservative estimates of 0.1 for fusion formation, 0.75 for dT purification, 0.9 for desalting, 0.9 for reverse transcription, and 0.5 for loss of material to tubes, tips, etc. have been previously determined and are reasonable estimates for yields of these steps. In order to experimentally determine the efficiencies of these steps, a ^{32}P-labeled template is needed and the efficiency visualized by gel electrophoresis (for fusion formation and reverse transcription) or determined by scintillation counting (for dT purification, desalting, and overall nonspecific loss of material).
40. The reaction can be annealed by heating to 95°C for 1–2 min, then cooling on ice. Do not heat for much longer as heating in the presence of magnesium can result in mRNA degradation. Annealing does not seem to increase the ligation efficiency for short (<200 nt) templates, however, in some cases has increased the ligation efficiency for longer (>400 nt) templates. The ratio of mRNA:splint:pF30P also does not seem to make a difference in the amount of ligated product obtained. RNase inhibitors can be also added to the ligation reaction, however, in our hands are not necessary.
41. Gel purification of the splint-mediated ligation is necessary to avoid the RNase H activity found in the rabbit reticulocyte lysate [37].
42. For templates longer than 400 nt, it is often difficult to separate the ligated and unligated products. In this case, dT-chromatography can be used after gel purification to separate the ligated and unligated products. If *E. coli*-based systems are used for translation, dT-chromatography can be used to purify the product directly from the ligation reaction [38].
43. For preparation of large libraries, several milliliters of translation must be performed. In these cases, it is more economical to prepare the lysate according to the procedure of Jackson and Hunt [39]. While the entire large-scale reaction can be performed hot, we tend to avoid this as it is more difficult

to work with a large volume of very radioactive material, it is unnecessarily expensive, and generates a large volume of radioactive waste. The most direct way of measuring and following the material through the multiple selection steps is to spike in a small amount of a ^{32}P-labeled template, however, this requires working behind a shield and is inconvenient.

44. Use extreme care when working with RNase as it is very difficult to remove if it contaminates the laboratory. Use gloves and change them frequently, use filter tips, and work carefully.
45. We recommend preparing the target beads fresh for every round of selection as this prevents loss of activity and gives more consistent results. However, this is target-dependent and if the immobilized target remains active after storage at 4°C, a larger batch can be prepared.
46. We find that 100 pmol of target per binding reaction is a good starting point for selection. Increasing the amount of target will typically increase overall binding and reduce the selective pressure on the library while decreasing the amount of target will decrease overall binding and increase selective pressure on the library. We recommend adding more target in the first round of selection to ensure a binder is not lost, as there are so few copies of a sequence in the first round.
47. It is possible to divide the samples among additional filters, however, doing so will increase the amount of material lost due to increased holdup.
48. The fusions can be further purified with a peptide-based purification scheme (e.g., FLAG, His_6 [26], or thiopropyl sepharose [37]), which can increase enrichment by reducing the amount of mRNA without peptide attached in the sample. This step is recommended if the fusion formation efficiency is low, as in the case for selections of proteins larger than 100 amino acids.
49. A typical yield for a 25 μL translation is 100,00 cpm. If less than 100,000 cpm are purified per 25 μL translation, consider retranslating and/or repurifying the library. A common cause of low counts is the incomplete desalting of the mRNA-F30P template, resulting in low translation yields.
50. The no target bead sample is an essential control since selection of ligands to the matrix or neutravidin is often more likely to occur before target binding. If nonspecific binding is seen, we recommend going back one to two rounds and switching the immobilization matrix as described in **Note 5**). Pool 0 binding should be low to both the target and the matrix (<0.1% binding). If the matrix binding for pool 0 is >0.3%, consider redesigning the library or testing different buffer and blocking reagents to reduce binding.

51. Alternatively, the dT elution can be desalted with an appropriately sized Amicon Centrifugal filter, though this is more time consuming.
52. The generic SSIV protocol includes DTT, however, DTT can be omitted in the reverse transcription reaction. DTT should be omitted when working with a disulfide-cyclized library or if the library and/or target contains disulfide bonds (e.g., with an antibody or nanobody library).
53. The generic SSIV protocol includes a 65°C heating step. We recommend omitting this step for protein libraries.
54. In some cases, a buffer exchange is required between reverse transcription and the affinity selection step.
55. It is also possible to perform a negative selection step (preclear) in an attempt to reduce isolation of matrix-binding sequences. To do this, incubate the RT reaction as described, except add beads containing no target. Up to five consecutive negative selection steps may be necessary since even in the best circumstances, only 80% of material is bound (as measured by the radioactive binding assay in Sect. 3.6, Step 10). Alternatively, perform the preclear in a column format, which we have observed to be slightly more efficient than a batch preclear. Generally, we find that preclearing is not sufficient to keep matrix binding sequences from being selected.
56. Alternatively, a Spin-X filter can be used to wash the beads. Adjust the wash volumes to 0.5–0.6 mL. In both cases, transferring the beads to a new tube after washing prevents carryover of any nonspecific sequences stuck to the original filter. If the library is sticking to the Spin-X filter (which can be determined by counting the filter in a scintillation counter), then the washing can be performed in a 1.7 mL tube.
57. It is important to perform a no template control reaction every round to detect contamination of PCR solutions. If a band is observed in the no template control, discard the primers and PCR solutions, retranslate the pool, and repeat the selection.
58. A 1 mL translation at 400 nM uses 400 pmol of input template. A 3% overall yield after dT purification, desalting, and RT results in 12 pmol entering the binding reaction. Binding of 0.1% results in 0.012 pmol of material on the beads after affinity selection. That 0.012 pmol is diluted to 1000 μL in the PCR reaction giving an initial concentration of ~0.000012 μM.

59. Performing three cycles fewer than calculated is to avoid over PCR of the library. However, it is not uncommon for the actual number of PCR cycles to exceed those calculated by three to ten rounds since the efficiency of the binding is not known. Thus, the number of cycles calculated represents a lower bound. As long as a band appears in the selected sample within 30 cycles of PCR, with no band observed in the negative control, the selection round was likely successful. Cycles for the first round of selection will depend on the size of the translation reaction while later rounds typically take 9–24 cycles (usually 18). If > 30 cycles are required for amplification, consider retranslating and reselecting.
60. Avoid over PCR of the library. Performing too many cycles can cause a shift in the size of the library but also has the effect of normalizing the relative proportions of different pool members, reducing the selective enrichment due to binding.
61. The volume of transcription can be decreased in later rounds to 250–500 μL.

Acknowledgments

This work is supported by NIH grant R01NS125769, the Michaelson Found Animals foundation, and the CHDI foundation.

References

1. Roberts RW, Szostak JW (1997) RNA-peptide fusions for the *in vitro* selection of peptides and proteins. Proc Natl Acad Sci U S A 94:12297–12302
2. Kamalinia G, Grindel BJ, Takahashi TT, Millward SW, Roberts RW (2021) Directing evolution of novel ligands by mRNA display. Chem Soc Rev 50:9055–9103
3. Takahashi TT, Austin RJ, Roberts RW (2003) mRNA display: ligand discovery, interaction analysis and beyond. Trends Biochem Sci 28:159–165
4. Mochizuki Y, Suzuki T, Fujimoto K, Nemoto N (2015) A versatile puromycin-linker using cnvK for high-throughput in vitro selection by cDNA display. J Biotechnol 212:174–180
5. Ishizawa T, Kawakami T, Reid PC, Murakami H (2013) TRAP display: a high-speed selection method for the generation of functional polypeptides. J Am Chem Soc 135:5433–5440
6. Frankel A, Millward SW, Roberts RW (2003) Encodamers: unnatural peptide oligomers encoded in RNA. Chem Biol 10:1043–1050
7. Fiacco SV, Kelderhouse LE, Hardy A, Peleg Y, Hu B, Ornelas A, Yang P, Gammon ST, Howell SM, Wang P, Takahashi TT, Millward SW, Roberts RW (2016) Directed evolution of scanning unnatural-protease-resistant (SUPR) peptides for in vivo applications. ChemBioChem 17:1643–1651
8. Li S, Millward S, Roberts R (2002) In vitro selection of mRNA display libraries containing an unnatural amino acid. J Am Chem Soc 124:9972–9973
9. Murakami H, Ohta A, Ashigai H, Suga H (2006) A highly flexible tRNA acylation method for non-natural polypeptide synthesis. Nat Methods 3:357–359
10. Ohuchi M, Murakami H, Suga H (2007) The flexizyme system: a highly flexible tRNA

aminoacylation tool for the translation apparatus. Curr Opin Chem Biol 11:537–542
11. Jalali-Yazdi F, Lai LH, Takahashi TT, Roberts RW (2016) High-throughput measurement of binding kinetics by mRNA display and next-generation sequencing. Angew Chem Int Ed Engl 55:4007–4010
12. Qi P, Gandhi YP, Zheng K, Jalali-Yazdi F, Ong JN, Takahashi TT, Kalia RK, Roberts RW (2025) A route to design novel functional peptides by applying a denoising diffusional model to mRNA display libraries. ChemBioChem 26:e202500302
13. Zhu B, Lane MD, Baller JA, Jagtap PD, Griffin TJ, Seelig B (2025) Comprehensive protease specificity profiling. bioRxiv 2024.11.06.622033. https://doi.org/10.1101/2024.11.06.622033
14. Howell SM, Fiacco SV, Takahashi TT, Jalali-Yazdi F, Millward SW, Hu B, Wang P, Roberts RW (2014) Serum stable natural peptides designed by mRNA display. Sci Rep 4:6008
15. Tsuboyama K, Dauparas J, Chen J, Laine E, Mohseni Behbahani Y, Weinstein JJ, Mangan NM, Ovchinnikov S, Rocklin GJ (2023) Mega-scale experimental analysis of protein folding stability in biology and design. Nature 620:434–444
16. Barrick JE, Takahashi TT, Ren J, Xia T, Roberts RW (2001) Large libraries reveal diverse solutions to an RNA recognition problem. Proc Natl Acad Sci U S A 98:12374–12378
17. Brody JR, Kern SE (2004) Sodium boric acid: a Tris-free, cooler conductive medium for DNA electrophoresis. Biotechniques 36:214–216
18. Ong JN, Grindel BJ, Rankin SA, Naylon SH, Srinivasamani A, Trusz GJ, Liang X, Uddin MN, Fuller L, Curran M, Roche SP, Takahashi TT, Roberts RW, Millward SW (2025) Using extension-based mRNA display to design antibody-like proteinogenic peptides for human PD-L1. Protein Sci 34:e70268
19. Gross GG, Junge JA, Mora RJ, Kwon H-B, Olson CA, Takahashi TT, Liman ER, Ellis-Davies GCR, McGee AW, Sabatini BL, Roberts RW, Arnold DB (2013) Recombinant probes for visualizing endogenous synaptic proteins in living neurons. Neuron 78:971–985
20. Olson CA, Roberts RW (2007) Design, expression, and stability of a diverse protein library based on the human fibronectin type III domain. Protein Sci 16:476–484
21. Keefe AD, Szostak JW (2001) Functional proteins from a random-sequence library. Nature 410:715–718
22. Wilson DS, Keefe AD (2000) Random mutagenesis by PCR. Curr Protoc Mol Biol 51:8.3.1-8.3.9. https://doi.org/10.1002/0471142727.mb0803s51
23. Stemmer WP (1994) Rapid evolution of a protein in vitro by DNA shuffling. Nature 370:389–391
24. Hammond PW, Alpin J, Rise CE, Wright M, Kreider BL (2001) In vitro selection and characterization of Bcl-X(L)-binding proteins from a mix of tissue-specific mRNA display libraries. J Biol Chem 276:20898–20906
25. Bartel DP, Szostak JW (1993) Isolation of new ribozymes from a large pool of random sequences [see comment]. Science 261:1411–1418
26. Cho G, Keefe AD, Liu R, Wilson DS, Szostak JW (2000) Constructing high complexity synthetic libraries of long ORFs using in vitro selection. J Mol Biol 297:309–319
27. Shimizu Y, Inoue A, Tomari Y, Suzuki T, Yokogawa T, Nishikawa K, Ueda T (2001) Cell-free translation reconstituted with purified components. Nat Biotechnol 19:751–755
28. Stormo GD, Schneider TD, Gold LM (1982) Characterization of translational initiation sites in *E. coli*. Nucleic Acids Res 10:2971–2996
29. O'Connor M, Dahlberg AE (2001) Enhancement of translation by the epsilon element is independent of the sequence of the 460 region of 16S rRNA. Nucleic Acids Res 29:1420–1425
30. Forster AC, Weissbach H, Blacklow SC (2001) A simplified reconstitution of mRNA-directed peptide synthesis: activity of the epsilon enhancer and an unnatural amino acid. Anal Biochem 297:60–70
31. Mills DR, Peterson RL, Spiegelman S (1967) An extracellular Darwinian experiment with a self-duplicating nucleic acid molecule. Proc Natl Acad Sci U S A 58:217–224
32. Liu R, Barrick JE, Szostak JW, Roberts RW (2000) Optimized synthesis of RNA-protein fusions for in vitro protein selection. In: Methods in enzymology. Academic Press, San Diego, London, pp 268–293
33. Ja WW, Roberts RW (2004) In vitro selection of state-specific peptide modulators of G protein signaling using mRNA display. Biochemistry 43:9265–9275
34. Cui J, Gizzi A, Stivers JT (2019) Deoxyuridine in DNA has an inhibitory and promutagenic effect on RNA transcription by diverse RNA polymerases. Nucleic Acids Res 47:4153–4168
35. Tabuchi I, Soramoto S, Suzuki M, Nishigaki K, Nemoto N, Husimi Y (2002) An efficient ligation method in the making of an in vitro virus for in vitro protein evolution. Biol Proced Online 4:49–54
36. Kurz M (2000) Psoralen photo-crosslinked mRNA-puromycin conjugates: a novel template for the rapid and facile preparation of

mRNA-protein fusions. Nucleic Acids Res 28:83e–883e
37. Barrick JE, Takahashi TT, Balakin A, Roberts RW (2001) Selection of RNA-binding peptides using mRNA-peptide fusions. Methods 23:287–293
38. Doshi R, Chen BR, Vibat CRT, Huang N, Lee C-W, Chang G (2014) In vitro nanobody discovery for integral membrane protein targets. Sci Rep 4:6760
39. Jackson RJ, Hunt T (1983) Preparation and use of nuclease-treated rabbit reticulocyte lysates for the translation of eukaryotic messenger RNA. Methods Enzymol 96:50–74
40. (2003) Procedures for gel preparation with the sequagel sequencing system. https://www.nationaldiagnostics.com/wp-content/uploads/2017/04/sequagel_ureagel_system_protocol.pdf
41. (2005) Microcon® Centrifugal filter devices user guide. Rev M. https://gannet.fish.washington.edu/seashell/bu-owl-halfshell/bu-git-repos/LabDocs/protocols/Commercial_Protocols/Millipore_Microcon_Filtration_Manuals.pdf

Part IV

Auxiliary Tools and Post-Selection Optimization

Check for updates

Chapter 13

AI-Driven Protein Research: From Prediction to Design

Guodong Min and Huan Peng

Abstract

Proteins are central to nearly all biological processes, mediating enzymatic catalysis, structural scaffolding, and molecular signaling. Deciphering how linear amino acid sequences encode three-dimensional conformations and biological functions has long been a defining challenge in molecular life sciences. Traditional structural biology approaches, such as X-ray crystallography and cryo-electron microscopy, have established the field, yet their high cost, labor intensity, and limited throughput restrict comprehensive coverage of the proteome. The exponential expansion of protein sequence databases, paired with advances in artificial intelligence (AI) and deep learning, has drastically accelerated our ability to predict, annotate, and even design proteins. In this mini review, we trace the evolution of AI-driven methods in protein research, from early residue-contact prediction using coevolutionary information to transformative breakthroughs, the rise of protein language models (PLMs), and the emerging era of generative design and functional modeling. Throughout, we highlight key conceptual advances and their translational implications for biomedical science and biotechnology.

Keywords Artificial intelligence, Protein structure prediction, Protein language model, Generative design, Molecular docking

1 Introduction

Proteins are the workhorses of life, orchestrating nearly every biological process, from enzymatic catalysis that drives metabolic pathways, to structural scaffolding that maintains cellular integrity, and molecular signaling that coordinates intercellular and intracellular communication. Unlocking the relationship between a protein's linear amino acid sequence, its three-dimensional (3D) structure, and its biological function is not only a foundational goal of molecular biology but also a prerequisite for advancing biomedicine and biotechnology. For decades, this "sequence-structure-function" paradigm has guided research, yet deciphering it has remained one of the most enduring challenges in the life sciences [1].

Traditional structural biology methods, including X-ray crystallography, cryo-electron microscopy (cryo-EM), and nuclear magnetic

Huan Peng and Theam Soon Lim (eds.), *Biomolecular Display Technologies*, Methods in Molecular Biology, vol. 3030, https://doi.org/10.1007/978-1-0716-5249-7_13,

resonance (NMR) spectroscopy, have been instrumental in resolving the structures of thousands of proteins, laying the groundwork for our understanding of molecular function [2, 3]. However, these techniques suffer from inherent limitations (Fig. 1). X-ray crystallography requires laborious crystal growth and is inefficient for membrane proteins or flexible complexes. Cryo-EM demands expensive instrumentation and specialized expertise, and NMR is restricted to small-to-medium-sized proteins. Collectively, these constraints have resulted in a stark mismatch between the exponential growth of protein sequence databases and the relatively slow expansion of experimentally determined structures, with less than 1% of known sequences having corresponding high-resolution structures [4]. This "structural coverage gap" has hampered efforts to fully exploit genomic data for biological discovery and translational research.

The advent of artificial intelligence (AI) and deep learning has emerged as a transformative solution to bridge this gap. Over the past decade, AI-driven methods have revolutionized nearly every facet of protein research, shifting the paradigm from labor-intensive experimental approaches to data-driven computational prediction,

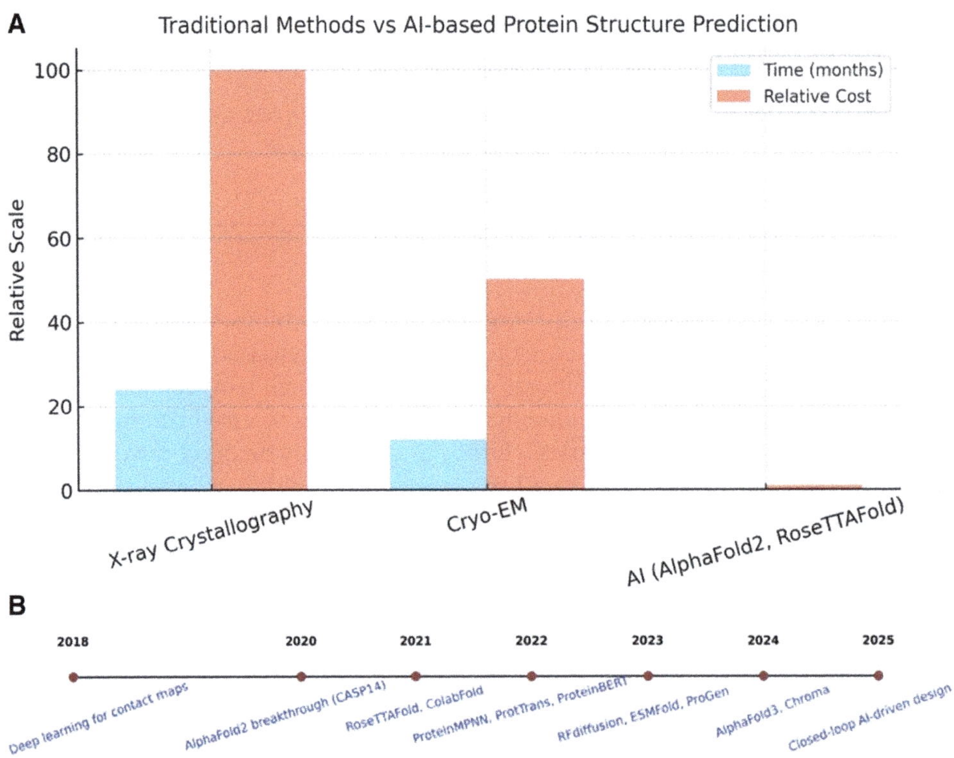

Fig. 1 (**A**) Comparison of time and relative cost between traditional protein structure determination methods (X-ray crystallography, cryo-EM) and AI-based structure prediction approaches. (**B**) Timeline of key artificial intelligence-driven methodological advances in protein structure prediction and design (2018–2025)

annotation, and design. What began with early attempts to predict residue–residue contacts using coevolutionary information [5] has evolved into a suite of powerful tools capable of predicting atomic-resolution structures, learning contextual sequence representations, generating de novo functional proteins, and modeling complex molecular interactions [6]. These advances have not only addressed longstanding limitations of traditional methods but also opened new avenues of research that were previously unimaginable, such as high-throughput proteome-wide structural modeling and the rational design of proteins with tailored properties.

In this mini review, we systematically trace the evolutionary trajectory of AI-driven protein research (Fig. 1), from its nascent stages to its current state-of-the-art. We begin by contextualizing early efforts in protein structure prediction and the pivotal role of deep learning in reshaping the field. We then focus on breakthrough technologies, including AlphaFold and its derivatives, which have redefined the accuracy and accessibility of structural prediction [7, 8]. Subsequent sections explore the rise of protein language models (PLMs) as a versatile tool for sequence analysis [9], the emergence of generative AI for de novo protein design, and advances in AI-driven functional annotation and ligand docking [10]. Finally, we discuss future directions, including the integration of dynamic modeling, closed-loop design paradigms, and multimodal data, that are poised to further transform the field [11]. By synthesizing key conceptual advances, methodological innovations, and translational applications, this review aims to provide a comprehensive overview of how AI is redefining our understanding and manipulation of proteins, and to highlight its potential to address pressing challenges in biomedicine and biotechnology.

2 Early Exploration and the Advent of Deep Learning

For decades, deciphering protein structure from sequence has been a cornerstone challenge in molecular biology. Prior to the advent of AlphaFold, most protein structure prediction methods relied heavily on evolutionary couplings and physics-based modeling. Early studies demonstrated that correlated mutations across homologous sequences could reveal residue–residue contacts, reflecting the coevolution of structurally or functionally coupled positions [5, 12]. For instance, Jones et al. developed PSICOV, which applied sparse inverse covariance estimation to predict structural contacts, representing a marked improvement over earlier statistical techniques by capturing subtle co-evolutionary signals [13]. Parallel to this, template-based strategies such as I-TASSER combined homology modeling with ab initio folding simulations, achieving moderate success in reconstructing tertiary structures for proteins with known homologs [14].

Tools like HHpred and Phyre2 further advanced template-based prediction by leveraging homology detection algorithms to identify distant structural relatives [15, 16].

The integration of deep learning reshaped this landscape. Neural networks were first deployed for contact map prediction, where convolutional and recurrent architectures enabled the capture of both local (short-range) and long-range sequence dependencies [17]. Ovchinnikov et al. showed that mining metagenomic data expanded sequence coverage, thereby enhancing structural inference for poorly conserved proteins [4]. Xu et al. further advanced the field by integrating deep learning to predict interresidue distances, a critical step toward more accurate structure modeling [18], and Yang et al. incorporated predicted interresidue orientations into prediction pipelines, refining structural constraints [19]. A pivotal advance came from Senior et al. [20], who introduced deep learning–derived potentials into structure refinement. This hybrid strategy bridged traditional physics-based methods with data-driven approaches by linking statistical sequence patterns to energy-like constraints. Collectively, these innovations laid the conceptual and methodological foundation for transformative systems like AlphaFold.

3 AlphaFold and the Breakthrough in Structure Prediction

2021 marked a watershed moment in protein structure prediction with the debut of AlphaFold2 (DeepMind). During the 14th Critical Assessment of Protein Structure Prediction (CASP14), AlphaFold2 achieved near-experimental accuracy, with predicted backbone positions deviating from experimental structures by <1 Å on average, an unprecedented level of precision (Fig. 2) [7]. The core innovation of AlphaFold2 resided in its hybrid architecture. It integrated multiple sequence alignments (MSAs), a rich source of evolutionary information, with attention-based neural networks that simultaneously reasoned over evolutionary patterns and geometric constraints inherent to protein folding. A dedicated structure module then transformed predicted interresidue distances and orientations into three-dimensional coordinates, yielding highly accurate models.

In parallel, Baek et al. introduced RoseTTAFold, a complementary tool with a three-track network design that enabled simultaneous information flow between sequence, MSA, and coordinate representations [21]. While slightly less accurate than AlphaFold2, RoseTTAFold offered substantial computational efficiency, facilitating rapid adoption by the broader research community. The impact of these breakthroughs was immediate and transformative. Tunyasuvunakool et al. used AlphaFold2 to model nearly the entire human proteome, generating >20,000 high-confidence structures and boosting proteome-level structural coverage from ~25% (based

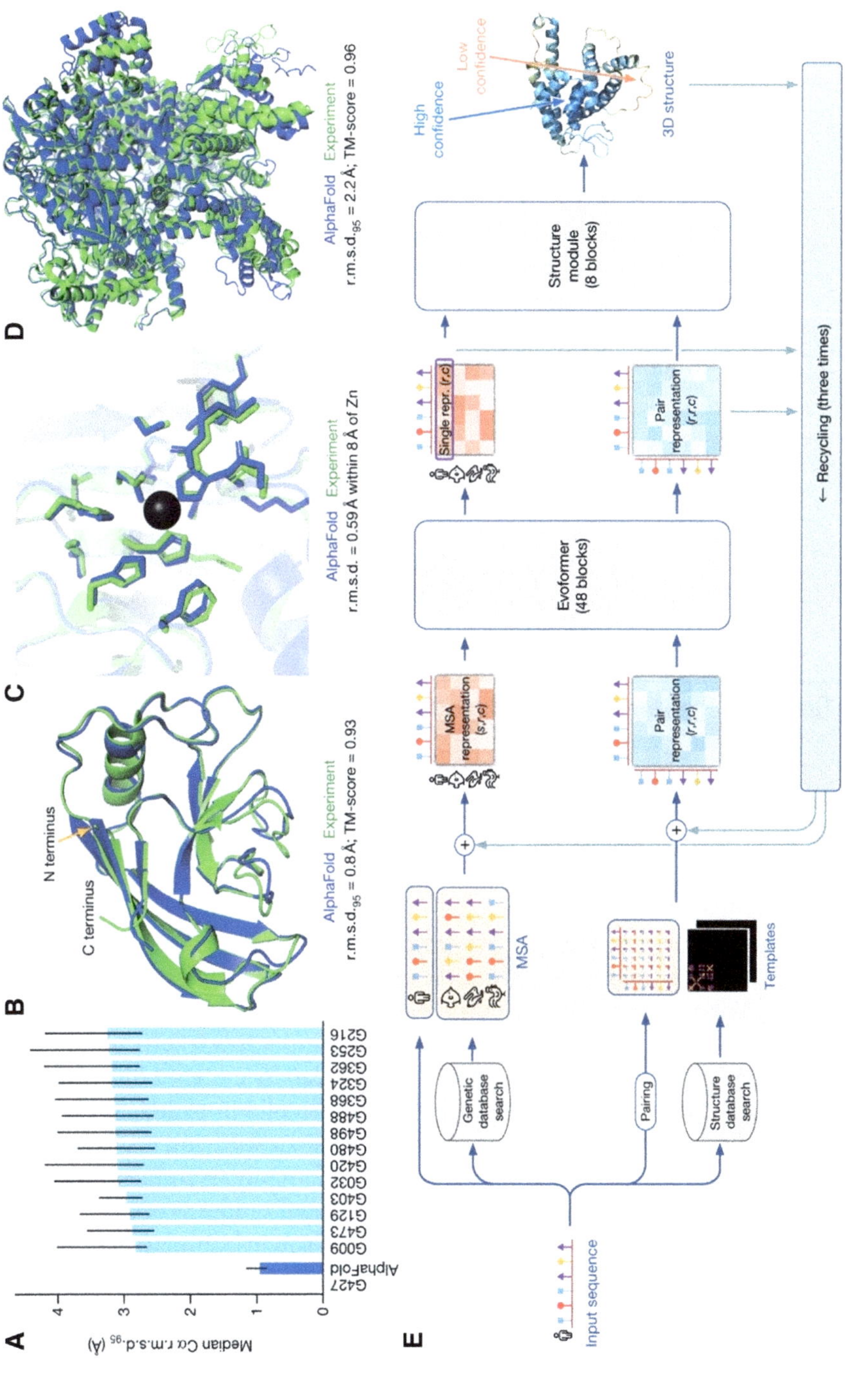

Fig. 2 AlphaFold2 Core Architecture, Prediction Accuracy Assessment, and Structural Consistency Between Predicted Models and Experimental Protein Structures. (Adapted with permission, Copyright © 2021, John Jumper et al. [7])

on experimental data) to nearly 60% [22]. This effort, combined with the launch of the AlphaFold Protein Structure Database [8], provided researchers with unprecedented access to reliable structural models, accelerating progress in immunology, virology, and drug discovery.

Extensions to complex systems soon followed. AlphaFold-Multimer adapted the framework for modeling protein complexes by incorporating symmetry-aware modules and interchain attention mechanisms, outperforming traditional docking methods in both speed and accuracy [14]. Most recently, AlphaFold3 expanded prediction capabilities to include proteins, nucleic acids, and small molecules in a unified framework, enabling modeling of intricate assemblies such as ribonucleoprotein complexes and drug–protein interactions with high precision [23].

Together, AlphaFold2 and RoseTTAFold transformed protein structure prediction from a specialized, low-throughput task into a broadly accessible tool. Platforms like ColabFold [24], which integrate these models into lightweight, cloud-based interfaces, democratized access by lowering technical and computational barriers. This shift ushered in an era where structural hypotheses can be generated rapidly and at scale, laying the groundwork for mechanistic studies and therapeutic innovation.

4 Expansion to Complex Systems and Proteomes

Building on the success of single-chain protein structure prediction, the field rapidly expanded AI-driven methodologies to tackle larger, more biologically relevant systems, from protein complexes to entire proteomes. A prominent example is AlphaFold-Multimer, which enhanced the original AlphaFold2 framework with interface-specific attention mechanisms and symmetry-aware modeling. This enabled accurate prediction of multimeric assemblies, including antibody–antigen complexes and homooligomers, outperforming conventional docking tools in both precision and computational efficiency.

AlphaFold3 represented a further leap by unifying the modeling of proteins, nucleic acids, and small molecules in a single framework [23]. This advance opened new avenues for studying mixed biomolecular systems, such as ribosomes, chromatin assemblies, and protein–drug complexes. For example, AlphaFold3 was used to predict the structure of the SARS-CoV-2 spike protein bound to neutralizing antibodies, providing critical insights into viral immune evasion and guiding therapeutic development. Efforts to broaden access to these tools have been equally impactful. ColabFold integrated AlphaFold and RoseTTAFold into a user-friendly, cloud-based platform, dramatically lowering technical barriers and enabling nonexperts to generate high-quality structural models with minimal computational resources [24]. This democratization accelerated adoption across academic labs and pharmaceutical companies, expanding the reach of AI-driven structural biology.

These developments extended AI's influence beyond individual proteins to the systems level. Protein family databases such as Pfam, CATH, and SCOPe have played a key role in organizing and analyzing large-scale structural data [25, 26], enriching our mechanistic understanding of cellular machinery and highlighting the value of making powerful algorithms broadly accessible.

5 The Rise of Protein Language Models

Parallel to structural prediction, a transformative paradigm emerged with the development of protein language models (PLMs). These models analogize amino acid sequences to natural language, learning contextual, sequence-derived representations from massive protein sequence databases. Rives et al. demonstrated that training a Transformer model on hundreds of millions of protein sequences enabled it to capture latent features related to structure and function [9]; when fine-tuned, these embeddings achieved state-of-the-art performance in downstream tasks such as secondary structure prediction and mutation effect estimation. Rao et al. validated the power of protein transfer learning with the TAPE benchmark [27], while Heinzinger et al. explored bidirectional LSTM models for capturing sequence context [28]. Brandes et al. introduced ProteinBERT, a Transformer tailored for protein sequence analysis (Fig. 3) [29]. ProteinBERT is a protein-specific model with a combined pretraining task and an efficient local-global architecture. Though smaller and faster than competing methods, this model delivers near or superior state-of-the-art performance across diverse protein property benchmarks, and enables efficient protein predictor training even with limited labeled data.

Subsequent advances expanded this framework. Rao et al.'s MSA Transformer enhanced sequence modeling by incorporating evolutionary alignments [30]. The ProtTrans suite, trained on billions of sequences by Elnaggar et al. showed that large-scale pretraining could extract generalizable representations applicable across diverse protein families [31]. Most notably, Lin et al. developed ESMFold, a PLM capable of predicting atomic-resolution structures directly from sequences without relying on MSAs, a critical departure from AlphaFold's framework and a major advance for proteins with limited homologous sequences [32]. Remarkably, ESMFold achieved performance comparable to AlphaFold2 on many proteins, highlighting the potential of sequence-only modeling. PLMs have also proven invaluable for studying fitness landscapes and mutation effects. Meier et al. reported that

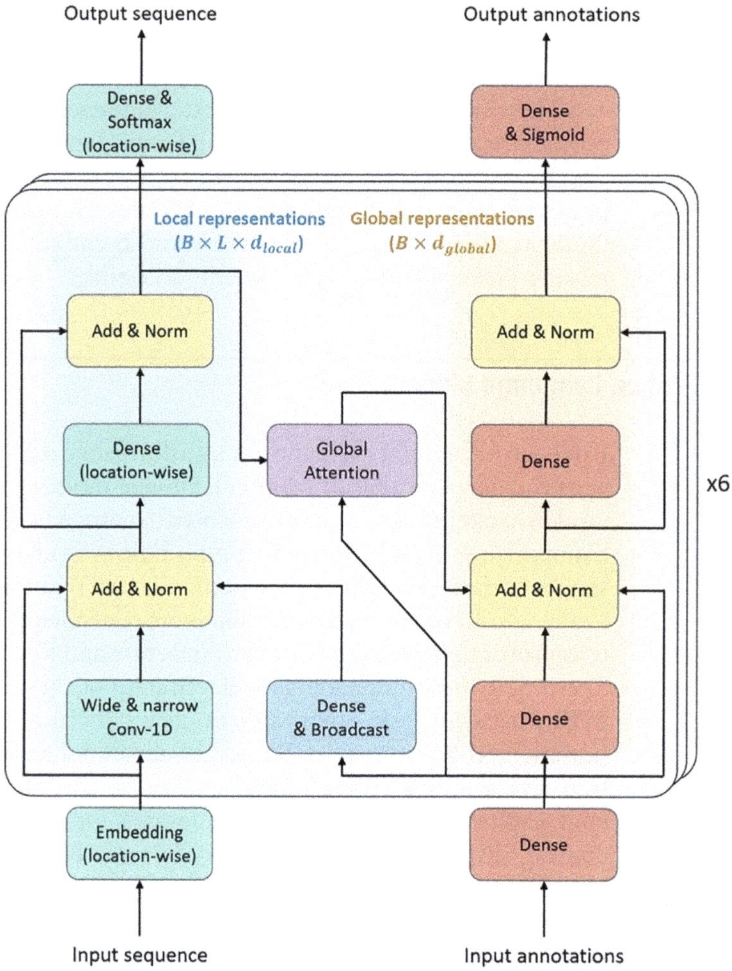

Fig. 3 Architecture of the ProteinBERT Model: dual-stream processing for input sequences and annotations, integrating local-global representation learning and stacked repeating module layers. (Adapted with permission, Copyright © 2022, Brandes et al. [29])

PLMs can predict mutation phenotypes in a "zero-shot" manner (without experimental training data), outperforming traditional approaches dependent on high-throughput screening [33]. Earlier work by Hopf et al. and Riesselman et al. laid the groundwork for this by leveraging sequence covariation and generative models to predict mutation effects [34, 35]. Hybrid frameworks such as TranceptEVE, which combine PLM priors with evolutionary information, further enhanced interpretability and performance [30]. Collectively, PLMs represent a versatile toolset for fundamental biology and applied protein engineering.

6 Generative Protein Design

Beyond prediction and analysis, AI has emerged as a transformative tool for generative protein design, enabling the de novo creation of proteins with tailored structures and functions. Early proof-of-concept studies introduced "deep network hallucination," where neural networks proposed novel amino acid sequences predicted to fold into stable structures [36]. Ingraham et al. explored graph-based generative models for protein design, pioneering approaches that integrate sequence and structural constraints [37]. Experimental validation confirmed that many AI-designed proteins were soluble, thermostable, and folded into the predicted structures, demonstrating the feasibility of AI-driven de novo design.

A major advance came with ProteinMPNN, a message-passing neural network developed by Dauparas et al. that designs sequences for predefined backbones [38]. ProteinMPNN achieved substantially higher native sequence recovery rates than traditional tools like Rosetta, making it a go-to method for designing sequences that fold into target structures, including complex assemblies such as protein nanoparticles. Hsu et al. further advanced inverse folding by leveraging millions of predicted structures to train models [39], while Norn et al. optimized conformational landscapes for sequence design [40].

Diffusion models have recently revolutionized the field. RFdiffusion adapted diffusion techniques to generate protein backbones, enabling the design of symmetric oligomers, binding proteins, and enzyme active-site motifs [41]. Trippe et al. explored diffusion probabilistic modeling for backbone generation [42], and Hsu et al. integrated RoseTTAFold into diffusion-based design pipelines. Meanwhile, large-scale language models like ProGen [43] and ProtGPT2 [10] generated functional protein sequences, including enzymes with low sequence identity to natural proteins, by learning sequence–function relationships from massive datasets. Nijkamp et al. extended this with ProGen2, enhancing sequence diversity and functional specificity [44]. The field continues to diversify, with tools like Chroma [45] enabling programmable, user-specified design objectives, and Ingraham et al. developing energy-based models for structure-guided design [37]. Together, these methods are transforming protein engineering from a trial-and-error process into a systematic, AI-guided endeavor.

7 Functional Modeling and Ligand Docking

AI has further revolutionized functional protein annotation and the prediction of molecular interactions, two critical areas for understanding protein function and advancing drug discovery. Tools like DeepFRI [46], based on graph convolutional networks, integrate

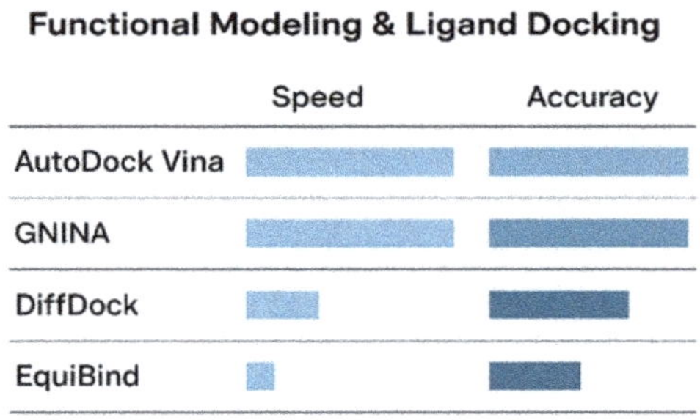

Fig. 4 Comparison of speed and accuracy across ligand docking tools for protein functional modeling

structural context to predict Gene Ontology (GO) terms with high accuracy, outperforming sequence-only methods. DeepGOPlus [47] enhanced functional annotation by combining multiple data sources, addressing the challenge of annotating proteins with few homologs.

In drug discovery, AI-based molecular docking has emerged as a powerful alternative to classical scoring functions. Early work by Wallach et al. with AtomNet demonstrated that convolutional neural networks (CNNs) could predict bioactivity by learning three-dimensional structural patterns [48]. McNutt et al. advanced this with GNINA 1.0, incorporating deep learning into docking scoring functions to improve binding pose prediction [11]. Recent innovations include EquiBind [49], which uses equivariant neural networks to preserve geometric symmetry during pose prediction, and DiffDock [50], which leverages diffusion processes to generate diverse, accurate binding poses. Beyond these docking-specific advances, related progress in molecular interaction modeling has also benefited the field. Gilmer et al. introduced neural message passing for quantum chemistry [51], and Xue et al. reported an SE(3)-equivariant framework for ternary complex prediction in targeted protein degradation [52]. These AI-driven tools frequently outperform traditional methods like AutoDock Vina, offering superior precision and faster throughput, accelerating in silico drug screening pipelines (Fig. 4).

8 Outlook

Looking forward, three interrelated directions stand out as particularly transformative for the future of AI-driven protein research. First, static structural models must be complemented by methods that capture protein dynamics. Efforts in this area include Boltzmann generators [53] and VAMPnets [54], which model conformational ensembles and slow dynamical processes, and Wang et al.'s machine learning–enhanced molecular dynamics sampling [55]. Husic et al. applied Markov state models to study slow conformational modes [56], while Doerr et al. introduced TorchMD for deep learning–accelerated molecular simulations [57], and Pantelopoulos et al. integrated AlphaFold with molecular dynamics to generate conformational ensembles. Integrating such dynamic modeling with AlphaFold-derived static structures could provide a holistic view of protein folding, allostery, and molecular regulation, critical for understanding how proteins function in native cellular environments.

Second, closed-loop design paradigms, coupling AI models with high-throughput experimental screening, are poised to expand. Machine learning–guided directed evolution [58] and informed training-set design have already demonstrated feasibility, with Alley et al.'s UniRep model and Wittmann et al.'s work enhancing data-efficient protein engineering [59, 60]. Biswas et al. further showed that deep learning enables low-N protein engineering, minimizing experimental effort [61]. Ultimately, fusing computational prediction, generative design, and automated experimentation could drastically reduce the cycle time for developing novel proteins.

Third, integrating multimodal data, including sequence, structure, expression context, and posttranslational modifications, will be essential to understand protein behavior in vivo. As AI methods continue to advance, they promise to deepen our fundamental knowledge of molecular biology while opening new frontiers in biomedicine (e.g., targeted therapeutics) and biotechnology (e.g., industrial enzymes).

References

1. Dill KA, MacCallum JL (2012) The protein-folding problem, 50 years on. Science 338(6110):1042–1046. https://doi.org/10.1126/science.1219021
2. Bai XC, McMullan G, Scheres SHW (2015) How cryo-EM is revolutionizing structural biology. Trends Biochem Sci 40(1):49–57. https://doi.org/10.1016/j.tibs.2014.10.005
3. Wüthrich K (2003) NMR studies of structure and function of biological macromolecules (Nobel Lecture). Angew Chem-Int Ed 42(29):3340–3363. https://doi.org/10.1002/anie.200300595
4. Ovchinnikov S, Park H, Varghese N, Huang PS, Pavlopoulos GA, Kim DE, Kamisetty H, Kyrpides NC, Baker D (2017) Protein structure determination using metagenome sequence data. Science 355(6322):294–297. https://doi.org/10.1126/science.aah4043
5. Marks DS, Colwell LJ, Sheridan R, Hopf TA, Pagnani A, Zecchina R, Sander C (2011) Protein 3D structure computed from evolutionary sequence variation. PLOS One 6(12):20. https://doi.org/10.1371/journal.pone.0028766
6. Eickholt J, Cheng JL (2012) Predicting protein residue-residue contacts using deep networks and boosting. Bioinformatics 28(23):3066–3072. https://doi.org/10.1093/bioinformatics/bts598
7. Jumper J, Evans R, Pritzel A, Green T, Figurnov M, Ronneberger O, Tunyasuvunakool K, Bates R, Zídek A, Potapenko A, Bridgland A, Meyer C, Kohl SAA, Ballard AJ, Cowie A, Romera-Paredes B, Nikolov S, Jain R, Adler J, Back T, Petersen S, Reiman D, Clancy E, Zielinski M, Steinegger M, Pacholska M, Berghammer T, Bodenstein S, Silver D, Vinyals O, Senior AW, Kavukcuoglu K, Kohli P, Hassabis D (2021) Highly accurate protein structure prediction with AlphaFold. Nature 596(7873):583–589. https://doi.org/10.1038/s41586-021-03819-2
8. Varadi M, Anyango S, Deshpande M, Nair S, Natassia C, Yordanova G, Yuan D, Stroe O, Wood G, Laydon A, Zídek A, Green T, Tunyasuvunakool K, Petersen S, Jumper J, Clancy E, Green R, Vora A, Lutfi M, Figurnov M, Cowie A, Hobbs N, Kohli P, Kleywegt G, Birney E, Hassabis D, Velankar S (2022) AlphaFold protein structure database: massively expanding the structural coverage of protein-sequence space with high-accuracy models.

Nucleic Acids Res 50(D1):D439–D444. https://doi.org/10.1093/nar/gkab1061
9. Rives A, Meier J, Sercu T, Goyal S, Lin ZM, Liu JS, Guo DM, Ott M, Zitnick CL, Ma J, Fergus R (2021) Biological structure and function emerge from scaling unsupervised learning to 250 million protein sequences. Proc Natl Acad Sci U S A 118(15):12. https://doi.org/10.1073/pnas.2016239118
10. Ferruz N, Schmidt S, Höcker B (2022) ProtGPT2 is a deep unsupervised language model for protein design. Nat Commun 13(1):10. https://doi.org/10.1038/s41467-022-32007-7
11. McNutt AT, Francoeur P, Aggarwal R, Masuda T, Meli R, Ragoza M, Sunseri J, Koes DR (2021) GNINA 1.0: molecular docking with deep learning. J Cheminform 13(1):20. https://doi.org/10.1186/s13321-021-00522-2
12. Ekeberg M, Lövkvist C, Lan YH, Weigt M, Aurell E (2013) Improved contact prediction in proteins: using pseudolikelihoods to infer Potts models. Phys Rev E 87(1):16. https://doi.org/10.1103/PhysRevE.87.012707
13. Jones DT, Buchan DWA, Cozzetto D, Pontil M (2012) PSICOV: precise structural contact prediction using sparse inverse covariance estimation on large multiple sequence alignments. Bioinformatics 28(2):184–190. https://doi.org/10.1093/bioinformatics/btr638
14. Yang JY, Yan RX, Roy A, Xu D, Poisson J, Zhang Y (2015) The I-TASSER suite: protein structure and function prediction. Nat Methods 12(1):7–8. https://doi.org/10.1038/nmeth.3213
15. Kelley LA, Mezulis S, Yates CM, Wass MN, Sternberg MJE (2015) The Phyre2 web portal for protein modeling, prediction and analysis. Nat Protoc 10(6):845–858. https://doi.org/10.1038/nprot.2015.053
16. Söding J, Biegert A, Lupas AN (2005) The HHpred interactive server for protein homology detection and structure prediction. Nucleic Acids Res 33:W244–W248. https://doi.org/10.1093/nar/gki408
17. Wang S, Sun SQ, Li Z, Zhang RY, Xu JB (2017) Accurate de novo prediction of protein contact map by ultra-deep learning model. PLOS Comput Biol 13(1):34. https://doi.org/10.1371/journal.pcbi.1005324
18. Xu JB (2019) Distance-based protein folding powered by deep learning. Proc Natl Acad Sci U S A 116(34):16856–16865. https://doi.org/10.1073/pnas.1821309116
19. Yang JY, Anishchenko I, Park H, Peng ZL, Ovchinnikov S, Baker D (2020) Improved protein structure prediction using predicted interresidue orientations. Proc Natl Acad Sci U S A 117(3):1496–1503. https://doi.org/10.1073/pnas.1914677117
20. Senior AW, Evans R, Jumper J, Kirkpatrick J, Sifre L, Green T, Qin CL, Zídek A, Nelson AWR, Bridgland A, Penedones H, Petersen S, Simonyan K, Crossan S, Kohli P, Jones DT, Silver D, Kavukcuoglu K, Hassabis D (2020) Improved protein structure prediction using potentials from deep learning. Nature 577(7792):706–770.
21. Baek M, DiMaio F, Anishchenko I, Dauparas J, Ovchinnikov S, Lee GR, Wang J, Cong Q, Kinch LN, Schaeffer RD, Millán C, Park H, Adams C, Glassman CR, DeGiovanni A, Pereira JH, Rodrigues AV, van Dijk AA, Ebrecht AC, Opperman DJ, Sagmeister T, Buhlheller C, Pavkov-Keller T, Rathinaswamy MK, Dalwadi U, Yip CK, Burke JE, Garcia KC, Grishin NV, Adams PD, Read RJ, Baker D (2021) Accurate prediction of protein structures and interactions using a three-track neural network. Science 373(6557):871–887. https://doi.org/10.1126/science.abj8754
22. Tunyasuvunakool K, Adler J, Wu Z, Green T, Zielinski M, Zídek A, Bridgland A, Cowie A, Meyer C, Laydon A, Velankar S, Kleywegt GJ, Bateman A, Evans R, Pritzel A, Figurnov M, Ronneberger O, Bates R, Kohl SAA, Potapenko A, Ballard AJ, Romera-Paredes B, Nikolov S, Jain R, Clancy E, Reiman D, Petersen S, Senior AW, Kavukcuoglu K, Birney E, Kohli P, Jumper J, Hassabis D (2021) Highly accurate protein structure prediction for the human proteome. Nature 596(7873):590–596. https://doi.org/10.1038/s41586-021-03828-1
23. Abramson J, Adler J, Dunger J, Evans R, Green T, Pritzel A, Ronneberger O, Willmore L, Ballard AJ, Bambrick J, Bodenstein SW, Evans DA, Hung CC, O'Neill M, Reiman D, Tunyasuvunakool K, Wu Z, Zemgulyte A, Arvaniti E, Beattie C, Bertolli O, Bridgland A, Cherepanov A, Congreve M, Cowen-Rivers AI, Cowie A, Figurnov M, Fuchs FB, Gladman H, Jain R, Khan YA, Low CMR, Perlin K, Potapenko A, Savy P, Singh S, Stecula A, Thillaisundaram A, Tong C, Yakneen S, Zhong ED, Zielinski M, Zídek A, Bapst V, Kohli P, Jaderberg M, Hassabis D, Jumper JM (2024) Accurate structure prediction of biomolecular interactions with AlphaFold 3. Nature 630(8016):24. https://doi.org/10.1038/s41586-024-07487-w
24. Mirdita M, Schütze K, Moriwaki Y, Heo L, Ovchinnikov S, Steinegger M (2022) ColabFold: making protein folding accessible to all. Nat Methods 19(6):679–682. https://doi.org/10.1038/s41592-022-01488-1
25. Mistry J, Chuguransky S, Williams L, Qureshi M, Salazar GA, Sonnhammer ELL, Tosatto SCE, Paladin L, Raj S, Richardson LJ, Finn RD, Bateman A (2021) Pfam: the protein

families database in 2021. Nucleic Acids Res 49(D1):D412–D419. https://doi.org/10.1093/nar/gkaa913
26. Orengo CA, Michie AD, Jones S, Jones DT, Swindells MB, Thornton JM (1997) CATH - a hierarchic classification of protein domain structures. Structure 5(8):1093–1108. https://doi.org/10.1016/s0969-2126(97)00260-8
27. Rao RS, Bhattacharya N, Thomas N, Duan Y, Chen X, Canny J, Abbeel P, Song YS (2019) Evaluating protein transfer learning with TAPE. In: 33rd Conference on Neural Information Processing Systems (NeurIPS), Vancouver, Canada, Advances in Neural Information Processing Systems. Neural Information Processing Systems (Nips), La Jolla 8–14 December 2019
28. Heinzinger M, Elnaggar A, Wang Y, Dallago C, Nechaev D, Matthes F, Rost B (2019) Modeling aspects of the language of life through transfer-learning protein sequences. BMC Bioinform 20(1):17. https://doi.org/10.1186/s12859-019-3220-8
29. Brandes N, Ofer D, Peleg Y, Rappoport N, Linial M (2022) ProteinBERT: a universal deep-learning model of protein sequence and function. Bioinformatics 38(8):2102–2110. https://doi.org/10.1093/bioinformatics/btac020
30. Notin P, Van Niekerk L, Kollasch AW, Ritter D, Gal Y, Marks DS (2022) TranceptEVE: combining family-specific and family-agnostic models of protein sequences for improved fitness prediction. https://doi.org/10.1101/2022.12.07.519495
31. Elnaggar A, Heinzinger M, Dallago C, Rehawi G, Wang Y, Jones L, Gibbs T, Feher T, Angerer C, Steinegger M, Bhowmik D, Rost B (2022) ProtTrans: toward understanding the language of life through self-supervised learning. IEEE Trans Pattern Anal Mach Intell 44(10):7112–7127. https://doi.org/10.1109/tpami.2021.3095381
32. Lin ZM, Akin H, Rao RS, Hie B, Zhu ZK, Lu WT, Smetanin N, Verkuil R, Kabeli O, Shmueli Y, Costa AD, Fazel-Zarandi M, Sercu T, Candido S, Rives A (2023) Evolutionary-scale prediction of atomic-level protein structure with a language model. Science 379(6637):1123–1130. https://doi.org/10.1126/science.ade2574
33. Meier J, Rao R, Verkuil R, Liu J, Sercu T, Rives A (2021) Language models enable zero-shot prediction of the effects of mutations on protein function. In: 35th Annual Conference on Neural Information Processing Systems (NeurIPS), null, ELECTR NETWORK, Advances in Neural Information Processing Systems. Neural Information Processing Systems (Nips), La Jolla 6–14 December 2021
34. Riesselman AJ, Ingraham JB, Marks DS (2018) Deep generative models of genetic variation capture the effects of mutations. Nat Methods 15(10):816–881. https://doi.org/10.1038/s41592-018-0138-4
35. Hopf TA, Ingraham JB, Poelwijk FJ, Schärfe CPI, Springer M, Sander C, Marks DS (2017) Mutation effects predicted from sequence co-variation. Nat Biotechnol 35(2):128–135. https://doi.org/10.1038/nbt.3769
36. Anishchenko I, Pellock SJ, Chidyausiku TM, Ramelot TA, Ovchinnikov S, Hao JZ, Bafna K, Norn C, Kang A, Bera AK, DiMaio F, Carter L, Chow CM, Montelione GT, Baker D (2021) De novo protein design by deep network hallucination. Nature 600(7889):547–552. https://doi.org/10.1038/s41586-021-04184-w
37. Ingraham J, Garg VK, Barzilay R, Jaakkola T (2019) Generative models for graph-based protein design. In: 33rd Conference on Neural Information Processing Systems (NeurIPS), Vancouver, Canada, Advances in Neural Information Processing Systems. Neural Information Processing Systems (Nips), La Jolla 8–14 December 2019
38. Dauparas J, Anishchenko I, Bennett N, Bai H, Ragotte RJ, Milles LF, Wicky BIM, Courbet A, de Haas RJ, Bethel N, Leung PJY, Huddy TF, Pellock S, Tischer D, Chan F, Koepnick B, Nguyen H, Kang A, Sankaran B, Bera AK, King NP, Baker D (2022) Robust deep learning-based protein sequence design using ProteinMPNN. Science 378(6615):49–55. https://doi.org/10.1126/science.add2187
39. Hsu C, Verkuil R, Liu J, Lin ZM, Hie B, Sercu T, Lerer A, Rives A (2022) Learning inverse folding from millions of predicted structures. In: 39th International Conference on Machine Learning (ICML), Baltimore, MD, Proceedings of Machine Learning Research. Jmlr-Journal Machine Learning Research, San Diego 17–23 July 2022
40. Norn C, Wicky BIM, Juergens D, Liu SR, Kim D, Tischer D, Koepnick B, Anishchenko I, Players F, Baker D, Ovchinnikov S (2021) Protein sequence design by conformational landscape optimization. Proc Natl Acad Sci U S A 118(11):7. https://doi.org/10.1073/pnas.2017228118
41. Watson JL, Juergens D, Bennett NR, Trippe BL, Yim J, Eisenach HE, Ahern W, Borst AJ, Ragotte RJ, Milles LF, Wicky BIM, Hanikel N, Pellock SJ, Courbet A, Sheffler W, Wang J, Venkatesh P, Sappington I, Torres SV, Lauko A, De Bortoli V, Mathieu E, Ovchinnikov S, Barzilay R, Jaakkola TS, Dimaio F, Baek M, Baker D (2023) De novo design of protein structure and function with RFdiffusion. Nature 620(7976):38. https://doi.org/10.1038/s41586-023-06415-8

42. Trippe BL, Yim J, Tischer D, Baker D, Broderick T, Barzilay R, Jaakkola T (2022) Diffusion probabilistic modeling of protein backbones in 3D for the motif-scaffolding problem. https://doi.org/10.48550/arXiv.2206.04119
43. Madani A, Ben K, Greene ER, Subramanian S, Mohr BP, Holton JM, Olmos Jr JL, Xiong CM, Sun ZZ, Socher R, Fraser JS, Naik N (2023) Large language models generate functional protein sequences across diverse families. Nat Biotechnol 41(8):1099–1109. https://doi.org/10.1038/s41587-022-01618-2
44. Nijkamp E, Ruffolo JA, Weinstein EN, Naik N, Madani A (2023) ProGen2: exploring the boundaries of protein language models. Cell Syst 14(11):15. https://doi.org/10.1016/j.cels.2023.10.002
45. Singh A (2024) Chroma is a generative model for protein design. Nat Methods 21(1):10. https://doi.org/10.1038/s41592-023-02155-9
46. Gligorijevic V, Renfrew PD, Kosciolek T, Leman JK, Berenberg D, Vatanen T, Chandler C, Taylor BC, Fisk IM, Vlamakis H, Xavier RJ, Knight R, Cho K, Bonneau R (2021) Structure-based protein function prediction using graph convolutional networks. Nat Commun 12(1):14. https://doi.org/10.1038/s41467-021-23303-9
47. Kulmanov M, Hoehndorf R (2020) DeepGOPlus: improved protein function prediction from sequence. Bioinformatics 36(2):422–429. https://doi.org/10.1093/bioinformatics/btz595
48. Wallach I, Dzamba M, Heifets A (2016) AtomNet: a deep, convolutional neural network for bioactivity prediction in structure-based drug discovery. Abstr Pap Am Chem Soc 251:1
49. Stärk H, Ganea OE, Pattanaik L, Barzilay R, Jaakkola T (2022) EQUIBIND: geometric deep learning for drug binding structure prediction. In: 39th International Conference on Machine Learning (ICML), Baltimore, MD, Proceedings of Machine Learning Research. Jmlr-Journal Machine Learning Research, San Diego 17–23 July 2022.
50. Corso G, Stärk H, Jing B, Barzilay R, Jaakkola T (2023) DiffDock: diffusion steps, twists, and turns for molecular docking. In: International Conference on Learning Representations (ICLR 2023). https://doi.org/10.48550/arXiv.2210.01776
51. Gilmer J, Schoenholz SS, Riley PF, Vinyals O, Dahl GE (2017) Neural message passing for quantum chemistry. In: 34th International Conference on Machine Learning, Sydney, Australia, Proceedings of Machine Learning Research. Jmlr-Journal Machine Learning Research, San Diego 6–11 August 2017
52. Xue FL, Zhang MH, Li SQ, Gao XY, Wohlschlegel JA, Huang WB, Yang Y, Deng WX (2025) SE(3)-equivariant ternary complex prediction towards target protein degradation. Nat Commun 16(1):15. https://doi.org/10.1038/s41467-025-61272-5
53. Noé F, Olsson S, Köhler J, Wu H (2019) Boltzmann generators: sampling equilibrium states of many-body systems with deep learning. Science 365 (6457):1001–1100. https://doi.org/10.1126/science.aaw1147
54. Mardt A, Pasquali L, Wu H, Noé F (2018) VAMPnets for deep learning of molecular kinetics. Nat Commun 9:11. https://doi.org/10.1038/s41467-017-02388-1
55. Wang YH, Ribeiro JML, Tiwary P (2020) Machine learning approaches for analyzing and enhancing molecular dynamics simulations. Curr Opin Struct Biol 61:139–145. https://doi.org/10.1016/j.sbi.2019.12.016
56. Husic BE, Pande VS (2018) Markov state models: from an art to a science. J Am Chem Soc 140(7):2386–2396. https://doi.org/10.1021/jacs.7b12191
57. Doerr S, Majewski M, Pérez A, Krämer A, Clementi C, Noe F, Giorgino T, De Fabritiis G (2021) TorchMD: a deep learning framework for molecular simulations. J Chem Theory Comput 17(4):2355–2363. https://doi.org/10.1021/acs.jctc.0c01343
58. Yang KK, Wu Z, Arnold FH (2019) Machine-learning-guided directed evolution for protein engineering. Nat Methods 16(8):687–694. https://doi.org/10.1038/s41592-019-0496-6
59. Alley EC, Khimulya G, Biswas S, AlQuraishi M, Church GM (2019) Unified rational protein engineering with sequence-based deep representation learning. Nat Methods 16(12):1315–1322. https://doi.org/10.1038/s41592-019-0598-1
60. Wittmann BJ, Yue YS, Arnold FH (2021) Informed training set design enables efficient machine learning-assisted directed protein evolution. Cell Syst 12(11):1026–1045. https://doi.org/10.1016/j.cels.2021.07.008
61. Biswas S, Khimulya G, Alley EC, Esvelt KM, Church GM (2021) Low-N protein engineering with data-efficient deep learning. Nat Methods 18(4):389–396. https://doi.org/10.1038/s41592-021-01100-y

Chapter 14

Engineering and Adapting Disulfide-Containing Proteins to Enable Intracellular Functionality

Elise Sylvander and Michael W. Traxlmayr

Abstract

Disulfide bonds are key structural components ensuring proper protein folding. Those bonds, however, do not form in the reducing intracellular environment, often resulting in misfolded, unstable proteins with subpar function. To enable intracellular functionality of such proteins, disulfide-free variants with restored stability and function should be engineered. Here, we present a method to substitute the cysteine residues with optimal amino acid combinations using site saturation mutagenesis and screening for improved disulfide-free variants using yeast surface display. We provide a detailed protocol to directly screen for thermal stability of proteins using conformationally specific ligands, and an alternative to harness the correlation between protein stability and expression levels in yeast. We also discuss different strategies for randomizing cysteine residues and approaches for handling proteins with multiple disulfide bonds.

Keywords Disulfide bond engineering, Disulfide bridges, Yeast surface display, Protein engineering, Protein stability

1 Introduction

1.1 Disulfide-Containing Proteins Are Unstable Intracellularly

Disulfide bridges (also known as disulfide bonds) are covalent bonds formed between the sulfur atoms of two cysteine residues in proteins. They are crucial for stabilizing protein structures and therefore greatly contribute to the function of said proteins [1]. Disulfide formation occurs through an oxidative process and thus does not take place in reducing environments such as the cytoplasm of cells. When expressed intracellularly, most disulfide-containing proteins have therefore suboptimal stability, poor folding and in the worst case are non-functional [2–5]. If such proteins must be expressed intracellularly for specific applications, protein engineering can be used to compensate for the loss of disulfide bonds by increasing protein stability and restoring their functionality.

To ensure that the protein will eventually function both extra- and intracellularly, fully disulfide-free proteins (i.e., with all cysteines

Huan Peng and Theam Soon Lim (eds.), *Biomolecular Display Technologies*, Methods in Molecular Biology, vol. 3030,
https://doi.org/10.1007/978-1-0716-5249-7_14,

substituted with other amino acids) should be designed and further stabilized. Here, we describe a method to randomize the cysteine positions by saturation mutagenesis and screen for optimal amino acid combination replacements using yeast surface display to select disulfide-free variants with regained stability and function. In comparison to just mutating the cysteines to a chosen set of amino acids (usually serine, valine, alanine [3, 4, 6–10]), this method allows for better cysteine replacements tailored to the conformation of the protein, i.e. enabling formation of salt bridges, hydrogen bonds, hydrophobic interactions, pi stacking, etc. that can stabilize the protein and help regain its proper conformation [5, 11, 12]. In addition, error-prone PCR (epPCR) and subsequent selection can still be used to introduce additional stabilizing mutations [6, 9].

1.2 Yeast Surface Display as High Throughput Screening Platform

Yeast-surface display is one of the most commonly used display methods for protein engineering [13, 14]. It has been successfully applied to optimize the affinity, stability, enzymatic activity, and expression of proteins [15–22]. It was also employed to introduce novel functions into proteins, such as enabling binding to new target antigens [23, 24], or engineering conditional binding of proteins in the absence or presence of a small molecule [25, 26].

Advantages of this system include the yeast eukaryotic post-translational machinery, the ability to screen libraries of very large sizes (up to 10^9 variants), and the short doubling time of yeast cells (2 h), which speeds up the directed evolution process. In addition, visual assessment of the engineering progress via flow cytometry enables precise control of the selection process.

This display technology is based on the anchoring of the protein of interest (POI) to the cell wall of *Saccharomyces cerevisiae* via the Aga1p—Aga2p a-agglutinin system. Aga1p is a yeast cell wall protein, tethered to the cell wall via a glycosylphosphatidylinositol anchor. The POI is fused to an Aga2p subunit, which forms disulfide bonds with Aga1p upon secretion and therefore covalently links the fusion construct to the cell wall. A hemagglutinin tag (HA tag) and c-Myc tag are typically also included N-terminally (HA tag) and C-terminally (c-Myc tag) of the POI to assess expression and full-length expression of the protein, respectively, by using fluorescently labelled antibodies and flow cytometry (Fig. 1) [13].

Since the fusion construct is introduced to the yeast cells on a plasmid, the yeast phenotype is directly linked to its genotype. In a yeast-display-based engineering campaign, yeast cells displaying variants of the desired phenotype are enriched in subsequent selection rounds until the library contains a limited number of clones displaying improved properties. The DNA pool of the library is then extracted and transformed into *Escherichia coli* for preparation and sequencing of individual plasmids.

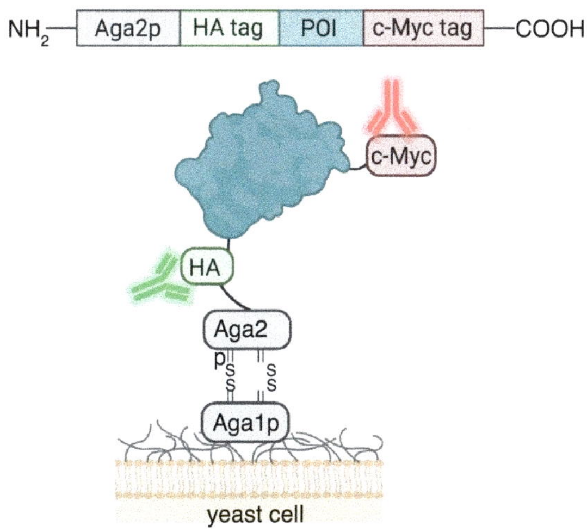

Fig. 1 Schematic of the yeast surface display platform. The protein of interest (POI) is usually fused to the C-terminus of Aga2p, which, upon expression, forms disulfide bonds with the Aga1p protein, anchoring the fusion construct to the yeast cell wall. HA and c-Myc-tags, fused to the N- and C-terminus of the POI, respectively, allow for expression detection by flow cytometry

1.3 How to Select for Thermostable Variants

Protein variants that are correctly folded on yeast and unstable mutants with improper conformations can be distinguished by analyzing their binding to a conformationally specific ligand, for example an antibody, an antigen, or an engineered binder (Fig. 2). The ligand should be added solubly and be detectable via flow cytometry, i.e., being directly conjugated to a fluorophore, containing an

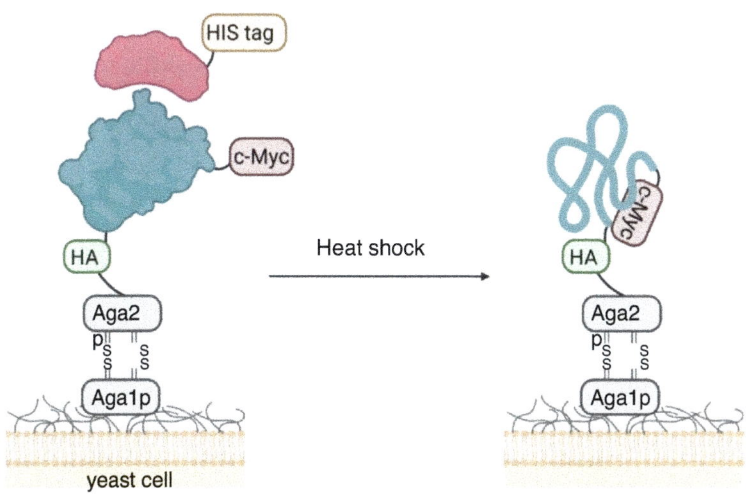

Fig. 2 Schematic of the detection of folded vs unfolded proteins (in blue) via binding to a conformationally specific ligand (in red). Unfolding can be promoted via heat shock. Here, the conformation-specific ligand has a HIS tag that allows for flow cytometric detection

expression tag or being recognized by a monoclonal antibody itself conjugated to a fluorophore. Using such a ligand enables to directly screen for thermal stability by subjecting the library to a heat shock that irreversibly denatures unstable proteins. Protein variants that are more resistant to irreversible thermal denaturation will retain binding to their conformationally specific ligand, allowing for fluorescence-activated cell sorting (FACS) and recovery [5, 27–29]. The duration and temperature of the heat shock should be carefully chosen so that most, but not all proteins, are denatured in yeast. Above a 30 min heat shock at 46°C or 10 min heat shock at 48°C, cell viability drastically reduces, i.e., the cells can still be sorted but not sub-cultured. In that case, the plasmids of the sorted library need to be extracted, PCR-amplified, and re-electroporated into yeasts to create a new library that can proceed to the next selection round [19, 20, 30, 31]. Importantly, above a 76°C and 85°C heat shock for 30 and 10 min respectively, the yeast cells lyse, preventing sorting and recovery of improved protein variants [19, 20]. However, those temperatures are generally sufficient to induce at least partial denaturation of most proteins.

An important prerequisite for this method is the irreversible denaturation of the protein displayed on yeast upon heat shock. If the denaturation is reversible, the protein can refold after heat shock and bind its ligand (Fig. 3). Thus, it is not possible to distinguish between thermostable variants that are not denatured at the temperature used for the heat shock, and unstable variants that refolded.

If conformation-specific ligands are unavailable, or if the protein of interest undergoes reversible denaturation, full-length protein expression levels can serve as a proxy for stability [1, 32, 33]. In unstable variants, the C-terminal c-Myc expression tag tends to be less abundant due to degradation of the POI in the endoplasmic reticulum and/or Golgi apparatus. By normalizing expression with the N-terminal HA tag, it is thus possible to distinguish proteins that are displayed but degraded from those that are exported as full-length versions. To push the system toward the selection of more thermostable variants, the temperature during induction of protein expression can be increased from 20°C to 37°C [5, 24, 27, 34]. *Saccharomyces cerevisiae* grows optimally at 30°C. By lowering the temperature to 20°C during the induction of protein expression, the translation process is slowed down, and cell stress is reduced, promoting proper folding of proteins. Increasing the temperature to 37°C has the opposite effect, resulting in misfolding of unstable proteins. Although selecting for increased protein expression level has been used successfully to stabilize a variety of proteins [27, 28, 32, 35–37], this method is not very sensitive and not always accurate. On the one hand, some unstable proteins can be displayed at high levels in a misfolded conformation [26, 34, 38, 39] and, on the other hand, there seems to be a stability threshold above which all proteins are

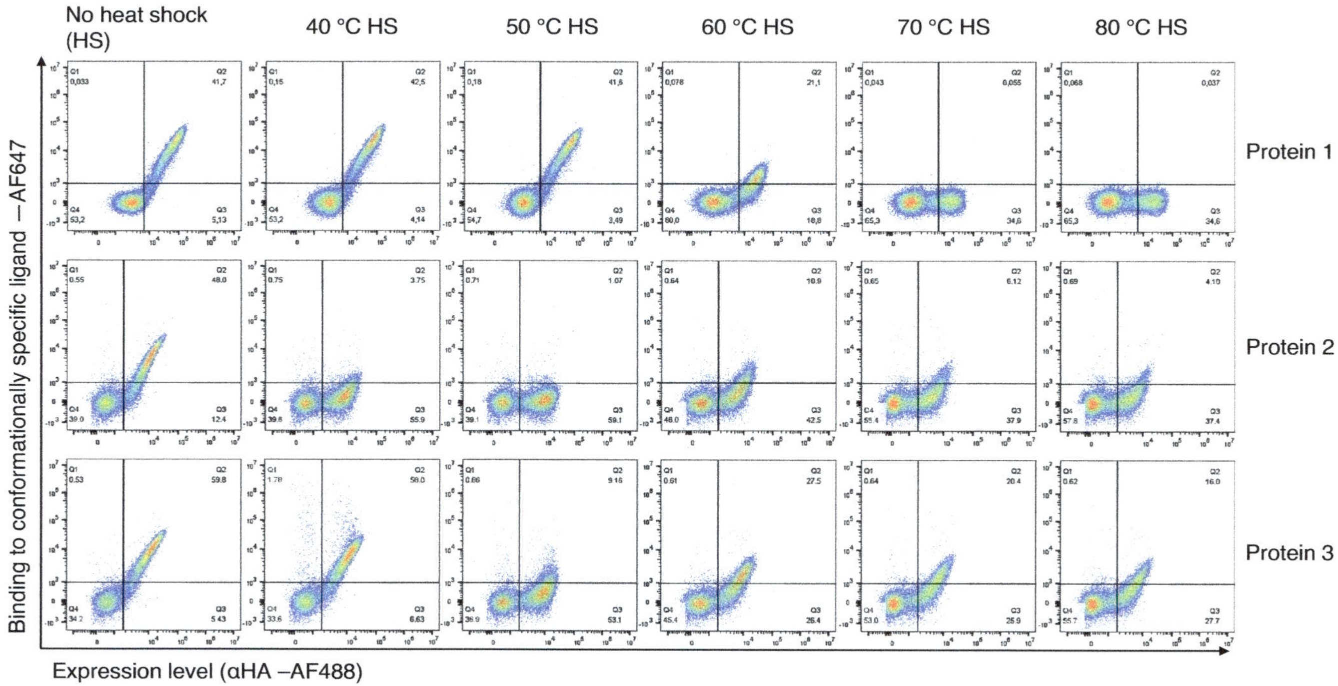

Fig. 3 Example of proteins showing irreversible vs reversible thermal denaturation. Yeast cells displaying the three proteins were subjected to a 10 min heat shock (HS) at the indicated temperature or stayed on ice ("no HS" condition). Protein 1 loses binding to its conformationally specific ligand upon higher HS temperatures, showing irreversible denaturation. Proteins 2 and 3 lose binding but regain it at higher temperatures, indicating some degree of reversible denaturation

efficiently displayed [5, 20]. We recommend only using this method if the prerequisites for the heat shock-based sorting are not met.

1.4 Degenerate Codons or Trimers to Randomize the Cysteine Residues

There are two possibilities to randomize the former cysteine positions.

The first one is to use primers with degenerate codons that encode for all amino acids. In this case, we recommend using the NNK codon instead of NNN, where N represents all four DNA bases and K represents only guanine and thymine. The NNN codon would include all three stop codons (TAA, TAG, and TGA) and would reduce the functional library diversity, compared to NNK, which only includes one stop codon (TAG). NNK primers are affordable and are usually delivered quickly by most vendors that offer oligonucleotides. However, their usage is associated with some limitations. First, there is a large codon-based bias in the amino acid distribution, since amino acids are encoded by one (methionine and tryptophane) to six codons (serine, leucine, arginine). Second, cysteines are included in the library. This complexifies the engineering process since variants containing cysteines would most probably have the highest thermostability and would be preferentially enriched during selections. To minimize this, a less restrictive gating strategy as well as a low number of selection rounds can be used, resulting in larger pools of variants that should be individually analyzed later on. Because of the codon bias mentioned above, this could result in a skewed enrichment of variants.

The other possibility is to use trinucleotide-based primers (e.g., from Ella Biotech), where defined codon mixtures are used during primer synthesis. This means that one codon is used per amino acid, removing codon bias, and the mixes can be customized to include only amino acids of interest and in ratios chosen by the customer. For our purpose, we excluded cysteines and stop codons and added every other amino acid in equivalent ratios. Since cysteines are excluded from the library, the engineering is more straightforward as more selection rounds can be performed and with stringent gating to enrich only in the best disulfide-free variants. The main disadvantages of trinucleotide primers are their high cost and the extended duration of synthesis.

1.5 Engineering Proteins with Multiple Disulfide Bonds

For proteins containing multiple disulfide bonds, randomizing all residues at once can impose excessive selection pressure and make it challenging—or even impossible—to recover variants with a restored native protein conformation through the right combination of amino acids. For example, for a protein with three disulfide bonds, we recommend first engineering separately the two disulfides that have the largest impact on protein stability. Then, create a third library where the first two bonds are restricted to a few optimal amino acid combinations each (not just one, to leave more flexibility) and fully randomize the two cysteines of the last bond [5]. To investigate the contribution of the different disulfide bonds to the stability of the protein, cysteines can be substituted with serines.

Depending on the importance of the disulfide bonds for the stability and/or function of the protein, it might not be sufficient to simply exchange the cysteines with optimal amino acid combinations, and therefore, the obtained variants might still be suboptimal. In this case, additional stabilizing point mutations can be introduced via error-prone PCR (epPCR) and subsequent selection rounds. This epPCR should be carried out early in the selection process. Indeed, the random point mutations might exert synergetic stabilizing effects with amino acid substitutions at cysteine positions that, on their own, might be suboptimal. A good starting point is after the first round of FACS selection, where the gating for highly thermostable variants is not very stringent, but all clearly dysfunctional proteins are excluded. In the case of proteins with multiple disulfide bonds, the epPCR should be carried out on the last, fully disulfide-free, library.

2 Materials

2.1 Cells and Plasmids

1. pCTCON2: The protein of interest is cloned into the pCTCON2 plasmid at the C-terminus of the anchor protein AGA2, between a N-terminal HA tag and a C-terminal c-Myc tag. The pCTCON2 vector also contains an ampicillin resistance cassette for transformation and selection in *Escherichia coli*, and a TRP1 gene (involved in tryptophan biosynthesis) for transformation and selection in EBY100 yeast cells. The vector can be obtained from Addgene [40].
2. EBY100: *Saccharomyces cerevisiae* strain (*GAL1-AGA1::URA3 ura3–52 trp1 leu2Δ1 his3Δ200 pep4::HIS2 prb1Δ1.6R can1 GAL)* in which Aga1 is under the control of a GAL promoter [13]. It also has a knocked-out TRP1 gene, which enables selection of yeast cells transformed with the pCTCON2 plasmid in selective medium containing no tryptophan. EBY100 cells are available at ATCC.
3. NEB 10-beta Electrocompetent *E. coli* C3020K (NEB).

2.2 Kits

1. Frozen-EZ yeast transformation II kit (Zymo Research).
2. Zymoprep Yeast Plasmid Miniprep II (Zymo Research).
3. GeneMorph II Random Mutagenesis Kit (Agilent).
4. Monarch® Spin PCR and DNA Cleanup Kit (NEB).
5. Monarch® Spin DNA Gel Extraction Kit (NEB).

2.3 Equipment

1. Electroporation cuvettes 1 mm (for *E. coli* cells) and 2 mm (for EBY100 cells; 400 μL volume) (VWR).

2. Gene Pulser Xcell Electroporation system (Bio-Rad).
3. SH800S cell sorter (SONY).
4. 96-well sequencing plates (Microsynth).
5. Thermocycler.
6. Thermomixer.
7. Photometer to measure optical densities at 600 nm (OD_{600}).

2.4 Reagents for Cloning and DNA Preparation

1. Restriction enzymes: NheI-HF, Sal I-HF, BamHI-HF (NEB).
2. Q5 polymerase (NEB).
3. 40 mM dNTPs (10 mM each, NEB).
4. 5× Q5 buffer (NEB).
5. 5× Q5 enhancer (NEB).
6. NNK primers or Trinucleotide primers for randomization of former Cys positions.
7. Flanking primers.

2.5 Reagents for Selections

1. Ligand: We usually recombinantly express the ligand fused to a HIS tag and use this for detection, or biotinylate the protein and use streptavidin to detect it.
2. Antibodies:
   - αHA-Alexa Fluor 647 or 488, clone 16B12, Biolegend (1:500).
   - αc-Myc - Alexa Fluor 647 or 488, clone 9E10, Thermo Fisher (1:200).
   - Streptavidin - Alexa Fluor 647 or 488, Thermo Fisher (1:400).
   - αPenta HIS- Alexa Fluor 647 or 488, Qiagen (1:40).

2.6 Yeast Media and Solutions

1. *SD-CAA medium* (selective growth medium, pH 4.5): 20 g/L dextrose (D-glucose), 5 g/L casamino acids (Becton Dickinson), 6.7 g/L yeast nitrogen base (Becton Dickinson), 11.85 g/L sodium citrate dihydrate, and 7.4 g/L citric acid monohydrate in ddH_2O. Sterilize by filtrating through a 0.2 μm filter into autoclaved bottles.
2. *SD-CAA agar plates* (selective plates, pH 6.0): 20 g/L dextrose (D-glucose), 5 /L casamino acids (Becton Dickinson), 6.7 g/L yeast nitrogen base (Becton Dickinson) in 0.1 × final volume ddH_2O. Sterilize by filtrating through a 0.2 μm filter into autoclaved bottles. In parallel, dissolve 8.56 g/L NaH_2PO_4 monohydrate, 5.4 g/L Na_2HPO_4 anhydrous, 182 g/L sorbitol and 15 g/L agar in 0.9 × final volume ddH_2O. Autoclave, cool

down to approximately 60°C, and add the filter-sterilized solution before pouring the agar plates.

3. *SG-CAA medium* (selective induction medium, pH 6.0): Dissolve 2 g/L dextrose (D-glucose), 20 g/L D-galactose, 5/L casamino acids (Becton Dickinson), 6.7 g/L yeast nitrogen base (Becton Dickinson), 8.56 g/L NaH_2PO_4 monohydrate, and 5.4 g/L Na_2HPO_4 anhydrous in ddH_2O. Sterilize by filtrating through a 0.2 μm filter into autoclaved bottles.
4. *YPD medium* (non-selective growth medium): 20 g/L peptone and 10 g/L yeast extract in 0.9 × final volume ddH_2O. Autoclave, cool down to approximately 50°C, and add filter-sterilized 20 g/L dextrose (D-glucose) in 0.1 × final volume ddH_2O.
5. *YPD agar plates* (non-selective plates): 20 g/L peptone, 10 g/L yeast extract, and 15 g/L agar in 0.9 × final volume ddH_2O. Autoclave, cool down to approximately 50°C, and add filter-sterilized 20 g/L dextrose (D-glucose) in 0.1 × final volume ddH_2O.
6. *PBSA* (staining buffer): 1 g/L bovine serum albumin (BSA) in 1 × PBS filter-sterilized through a 0.2 μm filter into autoclaved bottles.
7. *Lithium acetate:* 100 mM lithium acetate in ddH_2O. Sterilize by filtration through a 0.2 μm filter into autoclaved bottles. Can be kept at room temperature (RT) for months.
8. *DTT*: 1 M dithiothreitol in ddH_2O. Sterilize by filtration through a 0.2 μm filter into autoclaved bottles. Should be prepared freshly (on the day of use).

2.7 E. coli *Media and Solutions*

1. NEB outgrowth medium.
2. *Luria Broth (LB)*: 5 g/L yeast extract, 10 g/L peptone, 10 g/L NaCl in ddH_2O. Autoclave.
3. *Luria Broth agar (LB agar)*: 5 g/L yeast extract, 10 g/L peptone, 10 g/L NaCl, 13.5 g/L agar in ddH_2O. Autoclave.
4. *LB and LB agar with ampicillin*: Prepare the media as described above. After autoclaving, let it cool down and add 100 μg/mL ampicillin.

3 Methods

3.1 *Library Preparation*

Depending on where the cysteines are located in the gene, it might be necessary to build the library in multiple pieces. We recommend performing only one PCR with all the primers necessary for the

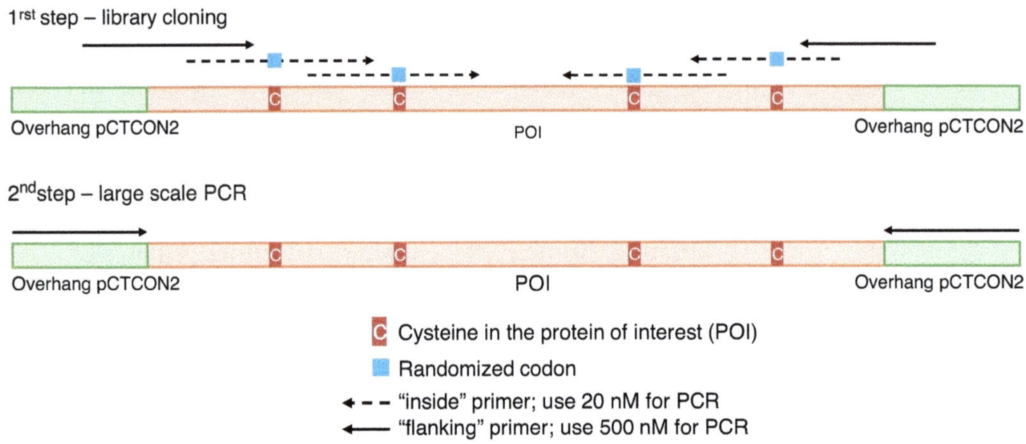

Fig. 4 Schematic for the generation of a library using multiple primers. The first PCR is an "all in one" PCR where all the primers are added at once at the indicated concentration

amplification. For this, use primers with overlapping sequences of similar annealing temperature and the same amount of reverse and forward primers. For primers inside the gene, use a concentration of 20 nM per primer. For the two flanking primers (one rev and one fwd) on the 3′ and 5′ terminus, use 500 nM (Fig. 4). This will help preferentially amplify full-length products.

As a template for the library creation, it is recommended to use a disulfide-free variant of the protein where cysteines were all mutated to serines, for example. Although a DpnI digestion will be performed on the PCR product to digest all plasmid DNA, there might still be some template sequence remaining, which will be further amplified in a large-scale PCR. It is important to prevent the disulfide-containing protein from appearing in the library.

1. Perform a PCR with a disulfide-free version of the protein of interest as template and the following reaction:
   - 10 μL 5× Q5 buffer.
   - 10 μL 5× Q5 enhancer.
   - 2.5 μL 10 μM flanking primer fwd (final concentration 500 nM).
   - 2.5 μL 10 μM flanking primer rev (final concentration 500 nM).
   - 1 μL of each 1 μM inside primers fwd (final concentration 20 nM each).
   - 1 μL of each 1 μM inside primers rev (final concentration 20 nM each).
   - 1 μL 10 mM dNTPs (final concentration 200 μM).
   - 0.5 μL Q5 polymerase (20 U/mL).
   - X μL 10 ng DNA template.

- Fill up to 50 µL with nuclease-free H_2O.

2. Amplify with the following conditions:
   - Initial denaturation at 98°C, 30 s.
   - 25 cycles of: 98°C for 10 s, X1°C for 30 s, 72°C for X2 s. X1 is the lowest annealing temperature of the primers used, and X2 is the elongation time based on the insert's length (30 s/kb).
   - Final extension at 72°C, 2 min.
   - Cool down to 4°C.

3. Digest the remaining plasmid DNA template with DpnI and incubate for 1 h at 37°C:
   - 50 µLDNA.
   - 5.6 µL10x CutSmartBuffer.
   - 1 µL*DpnI* (20 U).

4. Run the DpnI-digested PCR product on a preparative 1% agarose gel. Excise the band of the correct size and purify the DNA with a gel extraction kit. Elute in 20 µL.
5. Perform a large-scale PCR amplification. Large amounts of DNA are used to electroporate yeast. Prepare 2 × 100 µL PCR reaction per library of interest (200 µL total PCR product will be used for one electroporation). For 100 µL, use 50 ng DNA as template and the following:
   - 20 µL 5× Q5 enhancer.
   - 20 µL 5× Q5 buffer.
   - 5 µL 10 µM fwd primer (final concentration 0.5 µM). *See* **Note 1** for the sequence.
   - 5 µL 10 µM rev primer (final concentration 0.5 µM). *See* **Note 1** for the sequence.
   - 2 µL 10 mM dNTPs (final concentration 200 µM).
   - 1 µL Q5 polymerase (20 U/mL).
   - 50 ng DpnI digested DNA.
   - Fill up to 100 µL with nuclease-free H_2O.

6. Amplify as in Step 3.1.2.
7. Pool the 2 × 100 µL. Analyze 5 µL of the PCR product on a 1% agarose gel to make sure the library (band) is clean.

3.2 Ethanol Purification

Purify the amplified DNA via ethanol (EtOH) purification:

1. Add 0.1 × volume (19.5 µL) of sterile filtered 3 M sodium acetate pH 5.2 to the 195 µL DNA product. This buffer can be prepared in advance and stored for a few months at RT.

2. Add at least 2× volumes of 100% EtOH (429 μL). Incubate at RT for 2 min.
3. Centrifuge at 16,000×*g* for 5 min at RT. Discard the supernatant, add 500 μL of 70% EtOH, and mix briefly.
4. Centrifuge at 16,000×*g* for 5 min at RT. Discard the supernatant, add 500 μL of 100% EtOH, and mix briefly.
5. Centrifuge at 16,000×*g* for 5 min at RT. Remove the supernatant and let the DNA pellet dry under a laminar flow hood until all the EtOH evaporates. To speed-up this process, use a heat block at 48°C.
6. Dissolve the dried DNA pellet in 10 μL nuclease-free H_2O. Do not measure the DNA concentration; use all for the yeast electroporation.

3.3 Linearization of the Yeast-Display Vector for Electroporation

It is recommended to use a plasmid without the wild-type protein containing disulfide bonds as a template for the linearization of the vector. In case of incorrect enzymatic digestion, the disulfide-containing protein would be included in the library and would be preferentially enriched in the selection rounds. Therefore, either use a plasmid comprising an irrelevant protein or a variant of this protein where cysteines are mutated to other amino acids (e.g., serine).

1. Digest 200 μg of the pCTCON2 vector DNA with Sal I for 24 h at 37°C to linearize the vector (*see* **Note 2**):
   - X μL vector DNA.
   - 50 μL 10× CutSmartBuffer.
   - 30 μL (60 U) *Sal I-HF.*
   - Fill up to 500 μL with H_2O.
2. Digest with NheI and BamHI at 24°C to 37°C to excise the insert:
   - 500 μL Sal I digested pCTCON2.
   - 37.5 μL 10x CutSmartBuffer.
   - 15 μL (30 U) *NheI-HF.*
   - 15 μL (30 U) *BamHI-HF.*
   - Fill up to 875 μL with H_2O.
3. Add 5 μL of each enzyme to the final tube (Sal I, NheI, BamHI) and incubate for 24 h at 37°C.
4. Run the digested vector in multiple wells on a preparative 1% agarose gel. Excise the bands containing the linearized vector and purify the DNA with a gel extraction kit, using multiple columns. Adjust the concentration to 2 μg/μL.

3.4 Yeast Electroporation

Yeast cells are electroporated with the linear vector and the library of inserts. The inserts are flanked by homologous regions to the vector, facilitating homologous recombination in yeast. The following protocol typically yields of at least 10^7 transformants per electroporation.

1. Three days prior to electroporation, streak EBY100 yeast cells from a glycerol stock onto a YPD plate. YPD plates are non-selective and allow for the growth of EBY100 cells not transformed with a plasmid. Incubate the plate at 30°C.
2. One day prior to electroporation, inoculate a single colony of EBY100 cells into 30 mL YPD medium. Incubate overnight at 30°C, 180 rpm.
3. The next morning, measure the cell density via the optical density of the culture at 600 nm (OD_{600}). Dilute the culture to an OD_{600} of 0.2 in 100 mL YPD. 50 mL are sufficient for two electroporations. 100 mL will ensure having enough cells to electroporate the library as well as two controls (cells only and linearized vector only). For libraries with higher diversity, adapt the protocol according to **Note 3**.
4. When the OD_{600} reaches 1.3–1.5, pellet the cells in 2 × 50 mL tubes at 2000 × *g* for 5 min at room temperature (RT).
5. Discard the supernatant, resuspend the cell pellet in 0.5 × original volume (25 mL) of sterile filtered 100 mM lithium acetate.
6. Prepare freshly a solution of sterile filtered 1 M dithiothreitol in ddH_2O. Add to the cells to a final concentration of 10 mM (250 μL per tube).
7. Incubate the cells for 10 min at 30°C with shaking at 180 rpm.
8. In the meantime, add 1 mL YPD medium into three 1.5 mL tubes and incubate at 30°C. The cells will be rescued in this warm YPD medium later on.
9. Add 4 μg of linearized vector (Step 3.3) to the 10 μL of ethanol precipitated DNA library (Step 3.2.6). Also, add 4 μg linearized vector in an empty tube to be used as a negative control. Store on ice.
10. Chill sterile ddH_2O and three 2 mm electroporation cuvettes on ice.
11. After the 10 min incubation, pellet the cells (2000 × *g*, 5 min, 4°C), remove the supernatant, and place the cells on ice. All remaining steps should be carried out on ice and with chilled reagents and consumables.
12. Resuspend the cells in 0.5 × original volume (25 mL) of chilled sterile ddH_2O and pellet the cells (2000 × *g*, 5 min, 4°C).

13. Resuspend the cells in 300 µL chilled sterile ddH_2O. The total volume including the cell pellet should be 500 µL per 50 mL tube.
14. Add 250 µL cells into the 1.5 mL tube containing the linearized vector and library DNA, 250 µL into the tube containing only the linearized vector, and 250 µL into an empty tube.
15. Transfer the cells/DNA mixture into pre-chilled 2 mm electroporation cuvettes and keep on ice until electroporation.
16. Electroporate the cells with a Bio-Rad Gene Pulser Xcell with the square wave protocol and the following conditions: single pulse; 500 V; 15 ms pulse duration. Usual droop signals are 1%–3% for the negative control and 5%–9% for libraries. *See* **Note 4** if this is not the case. Other electroporators can be used but the conditions indicated here were optimized for the Bio-Rad Gene Pulser.
17. Immediately rescue the electroporated cells by flushing the cuvette with 1 mL pre-warmed YPD medium, mixing gently, and transferring them back to the pre-warmed 1.5 mL tube.
18. Incubate the cells in YPD at 30°C without shaking for 1 h.
19. Prepare a dilution series of the electroporated cells ranging from 10^{-3} (1:1000) to 10^{-6} and plate 100 µL on selective SD-CAA plates. For the negative controls, plating the 10^{-3} dilution is enough. Incubate the plates at 30°C for 3 days to allow for growth of transformants.
20. Centrifuge the rest of the cells at 2000 × *g* for 5 min. Make sure to discard as much of the YPD supernatant as possible to prevent growth of non-transformed cells. Resuspend the pellet in 100 mL selective SD-CAA medium.
21. Incubate the cells at 30°C, 180 rpm.
22. When the cells reach the saturation phase (OD_{600} of approximately 7), freeze the library. For this, pellet enough cells to cover at least 10× diversity (2000 × *g*, 3 min, RT). Resuspend the pellet in SD-CAA containing 15% glycerol and store at −80°C. If you do not know the diversity yet, for example, after an error-prone PCR library, freeze a few aliquots with 10^9 cells each. Store the rest of the library at 4°C.
23. After 2–3 days, count the colonies on the SD-CAA plates. When calculating the library diversity, consider the dilution factor and the ratio of the plated cells versus the original volume of the culture (100 µL vs 1 mL for one electroporation). Typically, at least 10^7 cells are transformed in one electroporation.

3.5 Yeast Culture and Induction of Protein Expression

For each yeast sub-culture and induction, i.e., after electroporation and between each selection round, it is crucial to cover at least 10× the library diversity (*see* **Note 5**). The fusion construct (Aga2p—protein of interest) is under the control of a galactose promoter on the pCTCON2 plasmid. Induction of protein expression is carried out by switching from a glucose- to a galactose-containing medium.

1. Measure the OD_{600} of the yeast library.
2. Dilute the culture to $OD_{600}=0.2$ in 10 mL SD-CAA. For larger libraries, this protocol can be modified according to **Note 6**.
3. When the culture reaches its exponential growth phase (OD_{600} 0.8–1), induce protein expression by centrifuging the entire culture at 2000 × *g*, 5 min, RT, discarding the supernatant, and resuspending the cell pellet in the same volume (10 mL) of SG-CAA. Incubate the library at 20°C overnight. The library can also be induced overnight at 37°C to increase misfolding and degradation of unstable proteins, thus lowering the expression levels of unstable protein variants.

3.6 Fluorescence Activated Cell Sorting Selections

Below is a protocol for heat shock-based cell sorting. For a selection based on expression level, skip the heat shock and the incubation with the ligand (Steps 4–12) and stain the cells with both anti-HA and anti-c-Myc antibodies.

1. Measure the OD_{600} of the culture.
2. Pellet the appropriate amount of culture (2000 × *g*, 3 min, 4°C). Make sure to cover at least 10× diversity, 100× if possible (*see* **Note 7**).
3. Resuspend the pellet in PBSA to 5×10^6–3×10^7 cells (depending on the diversity) in 700 μL in a 1.5 mL tube. Deposit the cells at the bottom of the tube and do NOT invert the tube (*see* **Note 8**).
4. Incubate on ice for at least 10 min.
5. Incubate in a thermomixer for 10 min while shaking (300 rpm) at the desired heat shock temperature (*see* **Note 9**).
6. Incubate immediately after on ice for at least 10 min.
7. If more than one tube was used for one library, pool them at this step. In the following steps of this protocol, it is assumed that the sample consists of one 700 μL aliquot with 5×10^6 cells. If this is not the case, adjust all volumes accordingly.
8. Centrifuge the aliquot (2000 × *g*, 3 min, 4°C) and discard the supernatant.
9. Resuspend the cells in PBSA containing the conformationally specific ligand.

10. Incubate at 4°C while shaking (300 rpm) for 30 min.
11. Centrifuge the cells (2000 × *g*, 3 min, 4°C), discard the supernatant, and wash with 1 mL PBSA.
12. Centrifuge the cells (2000 × *g*, 3 min, 4°C), discard the supernatant.
13. Resuspend in 50 μL PBSA (100 μL if the tube contains 3×10^7 cells) containing secondary reagents labeled with compatible fluorophores. For example, an anti-HA IgG to assess expression, anti-c-Myc IgG to assess full-length expression, anti-HIS IgG or streptavidin if the conformationally specific ligand is a His-tagged or biotinylated recombinant protein, respectively (*see* **Note 10**).
14. Incubate at 4°C while shaking (300 rpm) for 30 min.
15. Centrifuge (2000 × *g*, 3 min, 4°C), discard the supernatant and wash with 1 mL PBSA. Repeat this step.
16. Centrifuge (2000 × *g*, 3 min, 4°C), discard the supernatant, and store the cell pellet on ice.
17. Resuspend the cells right before sorting in PBSA, and transfer them to a FACS tube through a strainer.
18. Sort the yeast clones that are most positive for binding to the conformationally specific ligand (heat shock-based selection) or for high expression level. See Fig. 5 for gating examples.
19. If the heat shock temperature is low enough and viable cells can be recovered, sort the cells into 1 mL SD-CAA. After the sort, transfer into 10 mL SD-CAA and cultivate at 30°C, 180 rpm. When the cells are dense enough (OD_{600} of 7), freeze 10× diversity in SD-CAA containing 15% glycerol.
20. If no viable cells can be recovered after the sort due to high heat shock temperatures, sort the cells into 500 μL PBSA.
21. Centrifuge the cells in PBSA (2000×*g*, 15 min, 4°C). If less than 5×10^5 cells were sorted, add 5×10^6 non-transformed EBY100 yeast cells to facilitate pellet formation.
22. Pipette off the supernatant. Proceed with plasmid isolation.

3.7 Plasmid Isolation from Sorted Cells

Extract the plasmid DNA of the library using the Zymoprep Yeast Plasmid Miniprep II kit with the following modifications.

1. Centrifuge 3 mL culture or the dead yeast cells that were sorted into 500 μL PBSA at 600 × *g* for 2 min.
2. Add 200 μL Solution 1 and 6 μL Zymolyase to the pellet. Mix by flicking or mild vortexing and incubate at 37°C for 3 h.

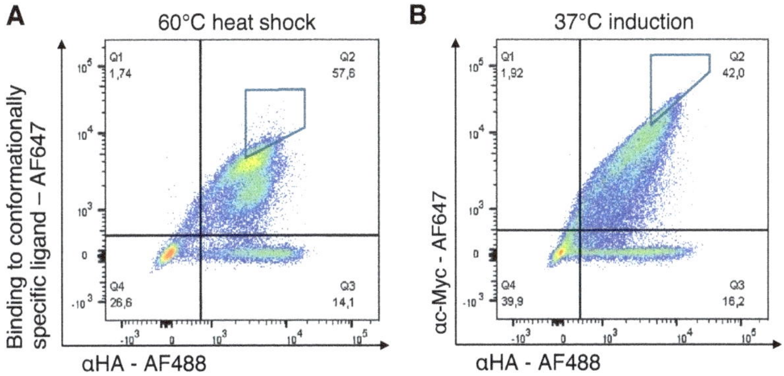

Fig. 5 Example of gating strategies for both heat shock (**A**) and expression-based (**B**) selection of a library. (**A**) The cells were incubated for 10 min at 60°C, incubated with a HIS-tagged conformationally specific ligand, and stained with αHIS and αHA antibodies. (**B**) Protein expression was induced at 37°C one day prior to the staining instead of the usual 20°C induction. Cells were stained with αc-Myc and αHA antibodies. The libraries sorted here were built with trinucleotide primers, allowing for stringent gating. If NNK primers are used instead, more permissive gating should be applied to avoid exclusive enrichment of disulfide-containing protein variants

3. Add 200 μL Solution 2 and mix gently.
4. Add 400 μL Solution 3 and mix gently.
5. Centrifuge at maximum speed for 10 min.
6. Transfer the supernatant to a new 1.5 mL tube, centrifuge at maximum speed for 3 min.
7. Transfer the supernatant to a Zymo-Spin-I column, centrifuge at maximum speed for 30 s and discard the flowthrough.
8. Add 550 μL Wash Buffer containing ethanol and centrifuge at maximum speed for 2 min.
9. Transfer the column to a 1.5 mL tube and centrifuge at maximum speed for 2 min to remove residual wash buffer.
10. Transfer the column to a new 1.5 mL tube, elute the DNA with 10 μL nuclease-free water and 1 min centrifugation step at maximum speed.

3.8 Insert DNA Amplification and Generation of a New Library

1. Use the entire 10 μL as a template for a large-scale PCR (2 × 100 μL) as described in Step 3.1.5.
2. Purify it via ethanol purification (Step 3.2) and electroporate it into new EBY100 cells (Step 3.3) to create the new library.
3. Perform the entire cycle until the enrichment of more thermostable variants in the library is clear, and proceed with library sequencing.

3.9 Library Sequencing

3.9.1 DNA Harvesting

1. Inoculate an overnight culture in SD-CAA.
2. The next morning, dilute to an OD_{600} of 0.2 and incubate at 30°C with shaking.
3. When the OD_{600} reaches 0.6–0.8, extract the plasmid DNA of the library using the Zymoprep yeast kit as described in Step 3.7.

3.9.2 Electroporation into *E. coli* 10-Beta Electrocompetent Cells

Electroporate the harvested DNA into *E. coli* 10-beta electrocompetent cells. One electroporation is used per library:

1. Place a 1 mm electroporation cuvette and 1.5 mL tube on ice per electroporation.
2. Pre-warm a 1.5 mL tube with 950 µL NEB outgrowth medium at 30°C to rescue the cells after electroporation.
3. Thaw the 10-beta cells on ice and mix by gently flicking the tube. One cell aliquot (100 µL) can be used for two electroporations (50 µL, preferred) to three electroporations (33 µL each). The protocol indicated here is for 50 µL cells but can be used as is if only 33 µL cells are used.
4. Transfer 50 µL cells to a pre-chilled 1.5 mL tube. Add 1 µL of the DNA harvested from the yeast library and mix gently.
5. Transfer the cell-DNA mix into a pre-chilled electroporation cuvette.
6. Electroporate with a Bio-Rad Gene Pulser Xcell and the following conditions: 2.0 kV; 200 Ω; 25 µF. Typical time constants range from 4.8 to 5.1 ms. If that is not the case, refer to **Note 4**. Other electroporators can be used but the conditions indicated here were optimized for the Bio-Rad Gene Pulser.
7. Immediately flush the electroporation cuvette with pre-warmed NEB outgrowth medium, mix gently, and transfer back to the warm 1.5 mL tube.
8. Incubate for 1 h at 37°C, 300 rpm.
9. Plate 10 µL, 100 µL, and the rest (890 µL) onto pre-warmed selective LB plates. The pCTCON2 vector has an ampicillin resistance gene used for antibiotic selection. Incubate the plates overnight at 37°C.

3.9.3 Library Sequencing

1. Prepare an LB agar copy plate: pipette 200 µL LB agar supplemented with 100 µg/mL ampicillin into each well of a 96-F well plate and let it solidify. The copy plate will be used to extract the desired plasmids by inoculating a liquid culture and performing a miniprep.

2. Prepare a 96-well sequencing plate by pipetting 50 μL LB supplemented with 100 μg/mL ampicillin per well. This amount is recommended for Microsynth sequencing plates and might be different for other companies.
3. Pick a single colony from the plates, inoculate first the copy plate and the same well of the sequencing plate. Incubate the copy plate overnight at 37°C, then store at 4°C until receiving the sequencing results.
4. Incubate the sequencing plate for 3–4 h at 37°C, 180 rpm, covered with a plastic or aluminum foil. It is also possible to skip this incubation step, but the company performing the sequencing should be made aware, so they include this step in-house.
5. Seal the sequencing plate and send it for sequencing with the desired pCTCON2 sequencing primer (5′ -CGTTTGTCAGTAATTGCGGTTCTC). 500 μL of 10 μM primer is sufficient for the full plate as well as repeated sequencing reactions if needed.
6. Align the DNA sequences of the variants with the original wild-type protein (*see* **Note 11**).

3.10 Single Clone Extraction and Transformation into EBY100 Cells

Clones with an interesting sequence should be analyzed individually and compared to find an optimal disulfide-free variant. For this, their DNA can be extracted from the copy plate and transformed into EBY100 cells.

3.10.1 Single-Clone Plasmid Harvest

1. Pick the colonies on the copy plates corresponding to the sequenced plasmids of interest. Inoculate individual overnight cultures in 3 mL LB supplemented with ampicillin.
2. Perform a miniprep the next day. Send the purified DNA for sequencing to confirm the identity of the chosen variant.

3.10.2 Transformation into EBY100 Cells

1. Prepare chemically competent EBY100 cells with the Frozen-EZ yeast transformation II kit according to the manufacturer's instructions. Store at −80°C in 50 μL aliquots.
2. Thaw a cell aliquot (50 μL) on ice or use a freshly prepared aliquot.
3. Mix 50 μL competent cells with 0.2–1 μg DNA. The DNA should be added in less than 0.1 × volume (5 μL). If needed, the transformation can be scaled down, using only 25 μL of competent cells. In this case, simply half the DNA amount (0.1–0.5 μg in 2.5 μL maximum) and EZ 3 volume (250 μL).
4. Add 500 μL EZ 3 solution and mix thoroughly by vortexing.
5. Incubate 45 min at 30°C, 300 rpm. Mix vigorously by vortexing 2–3 times during this incubation.
6. Spread 100 μL on an SD-CAA plate and incubate at 30°C for 2–3 days.

7. Pick a colony and inoculate 3 mL SD-CAA, incubate overnight at 30°C, 180 rpm.
8. The next day, prepare a glycerol stock and store the culture at 4°C or directly dilute and induce it for further analysis.

Detailed protocols to analyze single clone thermostability and obtain $T_{1/2}$ values (temperature of half-maximum irreversible denaturation, which correlates with the melting temperature T_m) are available elsewhere [19, 41].

3.11 epPCR to Further Stabilize the Protein

3.11.1 Harvesting the Library DNA

If the culture is not older than 1 month and stored at 4°C, simply inoculate an overnight culture of 10 mL SD-CAA medium with the library to an OD_{600} of 0.2. Make sure to cover at least 10× the diversity of the library (if the diversity is higher than 2×10^6, increase the culture volume).

If the culture is older, it is better to start from a glycerol stock. In this case:

1. Thaw the entire glycerol stock in 10 mL SD-CAA.
2. Prepare a dilution series ranging from 10^{-3} to 10^{-6} and plate 100 μL of each on SD-CAA plates. Incubate the plates at 30°C. Incubate the rest of the liquid culture at 30°C, 180 rpm.
3. Count the colonies on the plates 2–3 days later and calculate the new practical diversity of the library, considering the dilution factor and the ratio of the plated vs. the original culture volume (i.e., 100 μL vs. 10 mL in this case). This step is crucial to ensure that the freeze/thaw did not compromise the library diversity. It is acceptable if a minor fraction of the library dies during this step, since always at least 10× the library diversity is frozen.
4. When the culture reaches an OD_{600} or around 7, freeze the library again in SD-CAA with 15% glycerol. Store the new culture at 4°C.
5. In both cases, start with an overnight culture. The next day, extract the yeast DNA by performing a yeast miniprep as described above.

3.11.2 Performing the epPCR

Since a lot of genomic yeast DNA is extracted along with the plasmid DNA during the yeast miniprep, it is recommended to perform an initial PCR amplification of the insert on the yeast display vector. This clean DNA fragment, whose concentration can be accurately determined, will then be used as a template for the epPCR.

1. Perform the initial PCR in 50 μL with the following reaction:
   - 10 μL 5× Q5 enhancer (final concentration 1×).
   - 10 μL 5× Q5 buffer (final concentration 1×).
   - 2.5 μL fwd primer 10 μM (final concentration 0.5 μM).
   - 2.5 μL rev primer 10 μM (final concentration 0.5 μM).
   - 1 μL dNTPs 10 mM (final concentration 200 μM).
   - 0.5 μL Q5 polymerase (final concentration 20 U/mL).
   - 10 μL yeast miniprep DNA.
   - 13.5 μL nuclease-free H_2O.
2. Amplify according to the following conditions:
   - Initial denaturation at 98°C, 30 s.
   - 25 cycles of: 98°C for 10 s, X1°C for 30 s, 72°C for X2 s. X1 is the annealing temperature of the primers used, and X2 is the elongation time based on the insert's length (30 s/kb).
   - Final extension of 72°C, 2 min.
   - Cool down to 4°C.
3. Purify the DNA with a PCR and DNA cleanup kit. Elute in 20 μL nuclease-free H_2O.
4. Perform the epPCR with the GeneMorph kit in 50 μL with the following reaction (*see* **Note 12**):
   - 5 μL 10× Mutazyme II reaction buffer (final concentration 1×).
   - 1 μL 40 mM dNTP reaction mix (final concentration 200 μ M).
   - 0.5 μL primer mix (primer mix: 250 ng/μL each primer).
   - 1 μL Mutazyme II DNA polymerase (final concentration 2.5 U).
   - 500 ng target DNA.
   - Up to 50 μL nuclease-free H_2O.
5. Amplify according to the following conditions:
   - Initial denaturation at 95°C, 2 min.
   - 20 cycles of: 95°C for 30 s, X1°C for 30 s, 72°C for X2 min. X1 is the annealing temperature of the primers used—5°C and X2 is the elongation time based on the insert's length (1 min/kb, 1 min minimum).
   - Final extension of 72°C, 10 min.
   - Cool down to 4°C.

6. Run the digested vector on a preparative 1% agarose gel. Excise the band of the correct size and purify the DNA with a gel extraction kit. Elute in 20 μL and measure the concentration.
7. Use 50 ng of the epPCR product as a template for a large-scale PCR (2 × 100 μL, see Step 3.1.5) and proceed with the library generation as described above.

4 Notes

1. The same flanking primers are used for all PCRs (small and large scale as well as epPCR) except for the library construction (Step 3.1.1) and have the following sequence:
   Fwd: 5′-GGCTCTGGTGGAGGCGGTAGCGGAGGCGGAG-GGTCGGCTAGC
   Rev: 5′-CTATTACAAGTCCTCTTCAGAAATAAGCT-TTTGTTCGGATCC
2. The restriction site of this enzyme should be in the insert. For our template, we chose Sal-I but any enzyme can be used instead.
3. In case you need a library with a higher diversity, multiple electroporations can be carried out. In this case, simply increase all volumes accordingly, considering that 50 mL of culture is enough for two electroporations. The tubes containing cells electroporated with the same DNA library should be pooled after the 1 h incubation in YPD medium, before the serial dilutions and plating of the library (between Step 3.4.18 and Step 3.4.19). Make sure to also scale up the amount of library DNA prepared in Step 3.1.5, knowing that 200 μL of PCR is used for one electroporation.
4. If the droop values (for yeasts) or time constants (*E. coli*) during electroporation are completely out of the ranges indicated it could be due to bubbles in the electroporation cuvette, insufficient drying of the cuvettes, buffer salts that were not removed sufficiently, or dirty conductive surfaces on the sides of the cuvettes (do not touch those even with gloves). Also, ensure that the cells are properly deposited on the bottom of the cuvette.
5. For a protein with one disulfide bond where two cysteines are randomized, the theoretical library size is extremely small (20^2, i.e., 400 clones). In this case, only 4×10^3 cells would need to be passaged. Yeast cells are cultivated by diluting them to an OD_{600} of 0.2 in SD-CAA (i.e., 2×10^6 cells/mL; an OD_{600} of 1 corresponds to 10^7 cells/mL). For such a small library, only 2 μ L SD-CAA would be needed. To be able to cultivate the libraries in flasks and ensure optimal aeration and growth, we use

10 mL culture minimum, which is then sufficient for libraries up to 2×10^6 cells.

6. For large libraries with higher diversities, the culture volume to dilute to an OD_{600} of 0.2 would be too high. In this case, dilute the culture to an OD_{600} of one, making sure to choose a culture volume high enough to sample 10× the diversity. For example, for a library with a diversity of 5×10^8, you would need to passage 5×10^9 cells. Since an OD_{600} of one corresponds to a cell density of 10^7 cells/mL, you would need to dilute the cells in 500 mL SD-CAA. Here, protein expression is induced when OD_{600} reaches 4. Since it is a high cell density, do not induce the entire culture. Instead, only centrifuge 5×10^9 cells and resuspend the cells in 500 mL SG-CAA (this corresponds to an OD_{600} of 1). Incubate at 20°C overnight.
7. If the yeast plasmids need to be isolated after sorting and a new library is generated, some diversity will be lost. In this case, we recommend covering 100× diversity instead of 10× during FACS screening.
8. For larger libraries, up to 3×10^7 cells can be pelleted in one tube of 700 μL. 700 μL is the highest volume recommended if 1.5 mL tubes and a thermomixer are used for the heat shock to have a homogeneous heat distribution. Do not invert the tube before heat shock, and ensure that no cell suspension is in the lid or the top of the tube. The temperature of the lid may be different from that on the bottom of the tube, and the cells may be subjected to different thermal stress, skewing the library selection.
9. The incubation duration, like the temperature, is critical. If many samples are tested, we recommend splitting them into different batches of a maximum of five and using different timers to ensure all of them are incubated for the same period of time.
10. It is possible to follow the enrichment of interesting protein variants during the engineering process by sequencing the library at different time points in the selection process, for example, the naïve library and between crucial selection rounds. This is particularly useful if NNK primers were used to build the library and only the disulfide-containing WT-protein is recovered at the end.
11. We recommend using Alexa Fluor 488 and Alexa Fluor 647 conjugated detection reagents to measure expression of the protein on yeast and binding to the ligand, as their absorbance and emission spectra are clearly separated.
12. The error-prone PCR conditions are optimized to obtain specific mutation rates based on different parameters, such as the number of PCR cycles, the length of the insert, and the

amount of DNA used as template. The epPCR conditions indicated in this protocol were optimized to obtain an average of 1–2 mutations in an insert of 380 bp.

References

1. Teufl M, Zajc CU, Traxlmayr MW (2022) Engineering strategies to overcome the stability-function trade-off in proteins. ACS Synth Biol 11:1030–1039. https://doi.org/10.1021/acssynbio.1c00512
2. Gay JC, Eckenroth BE, Evans CM et al (2019) Disulfide bridge formation influences ligand recognition by the ATAD2 bromodomain. Proteins 87:157–167. https://doi.org/10.1002/prot.25636
3. Ramm K, Gehrig P, Plückthun A (1999) Removal of the conserved disulfide bridges from the scfv fragment of an antibody: effects on folding kinetics and aggregation. J Mol Biol 290:535–546. https://doi.org/10.1006/jmbi.1999.2854
4. Wörn A, Auf Der Maur A, Escher D et al (2000) Correlation between in vitro stability and in vivo performance of anti-GCN4 intrabodies as cytoplasmic inhibitors. J Biol Chem 275:2795–2803. https://doi.org/10.1074/jbc.275.4.2795
5. Sylvander E, Muñoz-López Á, D'Accardio G, et al (2025) Engineering human protein switches for functional control of CARs and transcription factors via oral drug administration. https://doi.org/10.1101/2025.10.17.683068
6. Colby DW, Chu Y, Cassady JP et al (2004) Potent inhibition of huntingtin aggregation and cytotoxicity by a disulfide bond-free single-domain intracellular antibody. Proc Natl Acad Sci U S A 101:17616–17621. https://doi.org/10.1073/pnas.0408134101
7. Rajpal A, Turi TG (2001) Intracellular stability of anti-caspase-3 intrabodies determines efficacy in retargeting the antigen. J Biol Chem 276:33139–33146. https://doi.org/10.1074/jbc.M101332200
8. Seo MJ, Jeong KJ, Leysath CE et al (2009) Engineering antibody fragments to fold in the absence of disulfide bonds. Prot Sci 18:259–267. https://doi.org/10.1002/pro.31
9. Schiefner A, Chatwell L, Körner J et al (2011) A disulfide-free single-domain V(L) intrabody with blocking activity towards huntingtin reveals a novel mode of epitope recognition. J Mol Biol 414:337–355. https://doi.org/10.1016/j.jmb.2011.09.034
10. Montoliu-Gaya L, Martínez JC, Villegas S (2017) Understanding the contribution of disulfide bridges to the folding and misfolding of an anti-Aβ scFv. Protein Sci 26:1138–1149. https://doi.org/10.1002/pro.3164
11. Hagihara Y, Matsuda T, Yumoto N (2005) Cellular quality control screening to identify amino acid pairs for substituting the disulfide bonds in immunoglobulin fold domains. J Biol Chem 280:24752–24758. https://doi.org/10.1074/jbc.M503963200
12. Drevelle A, Urvoas A, Hamida-Rebaï MB et al (2009) Disulfide bond substitution by directed evolution in an engineered binding protein. ChemBioChem 10:1349–1359. https://doi.org/10.1002/cbic.200800745
13. Boder ET, Wittrup KD (1997) Yeast surface display for screening combinatorial polypeptide libraries. Nat Biotechnol 15:553–557. https://doi.org/10.1038/nbt0697-553
14. Angelini A, Chen TF, de Picciotto S et al (2015) Protein engineering and selection using yeast surface display. Methods Mol Biol 1319:3–36. https://doi.org/10.1007/978-1-4939-2748-7_1
15. Cherf GM, Cochran JR (2015) Applications of yeast surface display for protein engineering. Methods Mol Biol 1319:155–175. https://doi.org/10.1007/978-1-4939-2748-7_8
16. Pepper LR, Cho YK, Boder ET, Shusta EV (2008) A decade of yeast surface display technology: where are we now?. Comb Chem High Throughput Screen 11:127–134. https://doi.org/10.2174/138620708783744516
17. Traxlmayr MW, Lobner E, Hasenhindl C et al (2014) Construction of pH-sensitive Her2-binding IgG1-Fc by directed evolution. Biotechnol J 9:1013–1022. https://doi.org/10.1002/biot.201300483
18. Traxlmayr MW, Kiefer JD, Srinivas RR et al (2016) Strong enrichment of aromatic residues in binding sites from a charge-neutralized hyperthermostable sso7d scaffold library. J Biol Chem 291:22496–22508. https://doi.org/10.1074/jbc.M116.741314
19. Traxlmayr MW, Shusta EV (2017) Directed evolution of protein thermal stability using yeast surface display. Methods Mol Biol 1575:45–65. https://doi.org/10.1007/978-1-4939-6857-2_4
20. Traxlmayr MW, Faissner M, Stadlmayr G et al (2012) Directed evolution of stabilized IgG1-Fc scaffolds by application of strong heat shock to libraries displayed on yeast. Biochim

Biophys Acta (BBA) - Proteins Proteomics 1824:542–549. https://doi.org/10.1016/j.bbapap.2012.01.006
21. Lipovsek D, Antipov E, Armstrong KA et al (2007) Selection of horseradish peroxidase variants with enhanced enantioselectivity by yeast surface display. Chem Biol 14:1176–1185. https://doi.org/10.1016/j.chembiol.2007.09.008
22. Chen I, Dorr BM, Liu DR (2011) A general strategy for the evolution of bond-forming enzymes using yeast display. Proc Natl Acad Sci U S A 108:11399–11404. https://doi.org/10.1073/pnas.1101046108
23. Dobersberger M, Sumesgutner D, Zajc CU et al (2024) An engineering strategy to target activated EGFR with CAR T cells. Cell Rep Methods 4:100728. https://doi.org/10.1016/j.crmeth.2024.100728
24. Teufl M, Mayer J, Holzer KE et al (2025) MiniCARbids: Minimalistic human binding domains specifically tailored to CAR T applications. https://doi.org/10.1101/2025.09.09.675083
25. Zajc CU, Dobersberger M, Schaffner I et al (2020) A conformation-specific ON-switch for controlling CAR T cells with an orally available drug. Proc Natl Acad Sci U S A 117:14926–14935. https://doi.org/10.1073/pnas.1911154117
26. Sylvander E, Salzer B, Emminger D et al (2025) Caffeine-regulated molecular switches for functional control of CAR T cells in vivo. https://doi.org/10.1101/2025.06.13.659487
27. Shusta EV, Holler PD, Kieke MC et al (2000) Directed evolution of a stable scaffold for T-cell receptor engineering. Nat Biotechnol 18:754–759. https://doi.org/10.1038/77325
28. Weber KS, Donermeyer DL, Allen PM, Kranz DM (2005) Class II-restricted T cell receptor engineered in vitro for higher affinity retains peptide specificity and function. Proc Natl Acad Sci U S A 102:19033–19038. https://doi.org/10.1073/pnas.0507554102
29. Aggen DH, Chervin AS, Insaidoo FK et al (2011) Identification and engineering of human variable regions that allow expression of stable single-chain T cell receptors. Protein Eng Des Sel 24:361–372. https://doi.org/10.1093/protein/gzq113
30. Pavoor TV, Wheasler JA, Kamat V, Shusta EV (2012) An enhanced approach for engineering thermally stable proteins using yeast display. Protein Eng Des Sel 25:625–630. https://doi.org/10.1093/protein/gzs041
31. Traxlmayr MW, Lobner E, Antes B et al (2013) Directed evolution of Her2/neu-binding IgG1-Fc for improved stability and resistance to aggregation by using yeast surface display. Protein Eng Des Sel 26:255–265. https://doi.org/10.1093/protein/gzs102
32. Shusta EV, Kieke MC, Parke E et al (1999) Yeast polypeptide fusion surface display levels predict thermal stability and soluble secretion efficiency. J Mol Biol 292:949–956. https://doi.org/10.1006/jmbi.1999.3130
33. Traxlmayr MW, Obinger C (2012) Directed evolution of proteins for increased stability and expression using yeast display. Arch Biochem Biophys 526:174–180. https://doi.org/10.1016/j.abb.2012.04.022
34. Kim Y-S, Bhandari R, Cochran JR et al (2006) Directed evolution of the epidermal growth factor receptor extracellular domain for expression in yeast. Proteins: Struct Funct Bioinf 62:1026–1035. https://doi.org/10.1002/prot.20618
35. Kieke MC, Shusta EV, Boder ET et al (1999) Selection of functional T cell receptor mutants from a yeast surface-display library. Proc Natl Acad Sci U S A 96:5651–5656. https://doi.org/10.1073/pnas.96.10.5651
36. Buonpane RA, Moza B, Sundberg EJ, Kranz DM (2005) Characterization of T cell receptors engineered for high affinity against toxic shock syndrome toxin-1. J Mol Biol 353:308–321. https://doi.org/10.1016/j.jmb.2005.08.041
37. Jones LL, Brophy SE, Bankovich AJ et al (2006) Engineering and characterization of a stabilized alpha1/alpha2 module of the class I major histocompatibility complex product Ld. J Biol Chem 281:25734–25744. https://doi.org/10.1074/jbc.M604343200
38. Esteban O, Zhao H (2004) Directed evolution of soluble single-chain human Class II MHC molecules. J Mol Biol 340:81–95. https://doi.org/10.1016/j.jmb.2004.04.054
39. Park S, Xu Y, Stowell XF et al (2006) Limitations of yeast surface display in engineering proteins of high thermostability. Protein Eng Des Sel 19:211–217. https://doi.org/10.1093/protein/gzl003
40. Chao G, Lau WL, Hackel BJ et al (2006) Isolating and engineering human antibodies using yeast surface display. Nat Protoc 1:755–768. https://doi.org/10.1038/nprot.2006.94
41. Zajc CU, Teufl M, Traxlmayr MW (2022) Affinity and stabilitystabilities analysis of yeast displayed proteins. In: Traxlmayr MW (Ed.) Yeast surface display. Springer US, New York, NY, pp 155–173

Chapter 15

High-Performance Computing in Tandem Mass Spectrometry (MS/MS) Peptide Identification

Chuang Li, Qiang He, Tao Chen and Yanhua Wen

Abstract

Tandem mass spectrometry (MS/MS) has become a cornerstone technology in large-scale proteomics, producing vast datasets that present considerable computational challenges for peptide identification. Conventional database-search-based approaches often exhibit limited efficiency, particularly as protein sequence repositories expand rapidly and experimental spectra grow increasingly complex. High-performance computing (HPC) offers a viable solution by supporting large-scale parallelization and algorithmic optimization. In this study, we introduce SW-Tandem, an efficient framework for peptide identification that implements parallelization of the spectrum dot product scoring algorithm on the Sunway TaihuLight supercomputer. Through the incorporation of memory-access optimization, double buffering, and vectorization techniques, SW-Tandem achieves marked improvements in computational performance while maintaining identification accuracy. Experimental evaluations reveal that SW-Tandem substantially accelerates peptide identification and surpasses existing state-of-the-art methods when deployed across multiple nodes. These findings underscore the potential of integrating HPC with algorithmic enhancements to advance large-scale bioinformatics research.

Keywords Bioinformatics, High-performance computing, MS/MS, Peptide identification, Parallel computing

1 Introduction

The extraction of non-obvious yet practically valuable knowledge from large-scale datasets has become increasingly critical across diverse scientific and industrial domains [1]. Bioinformatics, as a data-intensive discipline, exemplifies this trend. Over the past decades, vast amounts of biomedical information—including imaging data, biological signals, and multi-omics datasets—have been generated at unprecedented speed [2–6]. Once effectively analyzed, these resources carry tremendous potential for advancing healthcare, clinical diagnostics, and fundamental biological research, thereby drawing growing interest from both academic and industrial communities [7, 8].

Huan Peng and Theam Soon Lim (eds.), *Biomolecular Display Technologies*, Methods in Molecular Biology, vol. 3030,
https://doi.org/10.1007/978-1-0716-5249-7_15,

Within this context, tandem mass spectrometry (MS/MS) has emerged as an indispensable technique in high-throughput proteomics. Advances in mass spectrometry hardware now enable the acquisition of hundreds of thousands of spectra in a single experiment [9–12]. For example, in 2017, human protein expression profiling generated over 5.1 TB of raw data, while the rapid expansion of repositories such as PRIDE further illustrates the exponential increase in publicly accessible MS/MS datasets [13]. However, the sheer scale of these spectra introduces a pressing challenge: efficiently interpreting MS/MS data for peptide identification has become increasingly difficult, underscoring the need for computationally efficient and scalable solutions.

To meet this demand, HPC has been progressively incorporated into bioinformatics pipelines. Applications range from network and systems biology to large-scale medical imaging and sequence-based analysis tasks, including genomics and proteomics [14–19]. The central concept of HPC lies in aggregating clusters of interconnected computers or multiprocessor systems into a distributed infrastructure that integrates heterogeneous computational resources. Such architectures enable data-intensive bioinformatics workflows to achieve substantial performance improvements.

At the same time, the proliferation of hardware accelerators, such as graphics processing units (GPUs), field-programmable gate arrays (FPGAs), and Many Integrated Core (MIC) architectures, has introduced compact yet powerful alternatives for large-scale MS/MS data analysis. Compared with conventional computing clusters, these devices provide enhanced throughput while offering benefits in energy efficiency, spatial footprint, and cost-effectiveness, making them particularly appealing for sequence analysis tasks with heavy computational demands [20, 21].

HPC thus represents a holistic framework that unites advanced hardware accelerators with optimized software and programming models to resolve large-scale bioinformatics problems. Numerous HPC-enabled applications have already demonstrated success, including large-scale sequence analysis, gene and protein expression profiling, and investigations of cellular organization [22–25]. Among these, sequence analysis continues to attract particular attention due to its central importance in computational biology [26, 27].

In this work, we review recent advances in applying HPC to MS/MS data analysis. The following parts first introduce the background of tandem mass spectrometry, sequence analysis, and high-performance computing [28–30]. We then discuss HPC-enabled approaches for MS/MS data processing, with a particular focus on peptide database-search sequencing and de novo sequencing [31, 32]. Finally, we conclude with a summary of current progress and outline potential directions for future research.

2 Background

2.1 Tandem Mass Spectrometry (MS/MS)

The primary objective of proteomics is to comprehensively identify and characterize all proteins within a given system. Tandem mass spectrometry (MS/MS), in combination with liquid chromatography (LC), has become a central analytical technique in high-throughput proteomics. This approach is particularly effective for the identification, characterization, and comparative analysis of complex protein mixtures that may consist of thousands of distinct components. Figure 1 illustrates an example of an MS/MS spectrum, where the fragment ions are represented by peaks corresponding to their measured mass-to-charge ratios (m/z) and intensities. Ionization methods exert a pronounced influence on the likelihood of producing specific fragment ion types. For instance, in collision-induced dissociation (CID), six series of fragment ions are typically observed, including C-terminal x, y, and z ions as well as N-terminal a, b, and c ions, as depicted in Fig. 2.

A detailed process of the MS/MS approach to study complex protein mixtures is illustrated in Fig. 3.

Since intact proteins are generally unsuitable for direct mass spectrometric identification, they are first enzymatically digested into smaller peptides, most commonly using trypsin. To further reduce the complexity of the resulting peptide mixture, strong cation exchange chromatography can be applied during the digestion process. The peptides are then analyzed by liquid chromatography coupled with tandem mass spectrometry (LC–MS/MS spectra. Finally, computational algorithms are employed to interpret these spectra, thereby enabling the identification of the corresponding peptides and, ultimately, the proteins from which they are derived.

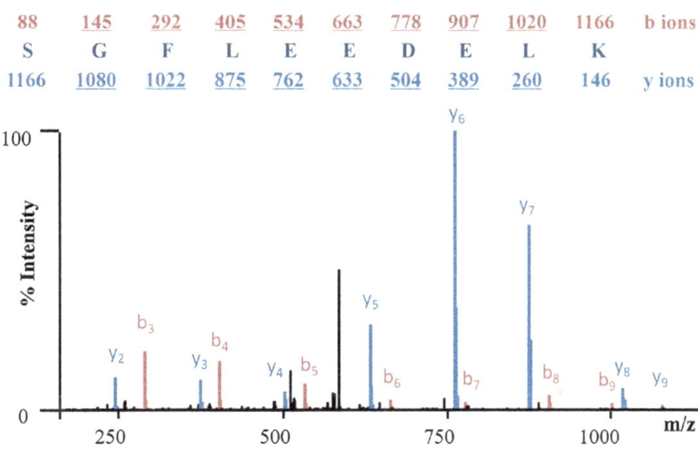

Fig. 1 An example of MS/MS spectrum

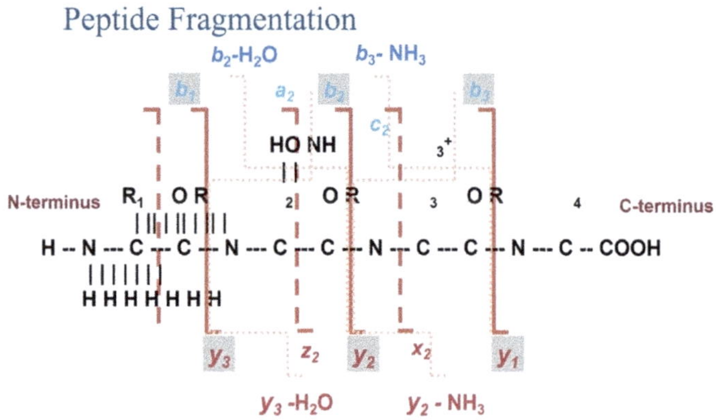

Fig. 2 The type fragments

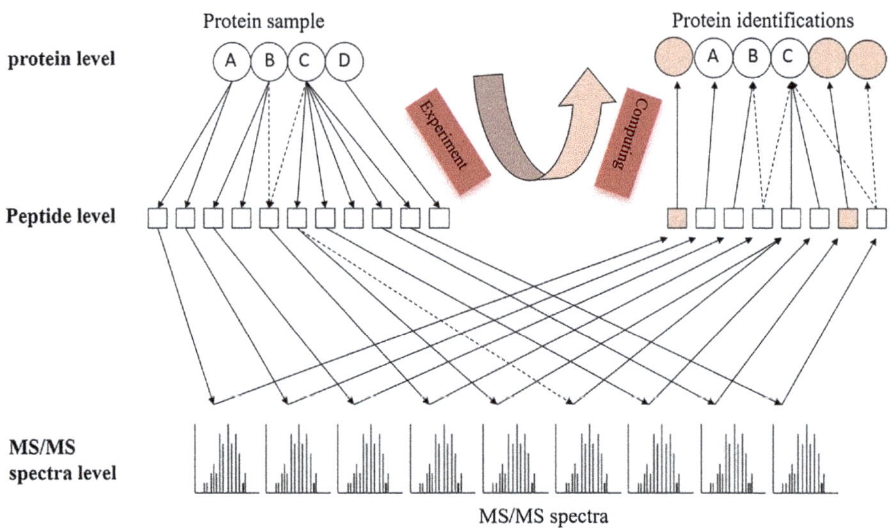

Fig. 3 The process of a high-throughput mass spectrometry-based protein identification method

2.2 MS/MS-Based Sequence Analysis

Computational approaches have long played a central role in biological research, particularly in the area of sequence analysis. In the field of proteomics, the high-throughput MS/MS shotgun strategy has emerged as the most effective and widely adopted computational framework for peptide identification. This method enables large-scale analysis of complex protein mixtures with both speed and accuracy, making it a cornerstone of modern proteomics research. As illustrated in Fig. 4, the shotgun workflow[33–35] typically consists of two major stages: the experimental stage, where peptide spectra are generated, and the subsequent sequence analysis stage, where computational methods are applied to interpret the spectra and identify the underlying peptide sequences.

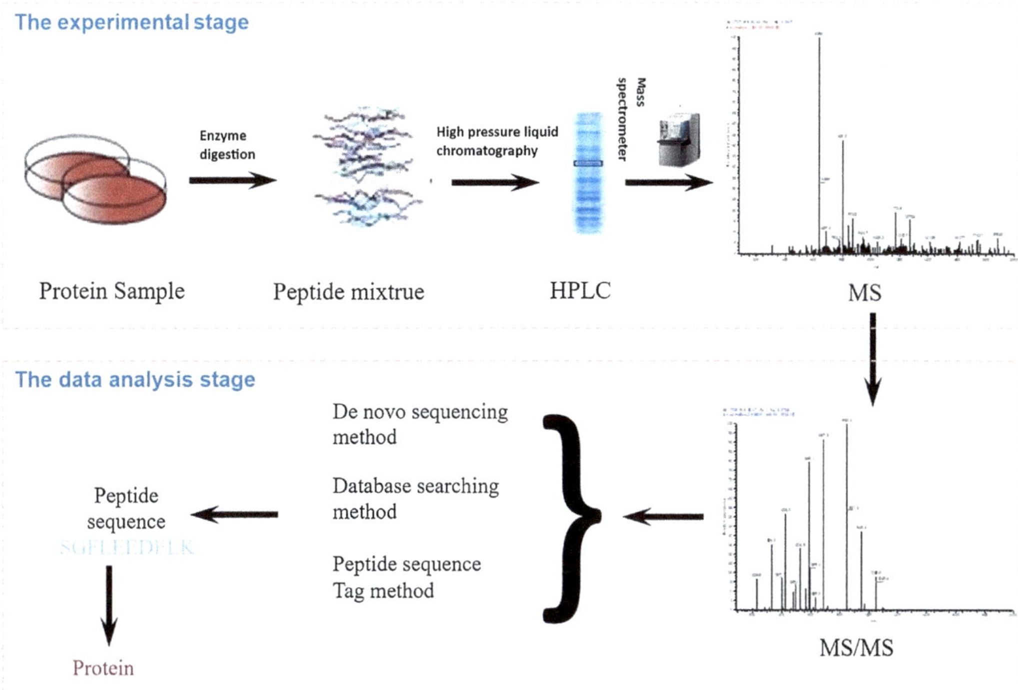

Fig. 4 Workflow of the shotgun method

Within the shotgun workflow, the sequence analysis stage plays a pivotal role in accurately identifying peptides and proteins. In this stage, the database search strategy remains the most widely applied approach, forming the basis for large-scale protein sequence and post-translational modification (PTM) analysis with high sensitivity, accuracy, and throughput. Prominent search engines such as SEQUEST, Mascot, and X!Tandem exemplify this methodology by matching experimental MS/MS spectra against peptide candidates derived from protein sequence databases [33]. A key limitation, however, is the strong dependence of this approach on the completeness and quality of existing protein repositories.

As an alternative, de novo peptide sequencing infers peptide sequences directly from MS/MS spectra without requiring reference databases [36]. Representative tools such as PEAKS and UniNovo demonstrate the utility of this approach, which has gained increasing attention in recent years as an indispensable technique for discovering novel proteins and PTMs.

Nevertheless, significant challenges remain in MS/MS sequence analysis. The exponential growth of spectral data has rendered large-scale analyses highly computationally intensive. Moreover, experimental noise and impurities in peptide mixtures often generate spurious peaks, while fragmentation mechanisms are still not fully understood [37–40]. These factors collectively reduce sequencing efficiency, increase the likelihood of misidentification, and complicate the discrimination among multiple candidate peptide sequences.

2.3 High-Performance Computing (HPC)

Scientific computing involves the design of numerical methods and mathematical models to address complex problems across engineering, natural sciences, and social sciences. In large-scale experiments and data-intensive studies, such models demand considerable computational resources to achieve both accuracy and efficiency. Traditionally, these requirements have been met by high-performance computing infrastructures such as clusters and supercomputers, which have long defined the state of the art in large-scale scientific computation.

With the rise of the big data era and the rapid proliferation of data-driven applications in fields such as genomics, medical imaging, and artificial intelligence, modern HPC architectures have increasingly evolved toward heterogeneous systems. These platforms integrate multi-core CPUs with diverse accelerators, including GPUs, FPGAs, tensor processing units (TPUs), and other domain-specific processors. Heterogeneous integration substantially enhances computational performance and energy efficiency, enabling data analysis and simulation at scales previously unattainable.

Among these accelerators, GPUs have emerged as the most widely adopted due to their suitability for massively parallel workloads. Modern GPU architectures incorporate specialized AI units such as tensor cores and leverage high-bandwidth memory to accelerate matrix and tensor computations, which are central not only to deep learning but also to large-scale bioinformatics tasks. In contrast, FPGAs offer reconfigurable hardware-level customization, making them particularly valuable in scenarios requiring low latency, high throughput, and energy efficiency, such as real-time signal processing and streaming bioinformatics pipelines.

Intel's MIC architecture, once embodied by the Xeon Phi product line, was discontinued in 2020. Although no longer actively deployed, its design principles, which include many core parallelism, wide vectorization, and x86 compatibility, have influenced subsequent advances in CPU and accelerator design. Rather than relying on standalone coprocessors, current HPC platforms increasingly incorporate these principles into integrated heterogeneous systems.

Recent developments in HPC have also emphasized performance–power efficiency, shifting the focus from raw FLOPS to energy-optimized computing. In this context, FPGAs and specialized accelerators are playing a growing role. Simultaneously, advances in programming models and software ecosystems are improving the usability of heterogeneous platforms, including automated load balancing, unified memory management, and domain-specific compiler technologies. Moreover, innovations in hardware integration and interconnects—such as high-bandwidth links, chiplet-based

2.5D/3D packaging, and near-memory or in-memory computing—are helping to mitigate data movement costs, which remain a critical bottleneck in large-scale workflows.

Collectively, these advances highlight the ongoing transformation of HPC from homogeneous supercomputers into heterogeneous, accelerator-driven platforms designed to meet the computational demands of modern scientific discovery and data-intensive applications.

3 MS/MS Data Peptide Identification

To efficiently handle large-scale proteomics data, SW-Tandem integrates three key optimization strategies—memory access optimization, double buffering, and vectorization—to fully exploit the computing power of the Sunway TaihuLight supercomputer [41]. The database-search-based peptide identification workflow in SW-Tandem is organized into four main phases, as illustrated in Fig. 5. In the first phase, the MS/MS spectra dataset is partitioned into appropriately sized subdatasets according to the total number of core groups (CGs), which are then distributed to the corresponding CGs for processing. In the second phase, the management processing element (MPE) performs an initial database search to obtain candidate peptide datasets and subsequently distributes each mass spectrum along with its candidate peptides to the computing processing elements (CPEs) [42]. In the third phase, the CPEs execute

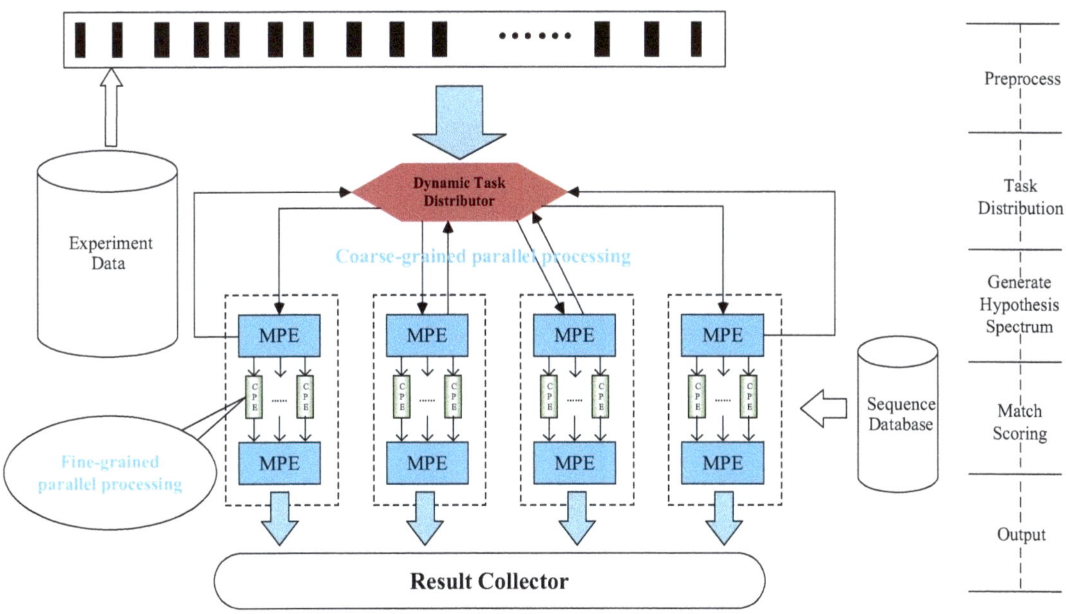

Fig. 5 Framework of dynamic task distribution.

the spectrum dot product algorithm in parallel, thereby accelerating the scoring process. Finally, in the fourth phase, the MPE collects and merges the output files generated by all CPEs within the same CG to produce the final peptide identification results [43].

Each CPE of Sunway TaihuLight is equipped with a user-managed Scratch Pad Memory (SPM), replacing traditional caches and enabling efficient data access. Through DMA intrinsics and collective communication, data can be asynchronously transferred between CPE SPMs and the MPE. For peak efficiency, transfers must be 128-byte aligned and sized in multiples of 128 bytes. Among the three supported DMA modes, SW-Tandem uses the single CPE mode, allowing each CPE to exchange data independently while overlapping computation and data fetching.

To further reduce overhead, SW-Tandem applies a double-buffering strategy: two buffers in the SPM enable one dataset to be processed while another is prefetched. This pipelined mechanism minimizes DMA latency and maximizes throughput, as illustrated in Algorithm 1.

Algorithm 1 The pseudocode of DMA double-buffering

Require: the group theoretical spectrum and experimental spectrum vectors.

Set: T: theoretical spectrum;

E: experimental spectrum;

H: hypothesis spectrum, the match theoretical spectra of the experimental spectra by unrefined research;

h_{i-m}, h^{i}_{i-m}: the m/z and intensity value of the m-th element of theoretical spectrum h_i;

e_{i-m}, e^{i}_{i-m}: the m/z and intensity value of the n-th element of experimental spectrume$_i$.

Ensure: the top one score of each experimental spectrum

for each $E_m \in E$
  search T, get H
    for each $H_j \in H$
    DMA_in h_{j-n+1}
      for each $h_{j-n} \in H_j$
      DMA_in E_{j+1}
        search h_{j-n} in E_j , get e_{j-l}
        DMA_in h_{j-n+1}, e_{j-l+1}
        SDP_score += dot(h_{j-n}, e_{j-l})
      DMA_out h_{j-n}, e_{j-l}
      end of for
    end for
end for

To fully exploit the computational potential of Sunway TaihuLight, each CPE is equipped with a 256-bit wide SIMD floating-point unit, capable of executing eight floating-point operations per instruction cycle. Although the processor provides specialized SIMD units and corresponding instructions, the automatic vectorization supported by the compiler system fails to generate sufficiently optimized binaries. Consequently, manual vectorization is required to achieve high performance. In the spectrum dot product (SDP) scoring algorithm, data dependencies appear in the innermost loops. To fully utilize the SIMD units, we restructure these dependency statements, remove the loop-carried dependencies, and apply inter-loop vectorization with manual loop expansion. Memory accesses are carefully aligned to 32-byte boundaries for optimal SIMD performance, while floatv4 data types require only 16-byte alignment. By explicitly controlling memory alignment and applying vectorized loop expansion, the SIMD vectorization achieves a peak performance of 67.21 Gflops.

We further evaluated the optimized SW-Tandem on a single SW26010 processor using a 580 MB MS/MS dataset containing 82,621 spectra. The optimized implementation achieved a 1.394× speedup compared with the unoptimized baseline, as summarized in Table 1.

MSFragger is recognized as a state-of-the-art database search engine that employs fragment ion indexing to significantly accelerate peptide identification. To assess the performance of SW-Tandem, we conducted a comparative evaluation against MSFragger. In these experiments, SW-Tandem was executed on a cluster equipped with SW26010 processors, whereas MSFragger was run on an Intel E5-26540 CPU, since it is not open source and does not support large-scale parallelization. As Table 2 presents the execution times of the two tools on three representative MS/MS datasets. The results demonstrate that SW-Tandem consistently outperforms MSFragger when utilizing six or more computing nodes, highlighting its superior scalability and efficiency in large-scale peptide identification tasks.

We evaluated SW-Tandem's accuracy by comparing its cosine values with X!Tandem and MR-Tandem (Table 3). All three tools produced identical results across datasets, confirming SW-Tandem's consistency with established methods.

Table 1
Computational time before and after optimization

Methods	Execution time (seconds)	Benefits
Before optimization	1553	0%
Memory-access-optimization	1391	10.1%
Double-buffering	1408	9.3%
Vectorization	1329	14.4%
With both optimization	1190	23.4%

Table 2
Comparison of performance between SW-Tandem and MSFragger

Search tools	Exp. 1	Exp. 2	Exp. 3
MSFragger	152 s	912 s	2801 s
SW-Tandem (1 node)	730 s	4264 s	12,051 s
SW-Tandem (3 nodes)	250 s	1480 s	3274 s
SW-Tandem (4 nodes)	198 s	1158 s	2690 s
SW-Tandem (5 nodes)	162 s	951 s	2290 s
SW-Tandem (6 nodes)	138 s	813 s	2299 s
SW-Tandem (7 nodes)	125 s	735 s	2077 s

Table 3
Accuracy analysis of SW-Tandem

Dataset	X1-Tandem	MR-Tandem	SW-Tandem
Exp. 1	0.99245	0.99245	0.99245
Exp. 2	0.98789	0.98789	0.98789
Exp. 3	0.96124	0.96124	0.96124

4 Conclusion

HPC has become indispensable for addressing the computational demands of peptide identification in tandem mass spectrometry (MS/MS). With the explosive growth of MS/MS data, conventional database-search-based approaches face critical challenges in efficiency and scalability, particularly when dealing with low signal-to-noise spectra, post-translational modifications, and sequence variations.

In this study, we introduced SW-Tandem, an HPC-based framework that parallelizes the spectrum dot product algorithm on the Sunway TaihuLight supercomputer. By incorporating memory access optimization, double buffering, and vectorization, SW-Tandem fully exploits the SW26010 many-core processor and achieves substantial performance improvements while maintaining accuracy. Furthermore, when deployed at scale, SW-Tandem outperforms MSFragger, underscoring the advantages of hardware-aware parallel optimization in large-scale proteomics.

In summary, SW-Tandem demonstrates that peptide identification can be significantly accelerated through architecture-specific optimizations and large-scale parallelization. Future research will focus on integrating HPC with deep learning and clustering-based strategies to further improve computational efficiency, robustness, and biological interpretability in proteomics workflows.

References

1. Ronneberger O, Fischer P, Brox T (2015) U-net: convolutional networks for biomedical image segmentation. International conference on medical image com puting and computer-assisted intervention. Springer, Cham, 234–241
2. Schindelin J, Rueden CT, Hiner MC, Eliceiri KW (2015) The image J. ecosystem: an open platform for biomedical image analysis. J Mol Reprod Dev 82(7–8):518–529
3. Shameer K, Badgeley MA, Miotto R, Glicksberg BS, Morgan JW, Dudley JT (2016) Translational bioinformatics in the era of real-time biomedical, health care and wellness data streams. J Brief Bioinform 118
4. Agarwal R, Dhar V (2014) Big data, data science, and analytics: the opportunity and challenge for IS research. Inf Syst Res 25(3):443–448
5. McLafferty FW (1981) Tandem mass spectrometry. J Sci 214(4518):280–287
6. Link AJ, Eng J, Schieltz DM, Carmack E, Mize GJ, Morris DR, Yates JR (1999) Direct analysis of protein complexes using mass spectrometry. J Nat Biotechnol 17(7):676
7. Nesvizhskii AI, Keller A, Kolker E, Aebersold R (2003) A statistical model for identifying proteins by tandem mass spectrometry. J Anal Chem 75(17):4646–4658
8. Hunt DF, Yates JR, Shabanowitz J, Winston S, Hauer CR (1986) Protein sequencing by tandem mass spectrometry. J Proc Natl Acad Sci U S A 83(17):6233–6237
9. Li C, Chen T, He Q, Zhu Y, Li K (2016) MRUniNovo: an efficient tool for de novo peptide sequencing utilizing the Hadoop distributed computing framework. J Bioinf 33(6):944–946
10. Sanbonmatsu KY, Tung CS (2007) High performance computing in biology: multimillion atom simulations of nanoscale systems. J Struct Biol 157(3):470–480
11. Ciresan DC, Meier U, Masci J, MariaGambardella L, Schmidhuber J (2011, July). Flexible, high performance convolutional neural networks for image classification. In: IJCAI Proceedings-International Joint Conference on Artificial Intelligence, vol 22(1), p 1237
12. Feng L, Datta A (2011) A generic mutual information based algorithm for spatial registration of multi-modal medical images. J Med Imaging Health Inform 1(2):131–138
13. Kalra PK, Kumar N (2014) Poisson's equation based image registration: An application for matching 2D mammograms. J Med Imaging Health Inform 4(1):49–57
14. Zhu X, Li K, Salah A, Shi L, Li K (2015) Parallel implementation of MAFFT on CUDA-enabled graphics hardware. IEEE/ACM
15. Zhu X, Li K, Salah A (2013) A data parallel strategy for aligning multiple biological sequences on multi-core computers. Comput Biol Med 43(4):350–361
16. Dorband J, Palencia J, Ranawake U (2003) Commodity computing clusters at goddard space flight center. J Space Commun 1(3):113–123. 21
17. Brightwell R, Fisk LA, Greenberg DS, Hudson T, Levenhagen M, MacCabe AB, Riesen R (2000) Massively parallel computing using com modity components. Parallel Comput 26(2–3):243–266. 22
18. El-Ghazawi TA, Kaewpijit S, Le Moigne J (2001, October) Parallel and adaptive reduction of hyperspectral data to intrinsic dimensionality. In: Cluster, p 102
19. Plaza A, Valencia D, Plaza J, Martinez P (2006) Commodity cluster-based parallel processing of hyperspectral imagery. J Parallel Distrib Comput 66(3):345–358
20. Plaza A, Plaza J, Valencia D (2007) Impact of platform heterogeneity on the design of parallel algorithms for morphological processing of high-dimensional image data. J Supercomput 40(1):81–107
21. Inoue T, Yamatani K, Itoh K, Ichioka Y (1993) Vector quantization for hyper spectral images using neural network. Opt Laser Technol 25(3):202
22. Plaza A, Valencia D, Plaza J (2008) An experimental comparison of parallel algorithms for hyperspectral analysis using heterogeneous and homogeneous networks of workstations. Parallel Comput 34(2):92–114
23. Ekanayake J, Fox G (2009) High performance parallel computing with clouds and cloud technologies. In: International conference on cloud computing. Springer, Berlin, Heidelberg, 20–38
24. Tehranian S, Zhao Y, Harvey T, Swaroop A, Mckenzie K (2006) A robust framework for real-time distributed processing of satellite data. J Parallel Distrib Comput 66(3):403–418
25. Gnerre S, MacCallum I, Przybylski D, Ribeiro FJ, Burton JN, Walker BJ, Berlin AM (2011) High-quality draft assemblies of mammalian genomes from massively parallel sequence data. Proc Natl Acad Sci U S A 108(4):1513–1518
26. Navarro J, Vera G, Ramos-Onsins S, Hernández P (2016) Improving bioinformatics analysis of large sequence datasets parallelizing tools for population genomics. In: European conference on parallel processing. Springer, Cwwham, 457–467
27. Botterill JJ, Fournier NM, Guskjolen AJ, Lussier AL, Marks WN, Kalynchuk LE (2014)

Amygdala kindling disrupts trace and delay fear conditioning with parallel changes in Fos protein expression throughout the limbic brain. Neuroscience 265:158–171
28. Macosko EZ, Basu A, Satija R, Nemesh J, Shekhar K, Goldman M, Trombetta JJ (2015) Highly parallel genome-wide expression profiling of individual cells using nanoliter droplets. Cell 161(5):1202–1214
29. Marcotte EM (2007) How do shotgun proteomics algorithms identify proteins?. Nature Biotechnol 25(7):755
30. Yang H, Chi H, Zhou WJ, Zeng WF, He K, Liu C, He SM (2017) Open-pNovo: de novo peptide sequencing with thousands of protein modifications. J Proteome Res 16(2):645–654
31. Sadygov RG, Cociorva D, Yates III JR (2004) Large-scale database searching using tandem mass spectra: looking up the answer in the back of the book. Nat Methods 1(3):195
32. Kapp E, Schütz F (2007) Overview of tandem mass spectrometry (MS/MS) database search algorithms. Curr Protoc Protein Sci 25–32
33. Eng JK, McCormack AL, Yates JR (1994) An approach to correlate tandem mass spectral data of peptides with amino acid sequences in a protein database. J Am Soc Mass Spectrom 5(11):976–989
34. Sadeh NM, Hildum DW, Kjenstad D, Tseng A (1999) Mascot: an agent-based architecture for coordinated mixed-initiative supply chain planning and scheduling. In: Workshop on agent-based decision support in managing the internet enabled supply-chain, at agents' 99
35. Bjornson RD, Carriero NJ, Colangelo C, Shifman M, Cheung KH, Miller PL, Williams K (2007) X!! Tandem, an improved method for running X! tandem in parallel on collections of commodity computers. J Proteome Res 7(1):293–299
36. Allmer J (2011) Algorithms for the de novo sequencing of peptides from tandem mass spectra. Expert Rev Proteomics 8(5):645–657
37. Ma B, Zhang K, Hendrie C, Liang C, Li M, Doherty-Kirby A, Lajoie G (2003) PEAKS: powerful software for peptide de novo sequencing by tandem mass spectrometry. Rapid Commun Mass Spectrom 17(20):2337–2342
38. Jeong K, Kim S, Pevzner PA (2013) UniNovo: A universal tool for de novo peptide sequencing. Bioinformatics 29(16):1953–1962
39. Bjornson RD, Carriero NJ, Colangelo C, Shifman M, Cheung KH, Miller PL, Williams K (2007) X!! Tandem, an improved method for running X! tandem in parallel on collections of commodity computers. J Proteome Res 7(1):293–299
40. Pratt B, Howbert JJ, Tasman NI, Nilsson EJ (2011) MR-tandem: Parallel X!tandem using hadoop MapReduce on amazon Webservices. Bioinformatics 28(1):136–137
41. Ye J, Zhao Z, Wu M (2008) Discriminative k-means for clustering. In: Advances in neural information processing systems, pp 1649–1656
42. Baumgardner LA, Shanmugam AK, Lam H et al. (2011) Fast parallel tandem mass spectral library searching using GPU hardware acceleration. J Proteome Res 10(6):2882–2888
43. Chuang L, Feng L (2020) High-Performance Computing in Tandem Mass Spectrometry (MS/MS) Data Processing. In: Application of omics, AI and blockchain in bioinformatics research, pp 123–140

Check for updates

Chapter 16

Post-Selection Methods for Analyzing mRNA Display Selections and Optimization of Hits

Pearl Qi, Colin M. Leaf, Richard W. Roberts and Terry T. Takahashi

Abstract

mRNA display enables the selection of peptide and protein ligands from libraries containing more than a trillion unique sequences. Identifying optimal target binders, however, requires extensive post-selection analysis and optimization, which is often more challenging than the selection itself. Here, we outline general strategies for analyzing mRNA display selections with the goal of advancing a small set of high-quality ligands for further study. We describe methods for sequencing and analyzing selection pools to identify potential binders, followed by experimental approaches to validate target binding and characterize ligand–target interactions. We present strategies for constructing second-generation libraries to improve initial hits, along with more specialized selection techniques for further improving binding affinity and/or protease resistance. Together, these methods provide a comprehensive strategy for post-selection analysis and the development of optimized ligands for downstream applications.

Keywords mRNA display, In vitro selection, Directed evolution, RNA-protein fusion, High-throughput sequencing, Protein engineering, Machine learning, Post-selection analysis

1 Introduction

The fundamental goal of mRNA display is to start with a library of billions to trillions of molecules and winnow it down to a handful of peptide or protein sequences that possess a desired function (Fig. 1a). mRNA display selections have yielded a significant number of impressive ligands that have found use as tools, diagnostics, and therapeutics [1–3]. While an mRNA display selection might seem straightforward, where one might need to merely perform several rounds of selection in order to identify a target-binding ligand, substantial post-selection analysis is required. Often, this analysis is more challenging and time-consuming than the selection itself. The goals of this analysis are twofold: first, to filter out non-target binding

Pearl Qi and Colin M. Leaf contributed equally to this manuscript.

Huan Peng and Theam Soon Lim (eds.), *Biomolecular Display Technologies*, Methods in Molecular Biology, vol. 3030,
https://doi.org/10.1007/978-1-0716-5249-7_16,

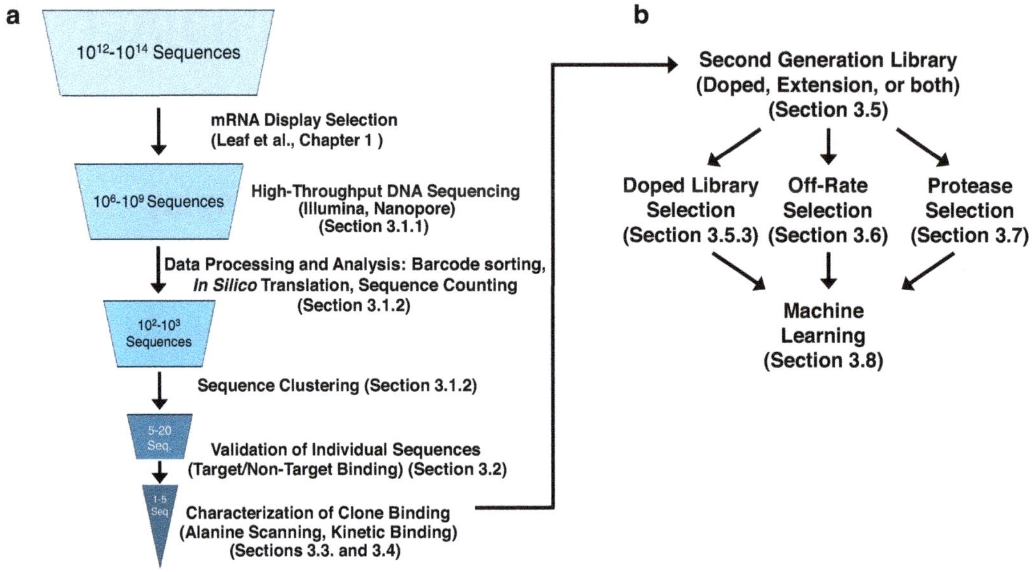

Fig. 1 (**a**) Overall strategy for an mRNA display selection followed by post-selection analysis. An mRNA display library typically begins with ~10^{12}–10^{14} unique sequences. After selection, this diversity is reduced to millions to billions of enriched sequences. High-throughput DNA sequencing enables the identification of these sequences. After data processing, hundreds to thousands of sequences are grouped by similarity, and 5–20 representative sequences are experimentally validated for target binding. Further characterization by Alanine Scanning and kinetic binding measurements provides a more detailed understanding of ligand-target interactions. Ultimately, one to five sequences are prioritized for additional experimental characterization. (**b**) These sequences can be used to design second-generation libraries for more specialized selections to optimize affinity and/or other important characteristics, such as protease resistance. These selections may be performed concurrently or consecutively to optimize multiple parameters or to obtain even higher affinity ligands. The results of these follow-up selections also provide excellent datasets for training machine learning models capable of generating novel, functional sequences not present in the original selection pool

sequences, and second, to validate, characterize, and improve target binders so that optimal sequences can be identified and advanced.

There is no definitive point at which a selection is complete. High-throughput sequencing technologies make sequencing of more than a single pool possible, allowing the analysis of multiple rounds of selection with exquisite depth. This allows the identification of millions of unique sequences and the ability to track those sequences across multiple rounds of selection. The challenge is to identify those sequences that not only have the desired functionality, but are most optimal. In general, testing for pool functionality before sequencing ensures that most sequences in the pool have the desired function and reduces the fraction of non-target binding sequences.

Processing of sequencing data is possible using publicly available scripts that extract amino acid sequences from the sequenced DNA, and sum their counts [4]. In this way, the clones that are most abundant can be identified, and if multiple pools are sequenced, round over round enrichment for each sequence can be calculated.

Here, we outline general strategies to refine an mRNA display library with a starting complexity of 10^{12}–10^{14} into a small number of optimal sequences (Fig. 1a). We describe preparation of libraries for high-throughput sequencing (Sect. 3.1.1) and subsequent analysis of the sequencing data to identify sequences for validation and testing (Sect. 3.1.2). Once these sequences are validated (Sect. 3.4), we present methods for alanine scanning (Sect. 3.5) and for determining binding kinetics (Sect. 3.6) to better characterize ligand-target interactions. These data can inform the construction of second-generation libraries (Fig. 1b), which can be used in more specialized selections to improve the initial ligands (Sects. 3.7–3.9). Finally, we describe approaches for integrating mRNA display with machine learning techniques to generate novel molecules (Sect. 3.10).

2 Materials

2.1 Library Preparation for Illumina Sequencing

1. A 5′ primer containing a unique 6–8 bp barcode (various suppliers) at 100 μM concentration. A unique primer/barcode is required for each sample (e.g., each round of a selection).
2. A 3′ primer containing a unique 6–8 bp barcode (various suppliers) at 100 μM concentration. This barcode should be different from that of the 5′ primer and should also be unique for each sample.
3. A 5′ universal primer for introducing Illumina adapters at 100 μM concentration. Generally, we use the sequence 5′ -AATGATACGGCGACCACCGAGATCTACACTCTTTC CCTA-3′, but users should confirm which sequence should be used with their sequencing provider.
4. A 3′ universal primer for introducing Illumina adapters at 100 μM concentration. Generally, we use the sequence 5′ -TCTGAACTCCAGTCACAACCGCGG ATCTCGTATG CCGTCTTCTGCTTG-3′. Similarly, users should confirm this sequence with their sequencing provider.
5. Taq DNA polymerase (various suppliers) or other thermostable polymerase (*see* **Note 1**). Store at −20 °C.
6. 10× PCR Buffer: 100 mM Tris-HCl, pH 9.0 at room temperature, 500 mM KCl, 20 mM $MgCl_2$, 1% (v/v) Triton X-100. Aliquot and store at −20 °C.
7. 10× dNTP solution (various suppliers): 2 mM of each dNTP, pH adjusted to 7–8. Aliquot and store at −20°C.
8. 20× SB: 200 mM NaOH, pH adjusted to 8.0 with boric acid [5].
9. 5× TBE Buffer: 445 mM Tris base, 445 mM boric acid, 10 mM EDTA, pH 8.0. Filter through a 0.45 μm filter to prevent precipitation. Store at room temperature.

10. Low-melt agarose for small DNA fragments (various suppliers).
11. 5× SB Loading Buffer: Add 2.5 mL of 20× SB, 2.5 mL of ddH_2O, 6.3 g of glycerol, and add bromophenol blue until dark purple (*see* **Note 2**).
12. 100 bp DNA ladder (New England Biolabs, cat# N3231L; various suppliers).
13. 10 mg/mL Ethidium bromide solution (various suppliers). Store in a dark bottle. Ethidium Bromide is a mutagen. Wear gloves and avoid exposure. Dispose of ethidium bromide waste accordingly.
14. Gel box for agarose gels (Bio-rad Sub-cell GT, cat# 1704466, or similar), including gel tray, 0.75 mm thick 15-well comb (*see* **Note 3**), preparative gel comb, and casting apparatus.
15. Agarose Gel Extraction Kit (Qiagen, or other vendor).

2.2 PCR of Individual Clones

1. DNA template encoding a clone for testing (various suppliers). Dilute to 1 μM. Store at −20°C.
2. 5′ primer for the DNA template. Typically, the 5′ primer is the sequence: 5′ - TAATACGACTCACTATAGGGACAAT TACTATTTACAATTACA-3'. Resuspend in ddH_2O and dilute to 100 μM. Store at −20°C (*see* **Note 4**).
3. 3′ primer for the DNA template. Resuspend in ddH_2O and dilute to 100 μM. Store at −20°C (*see* **Notes 4 and 5**).

2.3 Translation and dT Purification

1. Rabbit reticulocyte lysate (Promega, cat# L4960). The kit contains nuclease-treated reticulocyte lysate and amino acid mixtures. Alternatively, reticulocyte-rich rabbit blood can be purchased from Green Hectares (https://greenhectares.com) and nuclease-treated [6]. Store at −80°C.
2. ^{35}S-methionine, in vitro translation grade, >800 Ci/mmol (Revvity, Waltham, MA, or other supplier). Store at 4°C.
3. 2.5 M KOAc. Sterile filter. Store at −20°C.
4. 25 mM $Mg(OAc)_2$. Sterile filter. Store at −20°C.
5. 12.5× Translation buffer with methionine: 250 mM Hepes-KOH pH 7.6, 100 mM creatine phosphate, 25 mM DTT, 312.5 μM of each amino acid. Store at −80°C.
6. 12.5× Translation buffer without methionine: 250 mM Hepes-KOH pH 7.6, 100 mM creatine phosphate, 25 mM DTT, 312.5 μM of each amino acid except for methionine. This buffer is for use with ^{35}S-methionine for radiolabeling experiments. Store at −80°C.
7. 1 M $MgCl_2$. Sterile filter. Store at room temperature.
8. 2.5 M KCl. Sterile filter. Store at room temperature.

9. POROS Oligo $(dT)_{25}$ Affinity Resin (ThermoFisher Scientific, cat# A48605). Store at 4°C.
10. 1× Isolation Buffer: 100 mM Tris-HCl, pH 8.0, 1 M NaCl, 0.2% (v/v) Triton X-100. Sterile filter and store at 4°C.
11. RNase A, DNase, and protease-free (ThermoFisher Scientific, cat# EN0531).
12. Spin-X Filters, cellulose acetate, 0.45 μm (Corning; cat# 8163).

2.4 Validation of Clones by Radioactive Binding Assays

1. Neutravidin agarose (ThermoFisher Scientific, cat# 29200) or Streptavidin Agarose (ThermoFisher Scientific, cat# 20347) supplied as a 50/50 (v/v) slurry. Store at 4°C (*see* **Note 6**).
2. Selection target (*see* **Note 7**).
3. Selection buffer (see **Notes 8 and 9**).
4. 2 mM Biotin solution: 2 mM D-biotin dissolved in 1× PBS (137 mM NaCl, 2.7 mM KCl, 4.3 mM Na_2HPO_4, 1.47 mM KH_2PO_4). Sterile filter and store at 4°C.
5. Blocking buffer: 1 mL of selection buffer + 25 μL of 2 mM biotin solution (50 μM biotin, final concentration).

2.5 Alanine Scanning

1. Synthetic DNA encoding a clone for testing (various suppliers). Dilute to 1 μM.
2. Appropriate 5′ and 3′ primers (various suppliers) for the clone at 100 μM. Store at −20°C.

2.6 Evaluating the Kinetic Binding of Clones

1. A specific competitor: either a non-biotinylated selection target or other ligand that binds the same binding site as the library (*see* **Notes 10 and 11**).

2.7 Extension or Doped Library Design

1. Synthetic Library DNA (Integrated DNA Technologies or the Keck Oligo Facility at Yale).
2. Appropriate 5′ and 3′ primers (various suppliers) for the library at 100 μM. Store at −20°C.

2.8 Off-rate Selection

1. Synthetic DNA library (Integrated DNA Technologies or the Keck Oligo Facility at Yale).
2. Appropriate 5′ and 3′ library primers (various suppliers) at 100 μM. Store at −20°C.

2.9 Protease Selection

1. Protease, for example, trypsin or chymotrypsin (*see* **Note 12**). Immobilized proteases are preferred (e.g., Chymotrypsin agarose, Sigma cat# C9134) (but *see* **Note 13**). Sequencing-grade protease is recommended if it is important that a single protease is used for digestion.
2. Protease digestion buffer: 50 mM Sodium phosphate, pH 8.0 or similar.

3. Synthetic DNA library (Integrated DNA Technologies or the Keck Oligo Facility at Yale).
4. Appropriate 5′ and 3′ library primers (various suppliers) at 100 μM. Store at −20°C.

2.10 Machine Learning Training and Sequence Generation

1. Cloud computing resource (GPU). If no in-house cloud computing resource is available, Google Colab is a publicly available resource.

3 Methods

A critical step in an mRNA display selection is determining when the selection is complete. A hypothetical, ideal selection is shown in Fig. 2. The binding of each pool is measured to beads with (blue) and without (red) target. Background binding is low throughout the selection, and there are multiple successive rounds where binding increases, starting with Pool 4. This increase slows down between pools 7 and 8 and seems to plateau. Increasing selection stringency (e.g., selection at higher temperature or with reduced target concentration) can sometimes be used to delay this plateau and allow pool binding to keep increasing.

Such a plateau indicates that a pool has likely reached its peak affinity. Sequencing at this point is recommended, rather than increasing selection stringency further. Other common points to stop the selection are when net pool binding (binding to target minus binding to beads) to the target is observed, or following several successive rounds of binding increase.

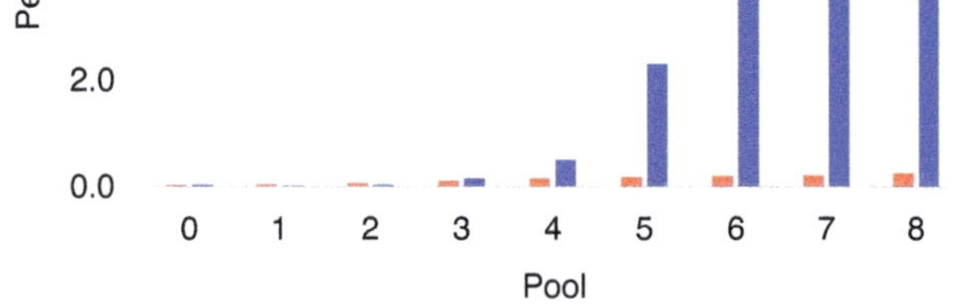

Fig. 2 A hypothetical example binding profile for an ideal mRNA display selection. Net binding to the target is seen relatively early (pool 4) and increases quickly. Binding to the solid support remains low throughout the selection. Binding plateaus between pools 7 and 8, indicating the pool is likely near its maximum affinity, and the selection should be sequenced

Radioactivity provides one of the most effective methods to monitor a selection, allowing one to assess the translation efficiency, binding to the target, and non-specific binding. In general, the radioactive counts from a 50 μL translation and binding to the target should increase over the course of a selection. The most common challenge encountered during selection is when the pool binds to the matrix rather than the target. Switching the solid support usually alleviates the problem, and switching when non-specific binding is observed, no matter how small, is usually the best course of action.

Sequencing is also an excellent non-radioactive method to monitor the selection, but time and cost are potential disadvantages. Sanger sequencing is fast and affordable but limited in the number of sequences. Although Sanger sequencing served as the primary method for sequencing selections for years, it has been largely supplanted by high-throughput sequencing technologies. High-throughput sequencing allows detailed tracking of over a million sequences across multiple pools. Illumina sequencing can return more than a billion sequences for a few thousand US dollars, though sequencing and data processing can take days to a week or two. Nanopore sequencing is affordable, and results are often returned overnight; however, sequence depth is not as great as Illumina sequencing.

If it is not feasible to use radioactivity to monitor the selection, and sequencing every round is prohibitively costly ((in terms of both cost and time), indirect measures must be used instead. Methods to monitor a selection indirectly include:

1. **Number of PCR cycles**. PCR cycles should remain constant and decrease as the pool binds the target with higher affinity.
2. **The quality of dsDNA and mRNA**. Synthesis of the nucleic acid should remain robust, and yields should remain constant or increase over a selection. The size of the nucleic acid and the number of products should also remain constant.
3. **Ligation efficiency**. Ligation efficiency should also remain constant or increase over the selection.

If any of these indirect measures show unfavorable trends, consider repeating that round of selection. If the measure remains poor for more than one round, consider sequencing the library and/or troubleshooting before continuing with the selection.

Once a decision to sequence the library at a large scale has been made, the library must be prepared for sequencing. First, one must decide which pools to sequence. High-affinity binders can be identified by sequencing only the final pool, but we recommend sequencing multiple rounds (ideally all rounds) so that enrichment of sequences (the increase in frequency of a sequence between consecutive rounds) can be calculated. Sequencing of multiple pools in the same run is achieved by appending identifying barcodes to each pool, combining the pools, and then sequencing all pools in a single run. Except in exceptional cases, every round of a selection can be sequenced concurrently, with more than 100 million reads per pool using Illumina sequencing.

Even with such sequencing depth, identifying successful binders from sequencing data is often challenging, especially from fully randomized libraries. First, binders should be grouped into families based on sequence homology. Families that consist of obvious non-target binders, such as known binders to the solid support used, should be discarded. Similarly, highly hydrophobic sequences should also be eliminated as these sequences will tend to non-specifically aggregate and/or be insoluble. The remaining families represent putative target binding sequences, which should be tested for binding to the target.

To verify these putative sequences for target binding, representative sequences from each family should be chosen, synthesized, and tested. While it is possible to chemically synthesize or express a putative binder and test binding via surface plasmon resonance (SPR) or other similar biophysical binding assays, we routinely use radioactive binding assays to test clones synthesized in an mRNA display format. These radioactive binding assays are a fast and easy way to verify these putative binders, with only a couple of days needed for binding results once the DNA template is received. Depending on resources, representative clones from multiple families should be tested via in vitro binding assays. A total of five to ten clones is a feasible number to test, however more can be tested if desired. Each clone must be tested for binding to both the target and the solid support to show binding specificity. If possible, several solid supports should be used to immobilize the target to show that binding is not artifactual. Sequences that show binding due to aggregation are also a concern and may be detected by testing binding under different detergent conditions [7].

To better understand the ligand-target interaction, alanine scanning can be used to determine the binding contributions of individual amino acids of the ligand. Such data can aid in the rational design of higher-affinity clones or for the design of a second-generation library. Kinetic evaluation of binders can help distinguish between candidates that appear similar and inform decisions regarding off-rate selections, which have yielded binders with affinities as low as single-digit pM [8].

Once binders to the target have been identified and verified, there are multiple potential strategies for improving these sequences. Typically, a second library is subsequently constructed based on a validated sequence identified by the original selection. This second library is then used in a second selection to obtain even higher affinity binders. The addition of a protease digestion step can also increase the protease resistance of the library.

Lastly, machine learning has been paired with mRNA display [9]. The results from an mRNA display selection provide excellent, high-quality training data for machine learning models. The use of machine learning techniques has allowed for the expansion of searchable sequence space well beyond 10^{14} sequences, as these models can generate novel sequences that are difficult to access by experimental methods.

3.1 Analysis of mRNA Display Selections Using High-throughput Sequencing

In order to sequence the DNA library from mRNA display selections, adapters compatible with Illumina sequencing must first be added. Both 5′ and 3′ adapters must be added to the library. Typically, these adapters are added by ligation using commercially available kits, and there are many protocols for doing so. However, we prefer to add these adapters by low-cycle PCR as we find it more robust. Though it is possible that additional cycles of PCR may bias the library, over the course of a selection, a library has typically gone through over a hundred cumulative PCR cycles, and a small number of additional cycles are unlikely to result in additional bias. We add unique 5′- and 3′- barcodes instead of the typical Illumina indexes and use these barcodes to de-multiplex samples. These barcodes are the first bases that are read during sequencing, and we find that the variability at the beginning of the sequencing run is important for high-quality sequencing results. In the first 4–7 cycles, the sequencing instrument is identifying the number and location of DNA clusters, and nucleotide diversity is critical during this process. We also add PhiX DNA (5%–15%) to the sample to increase nucleotide diversity (*see* **Note 14**). A typical DNA library, which has been prepared for Illumina sequencing by the addition of adapters and barcodes, is shown in Fig. 3.

With modern high-throughput sequencing platforms, millions of reads are easily accessible. While one million sequences is more than enough to analyze a selection, we typically sequence every round of the selection using multiple barcodes (where each round would typically have more than one million sequences). Additionally, it is possible to perform a selection multiple times under different conditions and then sequence these samples to determine the effect of changing conditions on the pool composition.

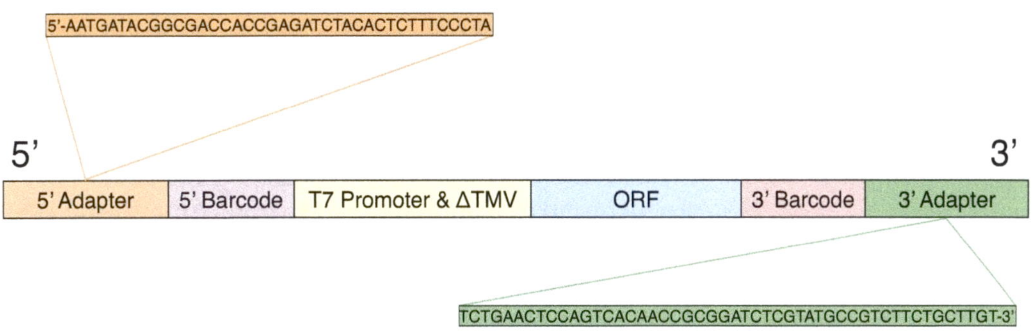

Fig. 3 Typical design of an mRNA display library sequence prepped for Illumina sequencing. Unique barcodes are added to the 5' and 3' ends of the DNA sequence allowing for the sequencing of multiple pools concurrently. Adapters that anneal to the sequences on the Illumina chips are added to the 5′ and 3′ ends

3.1.1 Preparation of Sequencing-Ready Libraries via Two-Step PCR Amplification

1. The first PCR step adds unique barcodes to the DNA template using a forward and reverse primer that both contain a unique barcode. These custom barcodes are used to distinguish different pools that are combined into the same final sequencing sample. The barcode is typically 6–8 bp and is inserted at the 5′ end of each primer, preceding a universal overhang that will serve as the priming site for the 2nd PCR. The remaining primer sequence anneals to the constant regions flanking the variable insert.
2. For each sample to be sequenced, prepare a PCR mix with 1 μL of each unique sequencing primer, 1 μL of library DNA, 10 μL of 10× dNTP, 10 μL of 10× PCR buffer, and 76 μL ddH_2O to a total of 99 μL.
3. Place the tube(s) on a PCR block and preheat the reaction to 94°C. Once the reaction(s) reach 94°C, add 1 μL of Taq to each tube. Perform 4–6 cycles of PCR at 94°C for 30 s, 55°C for 30 s, and 72°C for 45 s.
4. While the reaction is cycling, prepare a 2% agarose gel with the low-melting point (LMP) agarose. This protocol is for the Bio-rad mini-sub cell GT but can be adapted for other systems. Place the gel tray into the casting apparatus (or tape the ends). Weigh 1 g of LMP agarose, place it in a 125 mL Erlenmeyer flask, then add 50 mL of 1× SB buffer or 1× TBE buffer. Microwave until the agarose is dissolved, stirring occasionally. Caution is advised since the solution can easily boil over. Cool the flask under running tap water until it can comfortably be touched (~55°C), then add 2 μL of 10 mg/mL ethidium bromide. Before the gel hardens, pour the solution into the gel tray, place the comb into the gel, and allow it to harden (*see* **Note 15**).
5. After thermocycling is completed, remove the tube(s) from the thermocycler. Mix 1 μL of 100 bp DNA ladder with 1 μL of 5× SB Loading buffer and load on the gel. Mix 1 μL of 5× SB Loading buffer with 4 μL of PCR product and load on an adjacent lane (*see* **Note 16**). Run the gel for 4 min at 300 V if using SB buffer (or 7 min at 220 V for 1× TBE gels), then image the gel. Longer run times may be required for longer templates.
6. Evaluate the PCR reaction by comparing the density of the product band to that of the nearest band of the 100 bp DNA ladder. The PCR product should be roughly the same intensity as the corresponding band of the 100 bp ladder. Qualitatively, the PCR product should be one band of the correct size. Double-banding, smearing, incorrectly-sized products, or primer dimer all indicate that the PCR reaction should be optimized (see Leaf et al., Chap. 12 for more details).

7. If the quality of the DNA product is acceptable, pour a preparative agarose gel and gel purify the rest of the PCR reaction. Visualize the band using a handheld UV lamp and excise with a clean razor. Work quickly to minimize UV exposure. Be sure to wear proper Personal Protective Equipment (PPE), including gloves and eye and face protection.
8. Extract the DNA from the gel slice using a gel extraction kit according to the manufacturer's specifications. Elute with 15 μL of 10 mM Tris-HCl, pH 7.5, twice.
9. Perform a second PCR to add the full-length Illumina-compatible adapters using the 5′- and 3′- universal primers. These universal primers anneal to the overhangs introduced in the first PCR. For each sample, prepare 99 μL of a PCR mix with 1 μL of each universal primer, 1 μL of library DNA from step 8, 10 μL of 10× dNTP, 10 μL of 10× PCR buffer, and 76 μL ddH_2O. Heat the sample to 94 °C before adding the Taq polymerase.
10. Analyze the product via agarose gel, gel purify the sample, and extract the DNA as above (steps 5–8).
11. Determine the DNA concentration by UV absorbance. 1 OD260 = 50 μg/mL.
12. Dilute the DNA concentration to 50 nM (*see* **Note 17**). The A260/280 ratio should be >1.8.
13. Combine all samples that are intended for sequencing by adding 20 μL of each 50 nM sample to a single tube. If more or less sequence depth is desired for any one pool, adjust the volume added accordingly.
14. Concentrate the combined sample on a 10 K Amicon concentrator. Wash with 10 mM Tris–HCl, pH 7.5 at least five times (*see* **Note 18**). At this point, the sample is ready for Illumina sequencing.
15. We recommend submitting a small amount of this prepared sample for nanopore sequencing (e.g., https://plasmidsaurus.com) to confirm that the sample is prepared correctly before submitting the sample for the more expensive large-scale sequencing.

3.1.2 Post-Sequencing Data Analysis

Before the results of a selection can be analyzed, the results from the high-throughput sequencing must first be processed into peptide/protein sequences. Minimally, this process involves: (1) Extracting the DNA sequences from the sequencing datafile, (2) Sorting these DNA sequences according to barcode (and thereby each sample), (3) translating these DNA sequences into peptide or protein sequences, (4) Counting (i.e., determining the frequency) of each protein/peptide sequence in that sample, and (5) Sorting the protein/peptide sequences according to frequency.

The frequency of the peptide or protein sequences in a pool is often used as a metric to identify sequences for further study. Generally, a sequence with higher affinity will be observed more frequently than a sequence with lower affinity. However, while it can be tempting to assume that every high-abundance clone identified by sequencing is a successful binder, this is rarely the case. Care should be taken to judiciously choose which clones to test, as there could also be non-target binding sequences in the library, including sequences originating from primer dimers and matrix-binding sequences (e.g., neutravidin [10] or streptavidin-binding sequences [11]). Clones chosen for further study should then be rigorously validated and tested to show that any observed binding is not artifactual and is to the intended target, in its intended state.

1. Illumina files can be processed using scripts like EasyDIVER [4] that can demultiplex FASTQ files based on barcode sequences. These scripts can also translate the DNA reads into peptide/protein sequences and can count the number of times a peptide sequence is observed.
2. If multiple rounds or time points comparisons are available (e.g., using High Throughput Sequencing Kinetic (HTSK) analysis [8], it is often useful to normalize the data between samples. We use frequency in parts per million (ppm), which is calculated by taking the number of counts for a particular sequence and dividing by the total number of sequences in that sample, then multiplying by 1×106. Such comparisons are easily made in a spreadsheet application, or custom Python scripts can be written.
3. Using ppm, one can calculate the fold-enrichment for each peptide/protein sequence by taking the ratio of ppm from round_n and dividing by the ppm from $\text{round}_{(n\text{-}1)}$. Sequences that increase in frequency (thus ppm) going from round n-1 to round n are likely to be higher-affinity sequences (*see* **Note 19**).
4. Peptide/protein sequences can then be ranked by abundance and/or enrichment. Typically, selecting the most abundant sequences or those with the highest enrichment are good candidates to prioritize for further study.
5. Sequences that are clearly non-target binders should be eliminated. These include sequences which are known binders to the solid support used (e.g., if streptavidin was used to immobilize the target, sequences containing HPQ should be discarded [11]), sequences which consist of almost exclusively hydrophobic residues, truncated sequences that are only a few amino acids long, and any sequences containing stop codons. If the target has surface-exposed cysteines, sequences containing

an odd number of cysteines should be avoided, as these may have remained in the selection due to disulfide formation with the target.

6. Once obvious non-target binders have been eliminated, sort the remaining sequences into families by homology. Multiple sequence alignments are helpful to analyze and identify common motifs that can inform choices on which candidate sequences to choose for further study. Alignments can be manually produced or performed using web-based alignment tools (e.g., www.expasy.org). Custom-designed algorithms (e.g., Hammock [12]) can also be used for this purpose, as well as existing Python resources (e.g., Sequencematcher, Hamming distance, or Levenshtein distance).
7. Structural modeling or prediction tools (e.g., AlphaFold-Multimer [13]) can also be helpful to develop detailed models of peptide-target or protein-target complexes that allow prediction of specific interactions and binding interfaces. These models are useful for generating hypotheses and experiments for testing and rational design.
8. Choose 5–10 sequences for binding validation. Factors in choosing these sequences include high ppm or enrichment, favorable hydrophobicity, and homology with any natural peptide or protein binders. It is often worth testing representative sequences from different families.

3.2 PCR Amplification of Individual DNA Sequences

3.2.1 PCR Amplification of Clones

1. Design DNA templates that code for the clone(s) to be tested. Design corresponding 5′ and 3′ primers, and a splint for the selected clones. If more selection is planned for the original library, use a different 3′ primer than the original library (*see* **Note 5**). Typically, it is not necessary to gel purify the DNA templates of single clones unless the transcription or ligation steps fail.
2. Prepare a 500 μL PCR reaction mix for each clone. Each reaction mix consists of 5 pmol of ssDNA template, 5 μL of each 100 μM primer, 50 μL of 10× dNTP mix, 50 μL of 10× PCR mix, and 370 μL of ddH_2O. Each mix is then aliquoted into five 0.65 mL tubes.
3. Perform the PCR cycling and analysis as described in Sect. 3.1.1.
4. If the DNA quality is acceptable, perform phenol extraction, transcribe the DNA into RNA, and ligate the puromycin linker according to Leaf et al., Chap. 12, Sects. 3.2.4–3.4.

3.3 In Vitro Translation and dT Purification

This section details the preparation of a translation mix using rabbit reticulocyte lysate, though other translation mixes can be used. See Leaf et al., Chap. 12, Sect. 3.5 for a more detailed discussion.

1. For clone testing, only a hot translation with ^{35}S-methionine is necessary to perform radioactive binding assays. As there are normally multiple binding tests for a clone, the hot translation is generally at a larger scale than is needed for selection. Calculate the volume of translation necessary for the number of binding assays needed, assuming conservatively 200 k counts per 50 μL of hot translation, and the use of 100 k counts per binding assay. If replicates are needed, multiply the volume needed by three.
2. Prepare the translation reaction. The following protocol is for a total translation volume of 50 μL; adjust these volumes for different-sized translations. For each 50 μL hot reaction, add 2 μL of 10 μM ligated template, 2 μL of 2.5 M KOAc, 1 μL of 25 mM $Mg(OAc)_2$, 4 μL 12.5 × translation mix *without* Methionine, 2 μL in vitro translation grade ^{35}S-labeled methionine, 19 μL ddH_2O, and 20 μL of treated rabbit reticulocyte lysate. Incubate at 30°C for 1 h.
3. Add 4 μL of 1 M $MgCl_2$ and 14 μL of 2.5 M KCl per 50 μL of translation to facilitate fusion formation. Incubate at room temperature for 5–15 min. Alternatively, store at −20°C overnight.
4. While the sample is incubating in Step 3, aliquot 20% of the translation volume (10 μL) of the dT bead slurry into a 1.7 mL tube. Wash the beads three times with 1 mL isolation buffer (IB), spinning to pellet and discarding the supernatant each time. Resuspend washed beads in IB to a final volume of 1 mL per 50 μL translation.
5. Add 1 μL of 10 mg/mL RNase A (*see* **Note 20**) to the translation reaction.
6. Add fusion products to the dT slurry and rotate at 4°C for 1 h.
7. Before beginning the dT washing steps, fill two 1.7 mL tubes with ddH_2O and heat at 65°C.
8. Transfer the slurry-fusion mixture to a Spin-X column. Spin for 30 s at 1500×*g* and remove the filtrate. Repeat until all the solution is filtered. Wash the beads five times with 500–600 μL IB, spinning and removing the filtrate between washes.
9. Save the last wash and count in a scintillation counter. The last wash should be below ~2000 cpm. If not, continue washing until the cpm are below 2000.
10. Transfer the top cup of the Spin-X to a new 1.7 mL tube. Elute by adding 50 μL of 65°C water, incubating for 1 min,

then centrifuging. Repeat for a total of five elutions. Elution volume and number of elutions can be adjusted, but avoid using fewer than three elutions or lower volumes, as this may reduce yield. Count 1/10 volume of the eluent to determine the total cpm for the entire reaction (*see* **Note 21**).

3.4 Validation of Clones

While mRNA display is almost always capable of generating on-target binders, a sequence can survive and even come to dominate a selection even if it does not bind to the target. The largest source of these non-target binders is due to the selection of sequences that bind the solid support used to immobilize the target. It is important to validate putative binders for the target of interest and eliminate non-target binding sequences. We describe a protocol that uses radioactive binding assays to confirm that a sequence is an on-target binder. Experimental validation is essential as artifactual binders are frequently non-obvious and cannot be identified and filtered solely by inspection.

1. Binding should be tested to: (1) target immobilized on the solid support used during the selection, (2) target immobilized on a solid support **other** than what was used in the selection (*see* **Notes 22 and 6**), and (3) no target controls for both supports.
2. While the translation is incubating with dT beads, prepare the target/no target beads (*see* **Note 23**). For every binding reaction (both with and without target), use at least 10 μL of 50/50 bead slurry (e.g., Neutravidin or Streptavidin agarose). Add up to 100 μL of bead slurry (equal to ten binding reactions) in a 1.7 mL tube and wash with 3×1 mL of selection buffer. Add 1 mL of selection buffer and split the sample in half into two 1.7 mL tubes. For the target beads, add the desired pmol of target and incubate at 4 °C for 1 h, wash the beads three times with 1 mL of blocking buffer, then add 1 mL of blocking buffer and rotate at 4°C for another hour. For the no-target beads, add 1 mL of blocking buffer and rotate at 4°C. After incubation, divide the prepared beads into 1.7 mL tubes.
3. Prepare binding reactions by adding 100,000 cpm of hot fusions to the prepared beads, and add selection buffer to 1 mL. Incubate at 4°C for 1 h, transfer the solutions to a Spin-X filter and wash 3× with 700 μL of selection buffer. Count the supernatant, the washes, and the beads in a scintillation counter. Determine the percent binding by dividing the cpm left on the beads by the total number of cpm in the reaction (supernatant + washes + beads).
4. On-target binders should show significant binding regardless of support and should not show significant binding to solid support without a target.

5. If concerns of non-specific binding by aggregation exist, we recommend testing binding under different detergent concentrations, provided that the target is not affected by changes in detergent. Repeat the binding tests above with 0.1× or 10× detergent and compare binding under these conditions with that under standard detergent concentrations. Genuine binders should show consistent binding across detergent concentrations, while aggregators will show reduced binding with higher detergent concentrations.
6. Once clones have been validated using the radioactive binding assay, choose several sequences for chemical synthesis (for peptides) or expression (proteins) for further biochemical characterization. For example, binding can be characterized by surface plasmon resonance (SPR) or isothermal titration calorimetry. Sequences can also be tested in biological contexts, for example, sequences expressed inside cells can be screened for target binding [14].

3.5 Alanine Scanning

Alanine scanning is a well-established method to determine what positions in a peptide or protein ligand are important for binding [15]. In alanine scanning, a series of mutants, each with a single position in the ligand mutated to alanine, is constructed and tested for binding to a target. Once one or more clones from selection have been identified and successfully validated, alanine scanning can be used to identify the binding contributions of the individual amino acids of these sequences. This is achieved by constructing the different Ala mutants in an mRNA display format, testing the binding of each mutant, and comparing each mutant's affinity to that of the wild-type sequence. Those positions where mutation to Ala greatly decreases binding are likely to contribute greatly to the interaction with the target, while those that are not affected are less likely to significantly contribute to target binding. This information can be used in library design for subsequent selections and can also give insight into the binding mode of the ligand.

1. Obtain a template, 5′, and 3′ primers for the desired alanine mutants. If a particular amino acid is alanine in the wild type (WT) sequence, glycine can be substituted instead; however, the increased conformational flexibility of glycine makes this an imperfect replacement.
2. Prepare radiolabeled fusions and target beads as described in Sects. 3.2–3.4.
3. Evaluate the binding of alanine mutants to the target. When performing these experiments, it is essential to include the WT sequence as a control, as well as a sample without a target as a negative control (*see* **Note 24**).

4. Plot the binding of the alanine mutants normalized to the binding of the WT sequence. A mutant with a significant reduction in binding indicates that the position contributes significantly to binding.

3.6 Evaluating the Kinetic Binding of Clones

This section describes procedures for determining the kinetic binding constants (apparent association rate constant (k_{obs}) and dissociation rate constant (k_{off}) of peptide-protein complexes using immobilized targets and radiolabeled peptides. Although k_{obs} is not the true kinetic association rate constant (k_{on}), it provides a useful metric to allow comparison of how different sequences bind. In many cases, differences in binding affinity typically result from differences in k_{off} rather than large changes in k_{on}.

3.6.1 Determination of the Apparent Association Rate Constant

1. Perform translation of the clone of interest as in Sectis. 3.2 and 3.3 and prepare target beads as in Sect. 3.4. Beads with no target are not needed for this experiment.
2. Combine the dT-purified radiolabeled fusion mixture with the immobilized target and add blocking buffer to 1 mL. Ensure that the sample is well-mixed then immediately remove a 100 μ L aliquot of bead-peptide mixture and separate the beads from the supernatant by spinning the sample through a Spin-X column. Count the flow-through (unbound fraction) and the beads (bound fraction) to get the percent bound at the 0 sec time point. To ensure full recovery, wash the Spin-X cup twice with 500 μL ddH_2O when collecting the beads for scintillation counting.
3. Take additional 100 μL aliquots at other defined time points (e.g., 1, 2, 5, 10, 20, and 40 min). The optimal time points will depend on the actual rate of the reaction (*see* **Note 25**).
4. Analyze the on-rate data using an association kinetic model. GraphPad Prism or equivalent software (Excel) can be used for this analysis.
5. To determine the actual association rate constant (k_{on}), vary the concentration of target on beads and repeat the experiment with several concentrations of target. However, when comparing ligands, the apparent association rate constant k_{obs} is often enough to rank-order the binding of the clones.

3.6.2 Determination of the Off-Rate

1. Perform translation of the clone of interest and prepare target beads as in Sects. 3.2–3.4.
2. Combine the radiolabeled fusion mixture with the immobilized target and add blocking buffer to 1 mL. Incubate at 4 °C for 1 h (*see* **Note 26**) with tube rotation.
3. After incubation, ensure that the sample is well mixed and transfer to a Spin-X filter. Wash 3× with 700 μL of selection

buffer. Count the supernatant and the three washes in a scintillation counter. Resuspend the beads in 1 mL blocking buffer and count 1/10 of the resuspension to estimate the total counts present on the bead. Determine the percent bound by dividing the cpm on the beads by the total number of cpm in the reaction (supernatant + washes + beads).

4. Add 100-fold molar excess (relative to the immobilized target) of a non-biotinylated competitor to the beads (*see* **Note 27**) and add blocking buffer to a final volume of 1 mL. High levels of competitor are necessary so that any dissociation of fusion from the target is essentially irreversible (pseudo-first order conditions). Mix gently to avoid aggregation and maintain uniform suspension by rotating the sample (*see* **Note 28**).
5. At defined time points (e.g., 1, 5, 10, 20, and 60 min), remove a 100 μL aliquot of the bead-peptide mixture and immediately separate the beads from the supernatant using a Spin-X filter (*see* **Note 29**).
6. Measure the radioactivity of beads and supernatant to determine the fraction of peptide bound at each time point. To ensure recovery, wash the Spin-X cup twice with 500 μL ddH_2O to collect all beads.
7. Analyze the off-rate data using a one-phase exponential decay model to determine the dissociation rate constant (k_{off}) of binding. GraphPad Prism or equivalent software (Excel) can be used for this analysis.

3.7 Improving an Initial Hit by Synthesis of a Secondary Library and Reselection

Once a peptide or protein ligand has been identified and validated, the initial hit can be improved by creating a secondary library and performing additional rounds of selection. One option for generating such libraries is mutagenic PCR, which has been described in detail [16]. This approach is more suitable for protein libraries because mutations can be introduced throughout the entire coding region, including the constant regions (framework) and variable regions, from the initial selection. Mutations in either region can enhance the affinity, folding, stability, or other biophysical properties of the protein [17].

Mutagenic PCR introduces mutations at relatively low rates, which depend on the length of the amplified sequence. For proteins, this results in only a few changes in a sequence, which is beneficial since it reduces the likelihood of disruptive or destabilizing substitutions that could unfold the protein. In contrast, peptide sequences are short, and the number of mutations introduced via mutagenic PCR is even lower, limiting the sequence diversity that can be generated. Lastly, mutagenic PCR is constrained by the types of mutations that are possible; amino acid substitutions requiring two or three nucleotide changes are rare, further restricting accessible diversity.

For peptides, doping is often a better strategy for generating a secondary library (Fig. 4). In a doped library, specific positions can be targeted for mutagenesis, making this strategy particularly powerful when guided by the alanine-scanning data described in Sect. 3.5. The library is chemically synthesized such that each doped position predominantly codes for the wild-type residue, with a lower probability of encoding one of the other 19 amino acids. The mutation rate can be tuned accordingly to favor or disfavor the wild-type amino acid. Unlike polymerase-based (i.e., mutagenic PCR) methods, doped

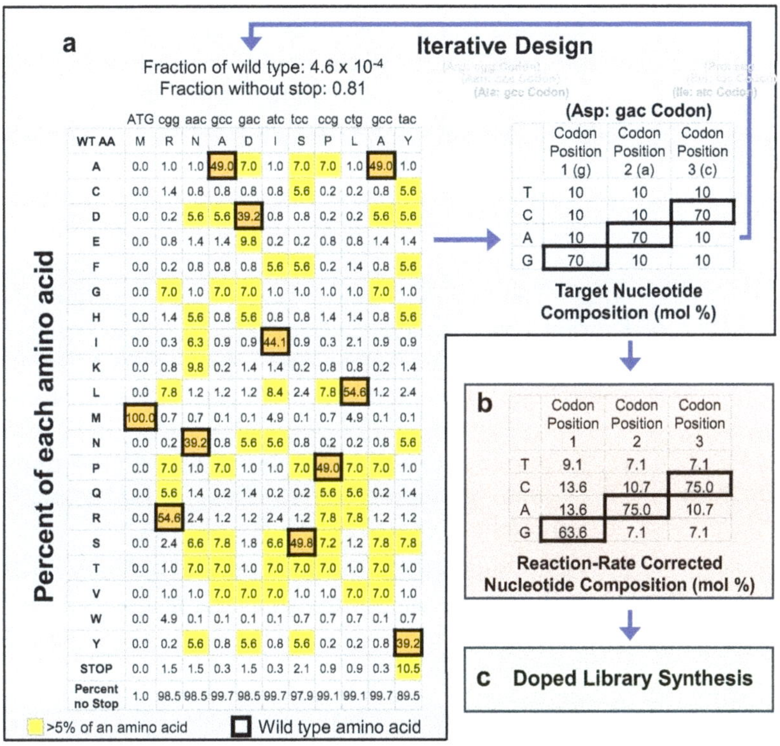

Fig. 4 (**a**) Design process for a doped library. Here, we show the process for doping an aspartic acid codon at 70% at the nucleotide level. The wildtype nucleotides are set to ~70%, with the three non-wildtype nucleotides set to 10% each (represented by lower-case text, e.g., "a" = 70% A, 10% C, 10% G, and 10% T). From these nucleotide percentages, the percentage of each amino acid is calculated for each position in the sequence. We begin by targeting a wild type amino acid frequency at each position of ~40%–50%. The frequencies of the wildtype amino acid at each position are multiplied to find the fraction of wildtype in the library. This process is iterative, and the target nucleotide composition may need to be changed several times to achieve the desired fraction of wildtype and balance of amino acids. A wildtype fraction between 10^{-4} and 10^{-8} is a good balance, depending on the strength and size of the initial binder. It is also important to calculate the fraction of the library without stop codons, as an excess of stop codons in the library will prevent a successful selection. (**b**) Once the desired nucleotide composition has been determined, the reaction-rate corrected nucleotide compositions are calculated. The percentage for each nucleotide is adjusted to compensate for the different reactivities of the phosphoramidites. (**c**) The adjusted nucleotide percentages are then used to synthesize a doped library for further selection

libraries do not suffer from mutational bias, and mutations that require two or three nucleotide changes that are exceedingly rare in mutagenic PCR can be generated using a doped library.

A critical factor to consider when making a doped library is the level of randomization: too much randomization results in what is essentially a naïve library, while not enough randomization will decrease the chances of finding beneficial mutations. We generally synthesize the library such that the wild type frequency is roughly 1 in 10^4 to 1 in 10^8 sequences (Fig. 4a). This level of randomization seems to be sufficient to balance these different factors and result in successful selections [18].

Another factor to consider is the number of residues that are randomized. When a larger number of positions are doped, a lower level of randomization is required. When fewer positions are doped, a higher level of randomization is needed. In practice, for short (~10–15 amino acid) peptides, a randomization level that results in ~40%–50% of the wild type amino acid is typically optimal.

Lastly, when ordering any doped library, design a new 3′ primer that has not been previously used by any sequence that binds the target. This includes the 3′ primer from the original library or any 3′ primer that was used to test clones. Any functional sequence that shares the same 3′ primer as the doped library will contaminate the doped library, making it difficult to identify higher-affinity sequences.

3.7.1 Designing a Second-Generation Library

1. Determine if the library should be created using mutagenic PCR or by doping and synthesis. If mutagenic PCR is used, follow the protocol as described in [16].
2. Determine which positions should be randomized. Consider keeping constant positions that the Alanine Scanning (Sect. 3.5) and/or high-throughput sequencing analysis (Sect. 3.1.2) indicate are essential.
3. Based on the number of positions that are targeted for randomization, determine the target nucleotide composition that will result in a wild type frequency of ~1 in 10^4 to 1 in 10^9 sequences (Fig. 4a). A good starting point is a target percentage of ~70% of the wild type nucleotides and 10% of the other remaining nucleotides (Fig. 4a). For example, for a codon GAC that encodes Asp, the G at the first position would be a mixture of 10% T, 10% C, 10% A, and 70% G. The second and third positions would similarly be adjusted to be 70% of the wild type nucleotides (A in the second position and C in the third) and 10% of the remaining nucleotides (Fig. 4a). While it is theoretically possible to change the target percentages for each codon, it is difficult to synthesize such a library and practically, every codon will use the same target nucleotide composition.
4. Calculate the amino acid composition based on the target nucleotide composition (Fig. 4a) for every position in the

peptide [19]. In the example above, a target of 70% for the wild type nucleotides for the GAC codon would result in ~39% of the wild type Asp residue, 5%–10% of seven other amino acids, and <5% for the remaining amino acids.

5. Multiply the wild-type probabilities from each position in the peptide to calculate the fraction of wild type in the library. In the peptide in Fig. 4, the wild-type fraction is 4.6×10^{-4}, or roughly 1/2000 sequences (*see* **Note 30**).
6. Calculate the fraction of the library that does not have stop codons. At each position, the fraction of sequences that do not have a stop codon is: (1 - stop codon frequency at that position). For example, at the last position of the peptide in Fig. 4a (Tyr), the fraction of amino acids that are not stop codons is $1-0.105=0.895$. Multiply the fraction without stop codons at each position over the entire peptide to get the fraction of sequences without stop codons (*see* **Note 31**).
7. Evaluate the doping of the library with respect to the wild-type amino acid percentages, non-wild-type amino acid percentages, the fraction wild-type sequences, and the fraction of sequences that are full-length (i.e., no stop codons). Optimizing these features often requires iterative adjustments to the target nucleotide composition, followed by evaluation of their effects on these benchmarks. For example, doping certain amino acids (e.g., Tyr and Trp) can produce a relatively higher fraction of stop codons (Fig. 4a). The peptide in Fig. 4a may also tolerate higher randomization (i.e., a lower fraction of wild type). Reducing the wild-type target nucleotide composition to 52% (with 16% for each of the remaining nucleotides) results in 20%–30% of the wild-type amino acids, a wild-type peptide frequency of 4.7×10^{-7} (1 in 1.2×106 sequences are wild-type), and a full-length fraction of the library of 0.726.
8. Once the target nucleotide composition is determined, the actual nucleotide composition that is ordered from the synthesis facility must be corrected for the different base reactivities (*see* **Note 32**). The phosphoramidites should be adjusted to account for the higher G and T reactivities: the bases should be mixed at a ratio of A:C:G:T = 3:3:2:2 [20]. Thus, for the example above, the first G will become 9.1% T, 13.6% C, 13.6% A, and 63.6% G (Fig. 4b). This reaction-rate corrected nucleotide composition is what is ordered from the synthesis facility (Fig. 4c).

3.7.2 Design of an Extension Library

Another strategy to increase binding affinity is to lengthen the peptide by extending either the N-terminus, the C-terminus, or both. This extension strategy has been used to change the binding specificity [21] or to increase the affinity of a peptide [8]. The critical factors in extension library design include how many amino acids to add and whether to extend from the N-terminus, the C-terminus, or both. Generally, the total number of additional random amino acids should not exceed ~9 ($20^9 = 5 \times 10^{11}$ possible sequences), which approaches the practical limit of what can be exhaustively searched using mRNA display.

The C-terminus is often the safest place to extend, as the original peptide was selected in the context of a constant C-terminus (encoded by the 3′ primer). The C-terminal end of the peptide was also the site of attachment to its encoding mRNA, reducing the likelihood that a C-terminal extension would cause an unfavorable steric clash. The N-terminus can often also be extended; however, there is a chance that in some contexts, such an extension could interfere with peptide binding.

1. Choose either the N-terminus, C-terminus, or both as the site to add additional random residues. Choose how many random amino acids to add to these sites. A total of six to nine random residues is a good starting point, as mRNA display can exhaustively search libraries of this complexity.
2. Extension can be combined with a doped library (Sect. 3.7.1). If a doped core is used, we recommend keeping the number of random amino acids lower (e.g., six random amino acids) to keep the overall library complexity lower.
3. Synthesize the library where X positions (where X = any of the 20 natural amino acids) are encoded by the NNS codon (where N = 20% T, 30% C, 30% A, and 20% G and S = 60% C and 40% G. These are reaction-rate corrected nucleotide compositions and are the ratios ordered from the DNA synthesis facility).

3.7.3 Selection with a Second-Generation Library

1. Purify the library and perform the selection as in Leaf et al., Chap. 12, Sects. 3.1–3.7. The first round should be performed as previously described, under relatively low stringency conditions, as the first round will contain only a few copies of any sequence in the library. Once the first round has been completed, the loss of any functional sequence is unlikely, and the selection stringency can be increased in subsequent rounds.
2. The selection should converge quickly, within 2–4 rounds, unless selection stringency is greatly increased.
3. Selection stringency can be increased by increasing temperature, decreasing the amount of target, or by using a selection for longer off-rates (Sect. 3.8).
4. Sequence and analyze the library as described in Sect. 3.1.

3.8 Improving Affinity Using an Off-Rate Selection

In order to select for higher-affinity sequences, the stringency during the selective binding step must be increased to separate sequences that bind with moderate affinity from those with even higher affinity. The number of targets can be decreased to increase the selective pressure on the library. However, at <10 nM, the target concentration is so low that the majority of binding events become diffusion-limited, making further enrichment based solely on equilibrium binding inefficient. Under such conditions, the selection no longer effectively distinguishes between sequences of similar affinity, as all high-affinity ligands bind rapidly to completion. To overcome this limitation, an off-rate selection strategy can be used.

In an off-rate selection, bound complexes first reach equilibrium with immobilized target, the beads are washed, and then a large excess of free competitor is introduced to prevent any dissociating sequence from rebinding. The key selective pressure arises from timed dissociation: peptides that dissociate slowly from the target remain bound to the beads, while faster-dissociating species are blocked from rebinding to the immobilized target by the competitor, and remain in the supernatant. By harvesting the beads after prolonged dissociation periods, sequences with the slowest dissociation rates are selectively enriched (Fig. 5). The off-rate selection requires a library that contains sequences with <10 nM affinity. A doped library (Sect. 3.7.1) or an extension library (Sect. 3.7.2) is well-suited for off-rate selections, as these libraries are more likely to contain high-affinity sequences that make the off-rate selection feasible. This strategy is not recommended for naïve libraries.

This approach follows the same general workflow as in Leaf et al., Chap. 12, with the addition of a defined dissociation step to discriminate based on kinetic stability.

1. Perform the first round of selection as described in Leaf et al., Chap. 12, Sect. 3.6.

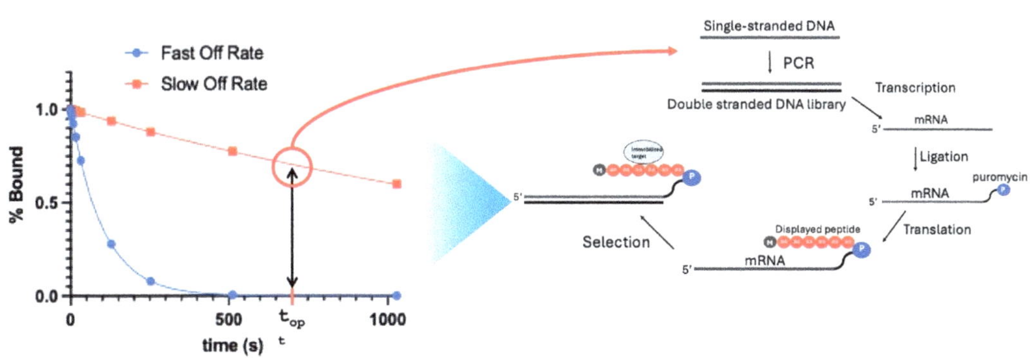

Fig. 5 Methodology for an off-rate selection. After allowing the mRNA-protein fusion to bind, the immobilized target is washed, and the competitor is added to prevent sequences that dissociate from the target from rebinding. At the time when there is the largest difference between the fast and slow off-rate populations, the beads are washed, and the remaining sequences are PCR amplified such that the resulting pool is enriched in higher affinity sequences

2. In the second round of selection, determine the off-rate of the initial pool as described in Sect. 3.6.1. Because the pool is a mixture of ligands with different off-rates, the dissociation should not fit a single exponential decay. The off-rate may instead be fit using a two-phase exponential model where the quicker off-rate describes the lower affinity population, and the slower off-rate describes the higher affinity population (Fig. 5).
3. To determine the optimal time for the off-rate selection, use the equation:

$$t_{opt} = \frac{\left[0.293 + 2.05\,Log(k_r) + \left(2.30 - 0.759 * \frac{1}{k_r}\right) * Log(S_r)\right]}{k_{off,wt}}$$

where $k_{\mathrm{off,wt}}$ is the off-rate of the lower affinity population, k_{r} is the ratio of the k_{off} from the lower affinity population to the k_{off} of the higher affinity population (or, the theoretical fold improvement that could be achieved), and S_{r} is the ratio of signal at $t=0$ to signal at $t=\infty$ [22].
4. Bind the cold library to the target beads, incubate for >1 h, and wash the beads as described in Leaf et al., Chap. 12, Sect. 3.7. After washing, add a100-fold molar excess (relative to the immobilized target) of a non-biotinylated competitor to the beads. Incubate for the time calculated in Step 3 to enrich in high-affinity sequences (Fig. 5) (*see* **Note 33**).
5. Wash the beads with selection buffer, and PCR amplify the sequences bound to the beads. Repeat these steps until the pool off-rate no longer improves.
6. Sequence and analyze the library as described in Sect. 3.1. Test individual clones as described in Sects. 3.2–3.4, and 3.6.

3.9 Protease Selection

To enrich sequences resistant to proteolytic degradation while retaining binding function, a protease challenge can be added before binding the library to target. This step applies selective pressure favoring sequences that remain intact after protease exposure and are still able to bind the target. The overall workflow is identical to a standard mRNA display selection (Leaf et al., Chap. 12, Sect. 3.7), with the addition of a protease digestion step prior to target incubation. This selection is best performed when a library already has detectable, reproducible binding to the target (>5% binding in the radioactive binding assay from Leaf et al., Chap. 12, Sect. 3.7) so that the protease digestion step can be optimized.

1. Perform a 100 μL cold translation and a 50 μL hot translation, dT purify, desalt, and reverse transcribe the sample as in Leaf et al., Chap. 12, Sect. 3.7.

2. Determine how the mRNA-peptide fusions will be purified from the protease. For immobilized protease, simple filtration through a 0.45 μm Spin-X filter can purify the sample. For non-immobilized protease, dT-based purification is recommended; if so, follow the protocol for dT purification as described in Sect. 3.4.
3. (Optional but recommended): Optimize the protease digestion step using the hot sample. Divide the hot sample into multiple tubes; we recommend a minimum of 50,000 cpm per tube. Add varying amounts of protease and/or vary the incubation time. Larger amounts of protease and longer incubation times result in more digestion (*see* **Note 34**). A good starting point for immobilized protease is 1 mg of immobilized beads (~2 Units) incubated with fusions for 5 min at room temperature (*see* **Note 35**). For solution-based protease, a good starting point is 2 μg of protease incubated with fusions for 15 min at room temperature. After digestion, purify the library away from the protease, then perform a binding assay as described above (Sect. 3.4). The binding after protease digestion should be reduced to below 50% of the non-digested sample; however, 10%–30% is recommended.
4. Add protease to the reverse-transcribed fusions and incubate to digest the sample. Remove the protease as determined in Step 2 and collect the flowthrough.
5. Perform a standard binding step followed by PCR amplification as described in Leaf et al., Chap. 12, Sect. 3.7, where the protease-treated pool is incubated with immobilized target under standard binding conditions. The beads are then washed to remove unbound material, and the remaining fusions are PCR amplified.
6. Perform additional rounds of selection, including the protease digestion and binding steps. Generally, as long as the pool is increasing in binding, we will continue to perform additional rounds of selection. When the binding no longer increases, that pool should be sent for high-throughput sequencing as described in Sect. 3.1.1. Alternatively, selection pressure can be increased by extending the digestion time, raising enzyme concentration, or using multiple proteases.

3.10 Generation of Novel Sequences Using a Denoising Diffusion Implicit Model (DDIM)

This protocol describes the generation of novel peptide sequences using a denoising diffusion implicit model (DDIM) trained on peptide-affinity data obtained from mRNA display selections (Fig. 6). The model learns the probability distribution of experimentally derived sequences and generates novel candidate sequences with similar or improved binding characteristics [9].

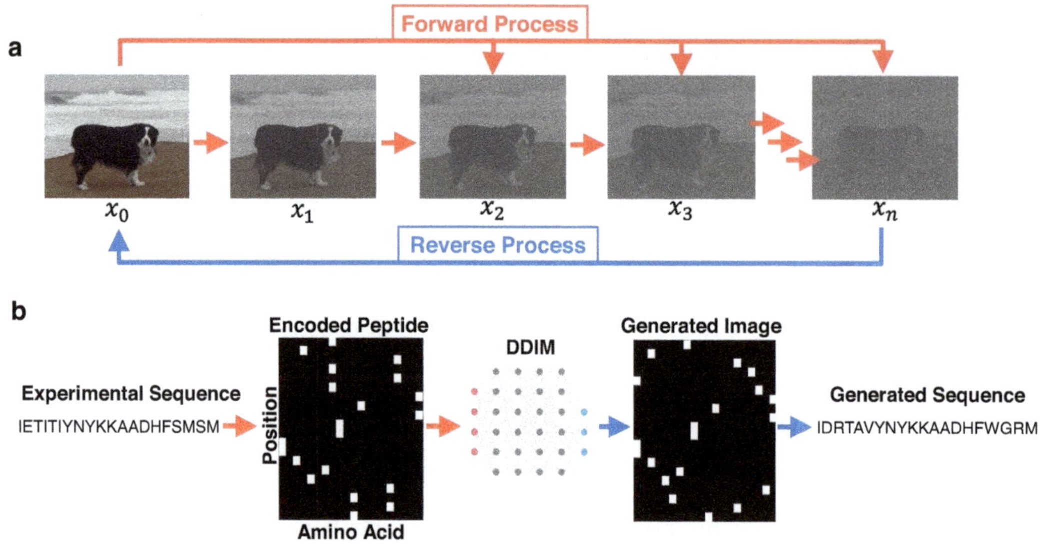

Fig. 6 (**a**) Diagram of the process of a denoising diffusion implicit model (DDIM). The DDIM forward pass is a non-Markovian process in which noise is gradually added to an image. In the reverse process, the model learns to remove noise step by step, which can be used to generate new data. (**b**) Overview of the methodology for the generation of novel peptides by a DDIM. Sequences from a selection are encoded as matrices, with one axis representing position and the other amino acids. At each position, the corresponding amino acid is represented as a white square. These images are used to train a DDIM, which will generate new images that, in turn, are decoded into novel peptide sequences

In order to train the model, a high-quality dataset of peptide sequences is needed. The dataset should be composed of sequences where most, if not all, of the sequences are functional. Generally, a later round of selection will be required for DDIM training, as opposed to an early round of selection (Pool 1 or 2), where the pool contains many sequences that are not functional. A later round pool that originates from a doped library (Sect. 3.7.3) is an excellent dataset for DDIM training.

3.10.1 Data Preparation

1. Obtain high-throughput sequencing data from the post-selection library.
2. Filter sequences to remove non-target binding sequences. This includes sequences that contain stop codons, that are not the correct length, and matrix-binding sequences. Retain sequences of the desired number of residues and sort the sequences according to frequency of occurrence. If there is obviously more than one family of sequences, sort the sequences by family.
3. Select the 15,000–50,000 most abundant sequences for model training. The ideal number depends on pool convergence and sequencing depth (*see* **Note 36**).

4. To be compatible with the DDIM, the peptide sequences first need to be encoded using one-hot encoding [23]. Encode each peptide sequence as an *L by 20* binary matrix, where L is the peptide length and the 20 columns correspond to the 20 natural amino acids (Fig. 6b). Each row contains a single "1" at the column corresponding to the amino acid present at that position, and "0" elsewhere. The initial methionine can be omitted before encoding and added back after generation if needed (*see* **Note 37**).
5. The DDIM also requires that the training data originate from a single probability distribution. To confirm this, calculate the pairwise energy distance between encoded sequences using the built-in Python function scipy.spatial.distance.energy_distance. A narrow clustering of energy distances near zero confirms the suitability of the dataset for DDIM training.
6. If energy distance shows multimodal separation, the dataset likely contains two or more sequence families. In this case, perform sequence-based clustering or unsupervised clustering on the sequences to identify individual families (*see* **Note 38**). Then train a separate DDIM for each family (see **Note 39**).

3.10.2 Training the DDIM

1. Train the model using the provided DDIM training script. This implementation follows Song et al. [24] and includes configurable parameters for the number of timesteps, learning rate, and noise schedule.
2. For default settings, use 50 diffusion timesteps and 5000 training iterations with mean-squared error (MSE) as the reconstruction loss.
3. Monitor both training and testing losses. The training is complete when both losses plateau and reach minima, which indicates convergence is achieved.

3.10.3 Generation of New Peptide Sequences

1. Use the trained model to produce continuous-valued matrices in the range [0, 1]. For each matrix, in each row, assign a value of 1 to the amino acid with the highest probability and 0 to all others.
2. Convert the resulting binary matrix back to an amino-acid sequence and add the conserved regions if required (*see* **Note 40**).

3.10.4 Analysis of DDIM-Generated Sequences

1. Assess the novelty and similarity of the generated sequences. First, compute Hamming distances between the generated sequences and their nearest original neighbors to quantify sequence diversity. A nearest original neighbor is the sequence from the training dataset that has the highest similarity (smallest Hamming distance) to a specific generated sequence.

2. Select a representative subset for subsequent experimental validation. Synthesize the selected sequences (Sects. 3.2 and 3.3) and determine binding (Sect. 3.4) or kinetic parameters (Sect. 3.6) and compare to wild type and/or nearest-neighbor controls.
3. Optionally, analyze the physicochemical properties of the sequences. Calculate hydrophobicity (GRAVY score), net charge, or molecular weight distribution to evaluate chemical diversity within the generated pool. A broader distribution indicates successful exploration of new regions of sequence space.
4. Optionally, other models such as recurrent neural networks (RNNs) or transformer-based architectures could be trained and used to predict the binding affinity of the generated peptides.

4 Notes

1. Plasmids for Taq, T4 DNA Ligase, T7 RNA Polymerase, and MMLV RNaseH^{-} Reverse Transcriptase are available on Addgene (https://www.addgene.org). Significant quantities of these enzymes can be purified making the overall process more affordable.
2. The amount of bromophenol blue added is not critical as it acts as an electrophoresis marker.
3. Thin 0.75 mm combs give better resolution but arc more difficult to load. Thicker 1.5 mm combs are easier to load, though they will give slightly worse resolution.
4. It is good practice to aliquot and store primers in small volumes since primers can easily be contaminated with template DNA.
5. The 3′ primer should be a different sequence than the 3′ primer used in the selection to avoid cross-contamination between the original library and sequences being tested. Any DNA template that is functional for binding to a target can and will contaminate a selection library that shares the same 3′ primer. If this happens, it is not possible to practically separate the functional contaminant from the library.
6. The target may be immobilized by other methods such as neutravidin acrylamide (Ultralink, ThermoFisher Scientific), streptavidin agarose, or other biotin-binding matrix. Covalent methods of immobilization include NHS-activated sepharose or agarose, epoxy-activated sepharose, or cyanogen bromide-activated sepharose.

7. Roughly 1–10 μg of a 30 kDa protein will be needed per binding assay (33–330 pmol). However, we recommend at least 1 mg of protein since, generally, a large number of binding assays are performed during analysis of functional sequences.
8. The selection buffer will depend on the specific requirements of the target. We have successfully used buffers such as 25 mM Hepes pH 7.5, 150 mM NaCl, 0.05% (v/v) Tween 20, 0.05% (w/v) Bsa, and 1 μg/mL tRNA. Buffers should have a buffering agent (e.g., Hepes, Tris, or phosphate), a monovalent salt (NaCl or KCl), a non-ionic detergent (Tween-20, NP-40, or Triton X-100), and Bsa and tRNA as blocking agents. Magnesium, reducing agents (DTT or β-mercaptoethanol), or protein specific requirements (such as GDP for G proteins [25]) can also be added, as needed.
9. We recommend using the same buffer as was used in the selection.
10. Both competitor and target must be stable for days or even weeks.
11. The competitor may be either a target with no biotin (so it cannot be immobilized) or a ligand that binds at the same site as the library. We find the non-biotinylated target to generally work more consistently, but because a 100-fold molar excess is needed for the competition, a significant amount of material is needed every round (~0.6 mg for a 30 kDa protein, sufficient for both a hot binding experiment and cold selection). In total, 5–10 mg of protein is likely needed. In theory, a biotinylated target incubated with free streptavidin/neutravidin in solution should also act as a competitor, allowing one to use the same protein as the target. However, we find that this blocked biotinylated target does not work as well as the authentically non-biotinylated target.
12. The choice of protease should reflect the intended application of the peptide. For example, use endopeptidases such as trypsin, LysC, GluC, or chymotrypsin to mimic intracellular or serum degradation conditions, or use specific proteases of interest to select for target-specific stability. Cocktails of proteases may also be used. Proteinase K is not recommended as a protease for peptide libraries as it digests too quickly, however it has been used successfully with protein libraries [26].
13. Some preparations of protease will be contaminated with other proteases or, in the case of trypsin, autolysis products that result in different specificity [27].
14. For protein libraries, a higher proportion (>15%) of PhiX DNA is recommended to achieve high-quality sequencing

results, as this increases nucleotide diversity during sequencing of constant regions.

15. Two combs can be added, and the 10 cm gel can be cut in half so that two gels can be made. These can be stored in a sealed plastic bag at 4°C for up to 2 weeks.

16. The gel can be more quickly loaded if 1 μL spots of 5× loading buffer (one spot per sample) are placed on a piece of parafilm. The PCR samples can then be mixed on the parafilm and loaded onto the gel.

17. To calculate the molecular weight of a library, 650 Da per base pair can be used.

18. Pure ddH_2O should not be used to wash the sample as it will denature the double-stranded DNA.

19. While it is not essential to sequence multiple pools, using enrichment and abundance together to identify clones for further study is often superior to using abundance alone.

20. Use extreme care when working with RNase, as it is very difficult to eliminate if it contaminates the laboratory. Use gloves and change them frequently, use filter tips, and work carefully.

21. A typical yield for a 25 μL translation is 100,00 cpm. If less than 100,000 cpm are purified per 25 μL translation, consider retranslating and/or repurifying the library. A common cause of low counts is the incomplete desalting of the mRNA-F30P template, resulting in low translation yields.

22. For example, if streptavidin was used for immobilization during the selection, switching to neutravidin is sufficient.

23. We recommend preparing the target beads fresh as this prevents loss of activity and gives more consistent results. However, this is target-dependent, and if the immobilized target remains active after storage at 4°C, a larger batch can be prepared.

24. For longer ligands, the number of binding assays involved in a complete alanine scanning can be daunting. In such cases, it is advisable to split the binding assays over multiple days to ensure binding data is of high quality. If splitting these experiments over multiple days, it is critical to include the wild-type binding to the target as a positive control and wild-type binding to beads with no target as a negative control for each day.

25. We recommend performing a scouting experiment to determine a rough rate of reaction so that the best spread of time points can be chosen for the experiment.

26. At very low target concentrations (< 10 nM, or <10 pmol of target on beads in 1 mL of buffer), the rate of reaction can be

very slow ,and incubation time may need to be extended to several hours or even days.

27. Either a non-biotinylated target or a specific competitor (e.g., a synthetic peptide) can be used as a competitor.
28. Alternatively, it is possible to wash the beads to prevent rebinding, for example, the experimental setups described in [28] and [29].
29. Time-point intervals should be chosen to sufficiently capture the early and late phases of the dissociation for accurate curve fitting.
30. The fraction wild type for the example in Fig. 4c is equal to $(1 \times 0.546 \times 0.392 \times 0.49 \times 0.392 \times 0.441 \times 0.498 \times 0.49 \times 0.546 \times 0.49 \times 0.392) = 4.64 \times 10^{-4}$.
31. The fraction of sequences without stop codons in Fig. 4c is equal to $(1 \times 0.985 \times 0.985 \times 0.997 \times 0.985 \times 0.997 \times 0.979 \times 0.991 \times 0.991 \times 0.997 \times 0.895) = 0.815$.
32. Some synthesis facilities (e.g., Integrated DNA Technologies) claim that they adjust for the different nucleotide coupling rates, so no adjustment would be necessary if ordering from these facilities.
33. Temperature can be used to change the off-rate to be manageable experimentally. For example, at 4°C, the off-rate will be slower than at room temperature.
34. Temperature is another variable that can be optimized, but room temperature reactions are preferable, and we recommend changing the amount of protease or incubation time rather than temperature.
35. Very small amounts of beads can lead to low reproducibility due to bead loss from holdup. Mixing inert, non-protease beads with the protease beads can reduce loss due to holdup.
36. The more diverse the pool, the more the sequences will be needed for model training. Higher counts for the sequences in the high-throughput sequencing dataset will also make the data more reliable.
37. Similarly, other conserved positions (e.g., those where virtually no variability is seen in the high-throughput sequencing data) can be omitted and added back after sequence generation as well. Generally, positions that are highly conserved (> 95% of a particular amino acid) are rarely worth optimizing, as it is rare for a different amino acid to replace the wild-type amino acid.
38. Unsupervised clustering groups on sequences based on similarity in their feature space without using any predefined

labels. Common algorithms include k-means and hierarchical clustering.

39. DDIM training will only be successful if the sequences in the training dataset belong to a single distribution.

40. Typically, tens of thousands of sequences can be generated per run, and more than 99% of these generated sequences are novel relative to the training data.

Acknowledgments

This work is supported by NIH grant R01NS125769, the Michaelson Found Animals Foundation, and the CHDI Foundation.

References

1. Iskandar SE, Bowers AA (2022) mRNA display reaches for the clinic with new PCSK9 inhibitor. ACS Med Chem Lett 13:1379–1383
2. Ong JN, Grindel BJ, Rankin SA, Naylon SH, Srinivasamani A, Trusz GJ, Liang X, Uddin MdN, Fuller L, Curran M, Roche SP, Takahashi TT, Roberts RW, Millward SW (2025) Using extension-based mRNA display to design antibody-like proteinogenic peptides for human PD - L1. Protein Sci 34:e70268
3. Tang G-Q, Tang Y, Dhamnaskar K, Hoarty MD, Vyasamneni R, Vadysirisack DD, Ma Z, Zhu N, Wang J-G, Bu C, Cong B, Palmer E, Duda PW, Sayegh C, Ricardo A (2023) Zilucoplan, a macrocyclic peptide inhibitor of human complement component 5, uses a dual mode of action to prevent terminal complement pathway activation. Front Immunol 14:1213920
4. Blanco C, Verbanic S, Seelig B, Chen IA (2020) EasyDIVER: A pipeline for assembling and counting high-throughput sequencing data from in vitro evolution of nucleic acids or peptides. J Mol Evol 88:477–481
5. Brody JR, Kern SE (2004) Sodium boric acid: a Tris-free, cooler conductive medium for DNA electrophoresis. Biotechniques 36:214–216
6. Jackson RJ, Hunt T (1983) Preparation and use of nuclease-treated rabbit reticulocyte lysates for the translation of eukaryotic messenger RNA. Methods Enzymol 96:50–74
7. Irwin JJ, Duan D, Torosyan H, Doak AK, Ziebart KT, Sterling T, Tumanian G, Shoichet BK (2015) An aggregation advisor for ligand discovery. J Med Chem 58:7076–7087
8. Jalali-Yazdi F, Lai LH, Takahashi TT, Roberts RW (2016) High-throughput measurement of binding kinetics by mRNA display and next-generation sequencing. Angew Chem Int Ed Engl 55:4007–4010
9. Qi P, Gandhi YP, Zheng K, Jalali-Yazdi F, Ong JN, Takahashi TT, Kalia RK, Roberts RW (2025) A route to design novel functional peptides by applying a denoising diffusional model to mRNA display libraries. Chembiochem 26:e202500302
10. Meyer SC, Gaj T, Ghosh I (2006) Highly selective cyclic peptide ligands for NeutrAvidin and avidin identified by phage display. Chem Biol Drug Des 68:3–10
11. Skerra A, Schmidt TGM (2000) [18] Use of the strep- tag and streptavidin for detection and purification of recombinant proteins. Methods in enzymology. Elsevier, New York, pp 271–304
12. Krejci A, Hupp TR, Lexa M, Vojtesek B, Muller P (2016) Hammock: a hidden Markov model-based peptide clustering algorithm to identify protein-interaction consensus motifs in large datasets. Bioinformatics 32:9–16
13. Evans R, O'Neill M, Pritzel A, Antropova N, Senior A, Green T, Žídek A, Bates R, Blackwell S, Yim J, Ronneberger O, Bodenstein S, Zielinski M, Bridgland A, Potapenko A, Cowie A, Tunyasuvunakool K, Jain R, Clancy E, Kohli P, Jumper J, Hassabis D (2021) Protein complex prediction with AlphaFold-Multimer
14. Gross GG, Junge JA, Mora RJ, Kwon H-B, Olson CA, Takahashi TT, Liman ER, Ellis-Davies GCR, McGee AW, Sabatini BL, Roberts RW, Arnold DB (2013) Recombinant probes for visualizing endogenous synaptic proteins in living neurons. Neuron 78:971–985

15. Clackson T, Wells JA (1995) A hot spot of binding energy in a hormone-receptor interface. Science 267:383–386
16. Wilson DS, Keefe AD (2000) Random mutagenesis by PCR. Curr Protoc Mol Biol Chapter 8:Unit8.3
17. Olson CA, Liao H-I, Sun R, Roberts RW (2008) mRNA display selection of a high-affinity, modification-specific phospho-IkappaBalpha-binding fibronectin. ACS Chem Biol 3:480–485
18. Kamalinia G, Grindel BJ, Takahashi TT, Millward SW, Roberts RW (2021) Directing evolution of novel ligands by mRNA display. Chem Soc Rev 50:9055–9103
19. Labean TH, Kauffman SA (1993) Design of synthetic gene libraries encoding random sequence proteins with desired ensemble characteristics. Protein Sci 2:1249–1254
20. Bartel DP, Szostak JW (1993) Isolation of new ribozymes from a large pool of random sequences [see comment]. Science 261:1411–1418
21. Austin RJ, Ja WW, Roberts RW (2008) Evolution of class-specific peptides targeting a hot spot of the Gαs subunit. J Mol Biol. 377:1406–1418
22. Boder ET, Wittrup KD (1998) Optimal screening of surface-displayed polypeptide libraries. Biotechnol Prog 14:55–62
23. Rumelhart DE, Hinton GE, Williams RJ (1986) Learning representations by back-propagating errors. Nature 323:533–536
24. Song J, Meng C, Ermon S (2020) Denoising diffusion implicit models. arXiv:2010.02502 [cs.LG]. https://doi.org/10.48550/arXiv.2010.02502
25. Ja WW, Roberts RW (2004) In vitro selection of state-specific peptide modulators of G protein signaling using mRNA display. Biochemistry 43:9265–9275
26. Nichols AL, Noridomi K, Hughes CR, Jalali-Yazdi F, Eaton JB, Lai LH, Advani G, Lukas RJ, Lester HA, Chen L, Roberts RW (2018) α1-FANGs: protein ligands selective for the α-bungarotoxin site of the α1-nicotinic acetylcholine receptor. ACS Chem Biol 13:2568–2576
27. Keil-Dlouhá V, Zylber N, Imhoff J-M, Tong N-T, Keil B (1971) Proteolytic activity of pseudotrypsin. FEBS Lett 16:291–295
28. Olson CA, Adams JD, Takahashi TT, Qi H, Howell SM, Wu T-T, Roberts RW, Sun R, Soh HT (2011) Rapid mRNA-display selection of an IL-6 inhibitor using continuous-flow magnetic separation. Angew Chem Int Ed Engl 50:8295–8298
29. Evenson WE, Lin W-ZS, Pang K, Czaja AT, Jalali-Yazdi F, Takahashi TT, Malmstadt N, Roberts RW (2020) Enabling flow-based kinetic off-rate selections using a microfluidic enrichment device. Anal Chem 92:10218–10222

Chapter 17

Tracking Synthetic Adhesins on Bacterial Surfaces with Immunofluorescence Microscopy

Sofía Fraile, Jaime Fernández de Córdoba, Víctor de Lorenzo and Esteban Martínez-García

Abstract

Programmable bacterial adhesion enables applications in biocatalysis, living materials, and targeted drug delivery. This functionality can be achieved through the expression of synthetic adhesins in bacterial cells. These molecules are hybrid proteins composed of four key elements: (i) a signal peptide for secretion; (ii) the beta barrel domain of an autotransporter for surface display; (iii) a nanobody module providing specific recognition and targeting capabilities; and (iv) an epitope tag for expression tracking and localization. This chapter describes a detailed protocol for visualizing these synthetic adhesins on *Escherichia coli* and *Pseudomonas putida* using indirect immunofluorescence combined with Super-Resolution Microscopy (SRM) techniques, such as STimulated Emission Depletion (STED). The workflow includes plasmid introduction into the bacterial cells, induction, immunostaining, and image acquisition to spatially track the adhesins on the cell surface.

Keywords Synthetic adhesins, Surface display, Bacterial cell surface, Immunofluorescence, Nanobodies, STED microscopy

1 Introduction

Engineering the outer membrane of Gram-negative bacteria to display synthetic adhesins enables the generation of cells with programmable adhesive properties. This approach supports applications including whole-cell biocatalysis [1–3], the development of living materials [4, 5], or even targeted therapeutic delivery [6–8]. Common strategies for surface display in Gram-negative bacteria involve the use of autotransporter systems (Type V secretion systems), such as the *Escherichia coli* Antigen 43 (Ag43) [9]. Typically, autotransporters consist of three modules: a signal peptide (SP), a passenger domain, and a beta-barrel translocation unit [10, 11]. Previous studies have shown that the passenger domain of autotransporters can be replaced with a DNA fragment encoding a heterologous protein for surface display

Huan Peng and Theam Soon Lim (eds.), *Biomolecular Display Technologies*, Methods in Molecular Biology, vol. 3030,
https://doi.org/10.1007/978-1-0716-5249-7_17,

[9, 12, 13]. Then, to construct a surface display system with an artificial adhesin, the Ag43 beta-barrel translocation domain is fused to a specific nanobody (VHHs), which function as the recognition/binding module. These synthetic constructs would enable researchers to reprogram bacterial adhesion properties [8, 12, 14]. Nanobodies serve as the adhesin module due to their ability to bind target antigens with high specificity and affinity, despite their single-chain architecture and small molecular size (~15 kDa) [15]. These antibodies originate from camelids [16] and sharks [17]. Besides, nanobodies targeting particular antigens, or entire cells, can be produced from immunized camelids using selected antigens or inactivated cells [18]. Moreover, the recombinant construct includes a *myc-tag* epitope along with the anchoring and nanobody modules [Fraile et al. *in preparation*], which facilitates verification of protein expression via western blot analysis and enables localization studies through indirect immunofluorescence techniques, as described in this protocol.

However, validating the correct translocation, folding, and localization of this chimeric protein remains a challenge. Conventional wide-field and confocal microscopy often lack the resolution given the small dimensions of bacterial cells (~1–2 μm). Traditional protein analysis methods, such as enzyme-linked immunosorbent assay (ELISA) and western blot, provide quantitative data but lack the ability to resolve spatial distribution. To address this limitation immunofluorescence (IF) is widely used for localizing and quantifying molecules within cells [19]. IF employs antibodies conjugated to fluorophores that emit light upon excitation, enabling high-resolution imaging and precise localization of proteins within cells. Within this technique, indirect immunofluorescence utilizes secondary antibodies labeled with fluorophores to enhance signal detection (since several secondary antibodies can attach to a primary antibody) [19].

Recent advances in fluorescence-based Super-Resolution Microscopy (SRM) have further expanded these capabilities, allowing researchers to investigate protein localization in bacterial cells at unprecedented detail. Because spatial mapping of proteins is critical for understanding numerous biological processes, SRM techniques, which surpass the diffraction limit of conventional light microscopy, are transformative. Among these, laser-scanning approaches such as STimulated Emission Depletion (STED) microscopy achieve resolutions as fine as 20–30 nm [20–22].

The selection of an appropriate fluorophore is a critical step in IF, as it directly influences signal intensity, photostability, and compatibility with imaging systems. Among these, Abberior-StarRED (a rhodamine dye also known as KK114; [23]) is an excellent choice for high-resolution applications due to its exceptional brightness, resistance to photobleaching, and optimal performance in super-resolution microscopy techniques such as STED [24]. Its emission spectrum minimizes overlap with commonly used fluorophores, enabling multiplexing while maintaining clear signal separation. These properties make Abberior-StarRED particularly suitable for precise localization studies where high contrast and durability under prolonged illumination are essential [25].

We describe below a protocol to visualize synthetic adhesins on the bacterial surface of *E. coli* and *Pseudomonas putida* using an indirect immunofluorescence technique combined with Super-Resolution Microscopy. This workflow relies on a specific detection system where the adhesin is tagged with a *myc-tag* epitope and targeted by a primary anti-*myc* antibody, followed by a secondary anti-mouse Abberior-StarRED antibody.

The following sections provide a step-by-step guide that goes from introducing the plasmid encoding the synthetic adhesin, followed by expression, sample preparation, immunostaining, and image acquisition.

2 Materials

2.1 Strains and Plasmids

The bacterial strains used in this protocol are: *Escherichia coli* MG1655-dTomate (F^- λ^- *ilvG rbf50 rph-1 galK*::*cat*-J23101→ *dTomato*; [6]) and *Pseudomonas putida* EM371-GFP [26].

This protocol employs two plasmids: pSEVA238 (Km^R; *oriV* pBBR1; *xylS*-P_m; [27] and pSEVA238-Ag43L-V_{fib} (Km^R; *oriV* pBBR1; *xylS*-P_m, which drives the expression of the Ag43β-V_{FIB1}-*myc* fusion protein; [Fraile et al. in preparation]). For this procedure, we used fluorescently labeled bacteria to clearly delineate their cellular contour, enabling precise visualization and localization of surface adhesins (*see* **Note 1**).

2.2 Bacterial Growth Media

1. **Liquid Medium**: LB broth was commonly employed for bacterial growth. The medium was prepared by dissolving 10 g/L tryptone, 5 g/L yeast extract, and 5 g/L NaCl in distilled water, followed by sterilization through autoclaving.
2. **Solid Medium**: LB agar plates were prepared by supplementing LB broth with 1.5% (w/v) agar prior to autoclaving. After sterilization, approximately 18–20 mL of molten medium was poured into 90 mm diameter Petri dishes under sterile conditions.

2.3 Chemicals Reagents and DNA Techniques

1. Kanamycin sulfate (PanReac AppliChem; A1493) was prepared as a stock solution at 50 mg/mL in water, sterilized by filtration, and stored at −20°C.
2. Gentamicin sulfate salt (Sigma-Aldrich; G1264) was prepared as a 10 mg/ml stock solution in water, filter sterilized, and kept at −20°C.

3. Chloramphenicol (Merck; C0378) was prepared as a 30 mg/ml stock solution in 100% (v/v) ethanol and kept at −20°C.
4. *m*-toluic acid (3-mBz; Merck T36609). This chemical functions as the inducer of the *xylS*-Pm expression module present in SEVA plasmids (cargo #8; [27]). Prepare a 0.5 M stock solution by weighing 34.03 g and dissolving it in 300 mL of H_2O. Add NaOH until fully dissolved, maintaining the pH between 7 and 7.5. Adjust the final volume to 500 mL with water, filter-sterilize, and store it at room temperature (RT). Use it at a final concentration of 1 mM.
5. Phosphate-buffered saline (PBS). Prepare a 10× stock solution containing 8 mM Na_2HPO_4, 1.5 mM KH_2PO_4, 3 mM KCl, and 137 mM NaCl, adjusted to pH = 7.0. Autoclave and store at RT.
6. Poly-L-lysine solution 0,1% (w/v) in H2O. (Sigma; P8920).
7. Bovine Serum Albumin (BSA; Sigma-Aldrich; A7906).
8. *E. coli* competent solution I: 10 mM sodium acetate, pH 5.6–6; 50 mM $MnCl_2$ and 5 mM NaCl. Filter sterilize, and store it at 4°C.
9. *E. coli* competent solution II: 10 mM sodium acetate, pH 5.6–6; 5 mM $MnCl_2$, 70 mM $CaCl_2$, and 5% (v/v) glycerol. Filter sterilize, and store it at 4°C.
10. 300 mM sucrose solution. Dissolve 25,6 gr of sucrose in H_2O to a final volume of 250 mL. Sterilize by filtration and store at RT.
11. Plasmid DNA was isolated using the QIAprep Spin Miniprep kit (Qiagen, Inc., Valencia, CA, USA) using manufacturer's instructions.
12. Blocking solution: a 2% (w/v) BSA prepared in 1× PBS. Filter, sterilize it, and store it at 4°C.
13. Myc-tag (9B11) mouse monoclonal antibody (Cell Signalling; #2276) as the primary antibody. For immunofluorescence use it at 1:50.
14. Abberior-StarRED, goat anti-mouse IgG StarRED (Abberior GmbH, Göttingen, Germany; STRED-1001) as secondary antibody. For immunofluorescence use it at 1:250.
15. Paraformaldehyde 16% (w/v) in distilled water (Electron Microscopy Sciences; Ref. 15710). To fix bacterial cells, use it at 4% (w/v) in 1× PBS.
16. Mounting medium ProLong Gold (Thermo Fisher Scientific; P36930).

2.4 Other Laboratory Materials

1. Centrifuge 5810 R (Eppendorf).
2. Benchtop centrifuge 5424 (Eppendorf).

3. 10 and 25 mL disposable serological pipettes (Costar).
4. 10 mL plastic test tubes.
5. Shaking incubator for liquid cultures.
6. Spectrophotometer (Ultrospec 2100 Pro; Biochrom, MA, USA).
7. Thermoblock.
8. Nanovue Spectrophotometer(GE Healthcare, IL, USA).
9. DNA gel electrophoresis system.
10. Vortex (Heidolph Max 2000; #541-19000-00).
11. 50 mL sterile tubes (VWR; #525-1099).
12. 1.5 mL reaction tubes (Sarstedt; #72.690.001).
13. 90 mm × 15 mm Petri dishes (∅ × h) (VWR; #P101VR20).
14. Sterile glass beads (∅ 3 mm) were used to spread bacterial cells on agar plates. After use, beads were cleaned using 70% (v/v) ethanol, dried, and autoclaved.
15. 24-well plates flat-bottom sterile (NuclonTM delta surface, Thermo Fisher Scientific).
16. 0.2 μm polyethersulfone (PES) filtration units (FisherbrandTM; Fisher Scientific).
17. 13 mm circular cover glass #1.5 H (high performance; VWR; 117530).
18. Microscope Slides Ground 45° frosted (EprediaTM ref: AB00000112E01MNZ10).
19. Filter forceps, blunt end, stainless steel (Merck; XX6200006P).
20. Type F Immersion oil (Leica Microsystems; 11 513 859).
21. Leica STELLARIS 8 STED 3X multispectral confocal nano and mesoscopy system.
22. Workstation with AMD Ryzen 9 7950X processor (16 cores, up to 4.5 GHz), 64 GB RAM, NVIDIA RTX 3060 with 12 GB VRAM (*see* **Note 2**).
23. Fiji (RRID:SCR_002285; [28]).
24. AIVIA software (version 14; Leica Microsystems).

3 Methods

This protocol outlines the complete procedure for visualizing a synthetic adhesin on the surface of bacterial cells. It comprises four key steps: (i) introducing the recombinant plasmid into the selected bacterial strain, (ii) inducing the expression of the synthetic adhesin, (iii) performing immunostaining of the bacterial cells, and (iv) visualizing

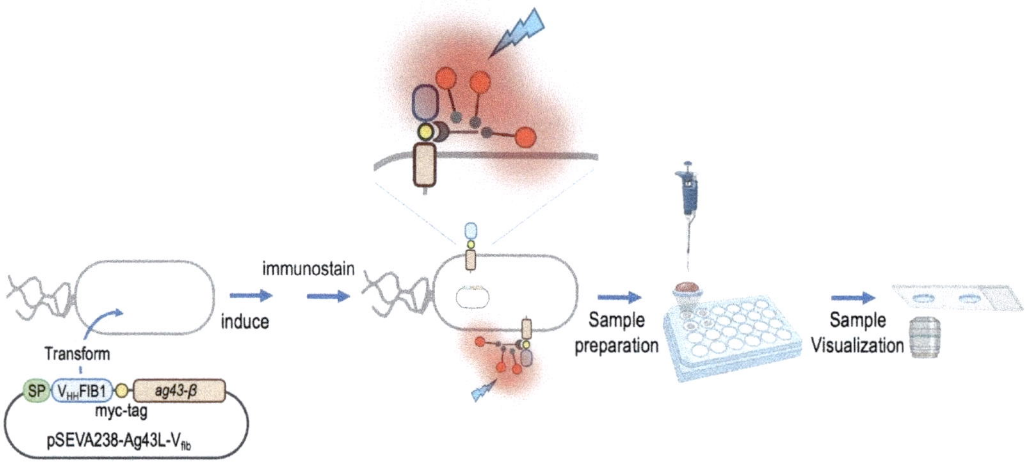

Fig. 1 Schematic representation of the protocol workflow. The process starts with the transformation of the plasmid harboring the recombinant adhesin. Next, the expression of the adhesin is induced. Then, cells are immunostained using a primary anti-*myc* antibody, followed by Abberior-StarRED as the secondary antibody. After sample and cover glass preparation, the labeled cells are visualized in a STED multispectral confocal microscope. Part of this image has been created with BioRender (https://BioRender.com)

the samples and analyzing the resulting images. A schematic representation of the process is shown in Fig. 1. As an example, the protocol is demonstrated using two fluorescently labelled bacterial variants of *E. coli* and *P. putida* EM371, each transformed with a recombinant plasmid designed to display a synthetic adhesin on the cell surface, tagged with the c-Myc epitope for detection.

3.1 Transformation of E. coli with the Adhesin Expression Plasmid

This section details the procedure for introducing a plasmid that conditionally expresses a recombinant adhesin into a fluorescently labeled variant of *E. coli* MG1655 [29]. The focus here is on plasmid delivery via transformation, specifically using chemically competent cells prepared in-house (*see* **Note 3**).

3.1.1 Preparation of E. coli Competent Cells

Preparation of chemically competent *E. coli* was performed as follows:

1. Inoculate 3 mL of LB medium in a 10 mL test tube using a frozen stock stored at −80°C.
2. Grow overnight at 37°C with shaking at 170 rpm.
3. Measure OD_{600} and dilute the culture to 0.01 in a 1 L flask containing 100 mL of LB.
4. Incubate at 37°C with shaking until OD_{600} reaches 0.4–0.5.
5. Chill the cells on ice for 10 min.
6. Centrifuge at 8200×*g* for 10 min at 4°C.
7. Decant the supernatant and add 20 mL of cold solution I.
8. Gently mix the cells while keeping them on ice.

9. Centrifuge again at 8200×*g* for 10 min at 4°C.
10. Remove the supernatant and add 2 mL of cold solution II.
11. Resuspend the cells carefully, maintaining them on ice.
12. Aliquot 100 μL of the suspension in pre-chilled 1.5 mL tubes.
13. Cells can be used immediately or stored at −80°C for months.

3.1.2 Transformation of E. coli Competent Cells

Once the competent cells have been prepared, the next step is to transform an aliquot of the *E. coli* chemically competent cells with two plasmid constructs: pSEVA238-Ag43L-V_{fib}, which encodes the synthetic adhesin, and pSEVA238, an empty vector serving as a negative control.

1. Add 50 ng of plasmid DNA to thawed cells.
2. Incubate the mixture on ice for 10 or 15 min.
3. Heat-shock the cells at 42°C for 90 s.
4. Immediately place the cells on ice for 5 min.
5. Add 900 μL of LB medium and incubate cells at 37°C for 1 h.
6. Plate appropriate dilutions on LB agar supplemented with kanamycin.
7. Incubate plates overnight at 37°C.
8. Pick a single colony and streak it onto a fresh agar plate.
9. Verify plasmid presence by performing a miniprep (*see* **Note 4**).
10. Confirm plasmid identity by agarose gel electrophoresis following HindIII digestion. Expected fragment size is approximately ~7.1 kb for pSEVA238-Ag43L-Vfib, and ~5 kb for the empty vector pSEVA238. For additional confirmation, plasmids can be sequenced using the standard SEVA primers available at https://seva-plasmids.com; [27] (*see* **Note 5**).
11. Store validated strains as frozen stocks at −80°C.

3.2 Transformation of P. putida EM371 with the Adhesin Expression Plasmid

3.2.1 Preparation of P. putida EM371 Competent Cells

This section presents the protocol for introducing a recombinant plasmid encoding the synthetic adhesin into a fluorescently labeled variant of *P. putida* EM371, a naked derivative of strain KT2440 [26], using electroporation as the delivery method (*see* **Note 6**).

1. Inoculate a 100-mL Erlenmeyer flask containing 20 mL of LB broth with *P. putida* EM371 from a frozen stock.

2. Incubate the culture overnight at 30°C with shaking at 170 rpm.
3. Transfer the overnight grown culture to a 50-mL centrifuge tube and pellet the cells by centrifugation at 3220×*g* for 10 min at RT.
4. Discard the supernatant, add 700 μL of 300 mM sucrose, gently resuspend the pellet, and centrifuge again at 9391×*g* for 2 min at RT. Repeat this step at least two times.
5. Finally, remove the supernatant and resuspend the pellet in 400 μL of 300 mM sucrose to obtain a concentrated suspension of electrocompetent cells.

3.2.2 Transformation of *P. putida* EM371 Electrocompetent Cells

Similarly to *E. coli*, the next step is to transform an aliquot of the competent cells with two plasmid constructs: pSEVA238-Ag43L-V_{fib} and pSEVA238.

1. Transfer 100 μL of the electrocompetent cells into a sterile 1.5 mL tube and add 100 ng of plasmid DNA. Mix gently and load the DNA-cell mixture into a 2-mm gap electroporation cuvette.
2. Insert the cuvette into the MicroPulser™ device, select program EC2, and electroporate.
3. Immediately after pulsing, add 900 μL of LB medium to the cuvette and transfer the content to a sterile 1.5-mL tube.
4. Incubate the cells at 30°C for 2 h with shaking at 170 rpm.
5. Plate appropriate dilutions of the recovered culture onto LB agar supplemented with kanamycin.
6. Incubate plates at 30°C overnight.
7. Pick a single colony and streak it on a fresh LB + Km agar plate.
8. Verify the presence of the correct plasmid using the same validation approach applied for *E. coli* (see Sec. 3.1.2).
9. Store validated strains as frozen stocks at −80°C.

3.3 Sample Preparation for Immunofluorescence Staining

Once the cells acquire the recombinant plasmid, the next steps include heterologous expression of the adhesins, preparation of the samples for immunostaining, and visualization using a confocal STED microscope to achieve high-resolution imaging.

The steps outlined in this section are: (i) induction of recombinant adhesin expression, (ii) preparation of the microscope cover glass for confocal microscopy, and (iii) preparation of the cells for immunostaining.

3.3.1 Expression of the Adhesins

1. Start the bacterial culture from the −80°C glycerol stock by inoculating 3 mL of LB plus kanamycin in a 10 mL test tube.
2. Grow overnight at 37°C with 170 rpm shaking.

3. Measure OD_{600} and adjust to 0.02 in 10 mL LB supplemented with kanamycin using a 50 mL flask.
4. Grow at 30°C with 170 rpm shaking until OD_{600} 0.8.
5. Add 20 μL of 500 mM 3-mBz (final concentration 1 mM).
6. Grow induced cells overnight at 30°C with 170 rpm shaking.

3.3.2 Cover Glass Preparation

1. Insert the 13 mm cover glass into a well of a 24-well plate (*see* **Note 7**).
2. Spot 80 μL of poly-L-lysine solution on the cover glass.
3. Incubate for 15 min at RT.
4. Wash the cover glass with 1x PBS.
5. Add 200 μL of 1× PBS to completely submerge the cover glass, then store it at 4°C to prevent drying for next day usage (*see* **Note 8**).

3.3.3 Cell Sample Preparation

1. Remove the 200 μL of 1× PBS from the well containing the cover glass.
2. Place 60 μL of overnight-grown cells directly on the cover glass (*see* **Note 9**).
3. Incubate for 10 min at RT.
4. Place the 24-well plate with the cover glass in it for 50 min on ice.
5. Remove the liquid from the well.
6. Wash twice with 60 μL of 1× PBS.
7. Add 60 μL of blocking solution (2% w/v BSA in 1× PBS).
8. Incubate for 30–60 min at RT without shaking.

3.4 Immunostaining of the Exposed Adhesins

This section describes the immunofluorescence staining protocol for the samples. The procedure involves indirect immunofluorescence using two antibodies. The first antibody targets the *myc-tag* epitope incorporated into the heterologous protein (*see* **Note 10**), while the second is a fluorescently labeled antibody that binds to the primary antibody (Fig. 1). After the bacterial cells have been immobilized on the cover glass and blocked, the sample is incubated with the primary antibody, followed by fixation and labelling with the secondary antibody. Both antibodies must be diluted according to several factors, including their specific characteristics. In this case, anti-Myc-tag is used as the primary antibody at an optimal dilution of 1:50, while the secondary antibody, Abberior-StarRED, is diluted at 1:250.

The detailed steps of this protocol are as follows:

1. Dilute 1:50 the anti-*myc* primary antibody in blocking solution (2% w/v BSA in 1× PBS).
2. Add 30 μL of the diluted primary antibody to a well containing the cover glass.

3. Incubate for 60 min at 4°C (*see* **Note 11**).
4. Wash three times with 60 μL of 1× PBS.
5. Add 30 μL of 4% (w/v) paraformaldehyde.
6. Incubate 20 min at RT.
7. Wash two times with 60 μL of 1× PBS.
8. Prepare the secondary antibody (Abberior-StarRED) at a 1:250 dilution in blocking solution (2% w/v BSA in 1x PBS).
9. Directly add 30 μL of the secondary antibody dilution to the cover glass.
10. Incubate the reaction in the dark for 90 min at RT.
11. Wash ten times with 60 μL of 1× PBS.
12. Place a 4 μL drop of ProLong on a microscope slide and carefully position the cover glass, bacteria-facing side down, onto the drop.
13. Leave the cover glass at RT in the dark for at least three days to allow the ProLong to fully polymerize (*see* **Note 12**).

3.5 Microscopic Visualization of Cell-Surface-Exposed Adhesins with Immunofluorescence

Next, proceed to visualize the samples using a Leica STELLARIS 8 STED 3× confocal microscope. The following steps detail the image acquisition process:

1. Focus the preparation sample using an appropriate filter for dTomato (Ex. 555 nm, Em. 580 nm) or for StarRed (Ex. 638 nm, Em. 655 nm) or for GFP (Ex. 480 nm, Em. 510 nm), with an HC PL APO CS2 100×/1.40 OIL objective.
2. Define the following parameters for confocal acquisition, in sequence 1:
    1. For *E. coli* MG1655 dTomato:
        1. Laser line 554 nm at 0.3% (approximately 0.4 μW at the objective back aperture).
        2. Hybrid detector S1 between 564 and 619 nm, operating in counting mode.
    2. For *P. putida* EM371-GFP:
        1. Laser line 490 nm at 10% (approximately 15 μW).
        2. Hybrid detector S1 between 500 and 560 nm, operating in counting mode.
3. Define the following parameters for STED acquisition, in sequence 2:
    1. Laser lines 637 at 5% (approximately 4 μW) and 775 STED at 10% (approximately 460 μW).
    2. Activate hybrid detector S3 in TauSTED operating mode, spectral range 648–750 nm. Tau background enabled; Tau strength 100; denoise level 50; time gate disabled.

4. Set image format to 1024 ×1024 pixels, scanning speed 200 Hz, zoom 4, and unidirectional mode, in order to obtain a pixel dwell time of approximately 3.9 μs and a pixel size of 28 nm. Activate the FLIM (Fluorescence Lifetime Imaging Microscopy) module to store fluorescence lifetime information.
5. Configure a step size of 183 nm and a pinhole of 151.6 μm.
6. Select fields of approximately 0.1 cell/μm² to ensure proper separation for subsequent analysis, and acquire Z-stacks of ~15 focal planes to cover the entire cell volume.
7. Once images are obtained, perform initial processing using the FLIM–TauSTED module of the Leica STELLARIS software. Fluorescence lifetime decay curves were recorded using the line profile tool, and files were exported in a format compatible with subsequent analysis.
8. To optimize image contrast, a blue LUT (Look-Up Table) was applied to the STED sequence. For the confocal acquisition, the GFP channel was displayed in green and the dTomato channel in red.

Figure 2 shows a representative image of the two samples *E. coli* and *P. putida* EM371.

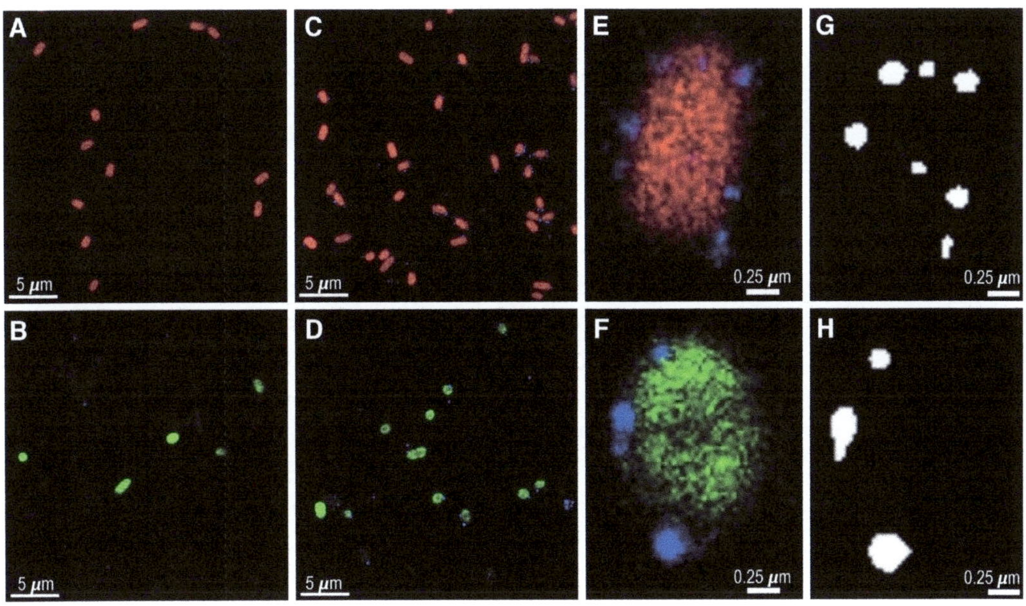

Fig. 2 Representative images of the *E. coli* and *P. putida* EM371 samples. In the image, *E. coli* cells are labeled in red, while *P. putida* EM371 is shown in green. The adhesin protein is visualized in blue, highlighting its localization. Panels (**A**) and (**B**) show *E. coli* and *P. putida* EM371 cells carrying the control plasmid pSEVA238. (**C**) and (**D**) depict *E. coli* and *P. putida* EM371 transformed with pSEVA238-Ag43L-V_{fib}. Pictures (**E**) and (**F**) provide a close-up view of individual cells of MG1655 and EM371 with the synthetic adhesin, respectively. Images G and H present the computational quantification of adhesins, mapped as white spots within the individual cells shown in (**E**) and (**F**)

3.6 Surface Adhesin Immunofluorescence Signal Quantification on the Cell Surface

Quantitative analysis can be performed using AIVIA software (Leica Microsystems), version 14.1 (*see* **Note 13**). For segmentation, the 3D Cell Analysis—Meshes recipe was used, enabling simultaneous segmentation of cells and synthetic adhesins (referred as vesicles in the software). In this example, the following parameters were applied:

- Cell segmentation (bacteria): image smoothing filter size 1; minimum cell intensity 7000; minimum and maximum diameters of 0.4 and 2 μm, respectively; minimum edge-to-center distance 1 μm.
- Vesicles (adhesins) segmentation: image smoothing filter size 1; minimum vesicle intensity 3500; minimum and maximum diameters of 0.1 and 0.5 μm; minimum edge-to-center distance 0.2 μm.

The resulting quantitative data can be exported in CSV or XLSX format for subsequent statistical analysis.

4 Notes

1. FM™ 4-64, FM™ 4-64FX, or CellMask™ (Thermo Fisher Scientific), which specifically labels cell membranes, can be used as an alternative to mark cellular boundaries when a fluorescent bacterial variant is not available.
2. The minimum computer requirements for smaller datasets include a 64-bit Microsoft Windows 10 or 11 Professional operating system, an Intel or AMD dual-core processor running at 2 GHz or higher, at least 8 GB of RAM, a hard disk with a minimum of 100 GB of free space, and an NVIDIA GeForce GTX 1060 graphics card with 6 GB of VRAM.
3. Plasmids can also be introduced into *E. coli* either by electroporation or by using commercially available competent cells.
4. Colony PCR can be employed to verify the presence of the plasmid using oligonucleotides designed to anneal within the plasmid backbone. Nevertheless, we strongly recommend confirming plasmid presence by visualizing it on an agarose gel.
5. Another option is to sequence the entire plasmid without requiring custom oligonucleotides, using the Plasmidsaurus service (https://plasmidsaurus.com/).
6. An alternative method for plasmid delivery into *P. putida* is conjugation, which can be performed through triparental mating using the *E. coli* helper strain HB101 carrying the pRK600 plasmid [30].
7. For same-day experiments, Parafilm can be used as an alternative to 24-well plates for placing the cover glass.

8. Although the experiment can be completed on the same day, for a clearer result, it is recommended to incubate the cover glass overnight at 4°C.
9. It is highly recommended to prepare samples in duplicate.
10. Alternative epitope tags, such as E-tag, can be incorporated into the target protein as substitutes for the *myc* tag, offering flexibility based on specific experimental requirements.
11. The incubation time can be adjusted within a range of 30–60 min, depending on the user's available time and experimental needs.
12. Samples for microscopic visualization should not be stored for longer than one week.
13. In this protocol, AIVIA software was used for quantification; however, users may choose any analysis software that meets their requirements.

Acknowledgments

The authors are indebted to the Advanced Light Microscopy facility of the CNB for superb technical assistance. This work was funded by NYMPHE (HORIZON-CL6-2021-UE 101060625) Contracts of the European Union and BIOEVO (PIE 202420E024) project of the Spanish National Research Council.

References

1. Tian Y, Yang Y, Ni M et al (2025) Surface display of eugenol oxidase and dioxygenase complex as a sustainable biocatalyst for efficient bioconversion of lignin-derived 4-n-propylguaiacol to vanillin. Microb Cell Fact 24(1):54
2. Han L, Zhao Y, Cui S et al (2018) Redesigning of microbial cell surface and its application to whole-cell biocatalysis and biosensors. Appl Biochem Biotechnol 185(2):396–418
3. Smith MR, Khera E, Wen F (2015) Engineering Novel and Improved Biocatalysts by Cell Surface Display. Ind Eng Chem Res 54(16):4021–4032
4. Wang S, Zhan Y, Jiang X et al (2024) Engineering microbial consortia as living materials: advances and prospectives. ACS Synth Biol 13(9):2653–2666
5. Liu H, Chittur PK, Kornfield JA et al (2024) Cohesive living bacterial films with tunable mechanical properties from cell surface protein display. ACS Synth Biol 13(11):3686–3697
6. Ting S-Y, Martínez-García E, Huang S et al (2020) Targeted depletion of bacteria from mixed populations by programmable adhesion with antagonistic competitor cells. Cell Host Microbe 28(2):313–321.e6. https://doi.org/10.1016/j.chom.2020.05.006
7. Timmis K, Timmis JK, Brüssow H et al (2019) Synthetic consortia of nanobody-coupled and formatted bacteria for prophylaxis and therapy interventions targeting microbiome dysbiosis-associated diseases and co-morbidities. Microb Biotechnol 12(1):58–65
8. Piñero-Lambea C, Bodelón G, Fernández-Periáñez R et al (2015) Programming controlled adhesion of *E. coli* to target surfaces, cells, and tumors with synthetic adhesins. ACS Synth Biol 4(4):463–473
9. Muñoz-Gutiérrez I, Moss-Acosta C, Trujillo-Martinez B et al (2014) Ag43-mediated display of a thermostable β-glucosidase in *Escherichia coli* and its use for simultaneous saccharification and fermentation at high temperatures. Microb Cell Fact 13(1):106
10. Clarke KR, Hor L, Pilapitiya A et al (2022) Phylogenetic classification and functional

review of autotransporters. Front Immunol 13:921272
11. Meuskens I, Saragliadis A, Leo JC et al (2019) Type V secretion systems: an overview of passenger domain functions. Front Microbiol 10:1163
12. Glass DS, Riedel-Kruse IH (2018) A synthetic bacterial cell-cell adhesion toolbox for programming multicellular morphologies and patterns. Cell 174(3):649–658.e616. https://doi.org/10.1016/j.cell.2018.06.041
13. Wentzel A, Christmann A, Adams T et al (2001) Display of passenger proteins on the surface of *Escherichia coli* K-12 by the enterohemorrhagic *E. coli* intimin EaeA. J Bacteriol 183(24):7273–7284
14. Fraile S, Briones M, Revenga-Parra M et al (2021) Engineering tropism of *Pseudomonas putida* toward target surfaces through ectopic display of recombinant nanobodies. ACS Synth Biol 10(8):2049–2059
15. Muyldermans S (2013) Nanobodies: natural single-domain antibodies. Annu Rev Biochem 82:775–797
16. Hamers-Casterman C, Atarhouch T, Muyldermans S et al (1993) Naturally occurring antibodies devoid of light chains. Nature 363(6428):446–448
17. Greenberg AS, Avila D, Hughes M et al (1995) A new antigen receptor gene family that undergoes rearrangement and extensive somatic diversification in sharks. Nature 374(6518):168–173
18. Muyldermans S (2021) A guide to: generation and design of nanobodies. FEBS J 288(7):2084–2102
19. Im K, Mareninov S, Diaz MFP et al (2019) An introduction to performing immunofluorescence staining. In: Yong WH (ed) Biobanking: methods and protocols. Springer, New York, pp 299–311
20. Carsten A, Wolters M, Aepfelbacher M (2024) Super-resolution fluorescence microscopy for investigating bacterial cell biology. Mol Microbiol 121(4):646–658
21. Dyba M, Jakobs S, Hell SW (2003) Immunofluorescence stimulated emission depletion microscopy. Nature Biotechnol 21(11):1303–1304
22. Hell SW, Wichmann J (1994) Breaking the diffraction resolution limit by stimulated emission: stimulated-emission-depletion fluorescence microscopy. Opt Lett 19(11):780–782
23. Kolmakov K, Wurm CA, Hennig R et al (2012) Red-emitting rhodamines with hydroxylated, sulfonated, and phosphorylated dye residues and their use in fluorescence nanoscopy. Chemistry 18(41):12986–12998
24. Wurm CA, Kolmakov K, Göttfert F et al (2012) Novel red fluorophores with superior performance in STED microscopy. Optical Nanoscopy 1(1):7
25. Kolmakov K, Winter FR, Sednev MV et al (2020) Everlasting rhodamine dyes and true deciding factors in their STED microscopy performance. Photochem Photobiol Sci 19(12):1677–1689
26. Martínez-García E, Fraile S, Rodríguez Espeso D et al (2020) Naked bacterium: emerging properties of a surfome-streamlined *Pseudomonas putida* strain. ACS Synth Biol 9(9):2477–2492
27. Martínez-García E, Fraile S, Algar E et al (2022) SEVA 4.0: an update of the standard European vector architecture database for advanced analysis and programming of bacterial phenotypes. Nucleic Acids Res 51(D1):D1558–D1567
28. Schindelin J, Arganda-Carreras I, Frise E et al (2012) Fiji: an open-source platform for biological-image analysis. Nature Methods 9(7):676–682
29. Blattner FR, Plunkett 3rdG, Bloch CA et al (1997) The complete genome sequence of *Escherichia coli* K-12. Science 277(5331):1453–1462
30. Kessler B, de Lorenzo V, Timmis KN (1992) A general system to integrate *lacZ* fusions into the chromosomes of gram-negative eubacteria: regulation of the P*m* promoter of the TOL plasmid studied with all controlling elements in monocopy. Mol Gen Genet 233(1-2):293–301

Index

Huan Peng and TheamSoon Lim (eds.), *Biomolecular Display Technologies*, Methods in Molecular Biology, vol. 3030, https://doi.org/10.1007/978-1-0716-5249-7,

R

S

T

V

Y

GPSR Compliance
The European Union's (EU) General Product Safety Regulation (GPSR) is a set of rules that requires consumer products to be safe and our obligations to ensure this.

If you have any concerns about our products, you can contact us on

ProductSafety@springernature.com

In case Publisher is established outside the EU, the EU authorized representative is:

Springer Nature Customer Service Center GmbH
Europaplatz 3
69115 Heidelberg, Germany

www.ingramcontent.com/pod-product-compliance
Ingram Content Group UK Ltd.
Pitfield, Milton Keynes, MK11 3LW, UK
UKHW051811290926
475987UK00009B/110
* 9 7 8 1 0 7 1 6 5 2 4 8 0 *